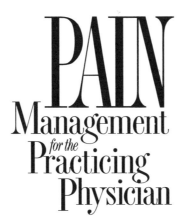

PAIN
Management
for the Practicing Physician

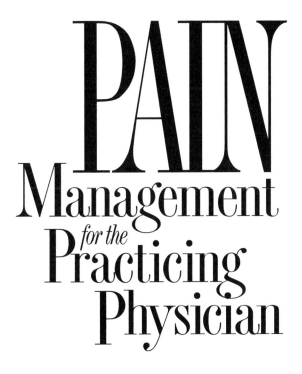

PAIN Management for the Practicing Physician

GORDON A. IRVING, MB, BS, MSc(Med), M.Med, FFA(SA)

Associate Professor
Department of Anesthesiology
University of Texas Medical School at Houston
Medical Director
University Center for Pain Medicine
and Rehabilitation at Hermann Hospital
Houston, Texas

MARK S. WALLACE, MD

Assistant Clinical Professor
Department of Anesthesiology
University of California, San Diego, School of Medicine
Co-Director
Pain Management Medical Group
Department of Anesthesiology
University of California, San Diego, Medical Center
San Diego, California

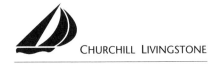

CHURCHILL LIVINGSTONE

Philadelphia, Edinburgh, London, Toronto, Montreal, Sydney, Tokyo

Library of Congress Cataloging-in-Publication Data

Pain management for the practicing physician / edited by Gordon A. Irving, Mark S. Wallace.
   p.   cm.
   Includes bibliographical references and index.
   ISBN 0-443-07913-7 (alk. paper)
   1. Pain. 2. Pain—Treatment. 3. Analgesia. I. Irving, Gordon A. II. Wallace, Mark S.
   [DNLM: 1. Pain—therapy. WL 704 P146585 1997]
RB127.P332356 1997
616'.0472—dc20
DNLM/DLC
for Library of Congress   96-35129
                                             CIP

Churchill Livingstone® is a registered trademark of Harcourt Brace & Company.
™ 𝕯 is a trademark of Harcourt Brace & Company.

Distributed in the United Kingdom by Churchill Livingstone, Robert Stevenson House, 1–3 Baxter's Place, Leith Walk, Edinburgh EH1 3AF, and by associated companies, branches, and representatives throughout the world.

Medical knowledge is constantly changing. As new information becomes available, changes in treatment, procedures, equipment and the use of drugs become necessary. The editors/authors/contributors and the publishers have, as far as it is possible, taken care to ensure that the information given in this text is accurate and up to date. However, readers are strongly advised to confirm that the information, especially with regard to drug usage, complies with the latest legislation and standards of practice.

The Publishers have made every effort to trace the copyright holders for borrowed material. If they have inadvertently overlooked any, they will be pleased to make the necessary arrangements at the first opportunity.

Acquisitions Editor: *Michael J. Houston*
Production Editor: *Rachel Klahr*
Production Supervisor: *Laura Mosberg Cohen*
Desktop Coordinators: *Robb Quattro and Barbara Ulbrich*
Cover Design: *Jeannette Jacobs*

Printed in the United States of America

First published in 1997   7 6 5 4 3 2

Contributions by

HUGH G. GALLAGHER, MB, BCh, FFARCS
Consultant Anaesthetist, South-East Dublin Department of Anaesthesia, St. Vincent's Hospital; St. Vincent's and St Columcille's Hospitals, Dublin, Ireland

DAVID V. NELSON, PhD
Assistant Professor, Departments of Anesthesiology and Psychiatry and Behavioral Sciences, University of Texas Medical School at Houston; Director of Psychological Services, University Center for Pain Medicine and Rehabilitation at Hermann Hospital, Houston, Texas

DIANE M. NOVY, PhD
Assistant Professor, Departments of Anesthesiology and Psychiatry and Behavioral Sciences, University of Texas Medical School at Houston; Attending Psychologist, University Center for Pain Medicine and Rehabilitation at Hermann Hospital, Houston, Texas

Preface

What book on pain would be best for a resident or medical student? What pain book gives practical advice on dealing with pain at the primary care physician level? How do you treat X, Y, or Z pain syndrome? These questions and others on pain management seem to have increased in number over the last few years, yet we found that a book that gives easy to follow advice for the non-pain specialist does not exist. So, combining our theoretical and clinical pain management knowledge, we decided to write *Pain Management for the Practicing Physician*. It is primarily designed for the physician or medical student not only to educate him or her in basic pain theory but also to present a logical and easy way to follow treatment plans for a large variety of pain syndromes.

Medicine is not an exact science and the treatment of pain is no exception. The decision trees, or algorithms, found in this book are not the final answer to treating everyone with a particular pain syndrome. Rather, they are a practical way of following a logical treatment plan that can be modified according to the experience of the physician and the effects on the patient. The clinical case discussions at the end of each chapter relate to patients and to the results that were obtained as the decision tree was followed. The reader will notice that, just as in real life, the patients in the clinical cases miss appointments, take medications at the wrong time, get significant side effects, and often are not cured. However, the patients are always encouraged to function as normally as possible and maintain a good quality of life without expensive investigations or invasive therapies. In addition, we have tried to keep the treatment plans time contingent. Chronic pain takes the physician out of the paradigm of cure and into the practical aspects of how to enable the patient to function and have a good quality of life despite pain. Telling the patient to "come back and see me in one month," and ordering passive, useless, and maybe damaging therapies in the meanwhile is of no value. Instead, a caring physician should form a logical treatment plan and discuss it with the patient, whose life appears to be on an emotional downward spiral. In this way, the physician has a good chance of preventing the patient from seeking multiple physician referrals, stronger analgesics, and perhaps unnecessary surgery.

This book is not intended to provide an in-depth discussion on pain management. It is intended as a practical approach to everyday encounters with pain patients. Some sections of this book are more in-depth than others. For instance, the section on the physiology and pharmacology of pain management may provide more information than needed for most physicians, but should answer the many questions that arise across specialties (including residents and medical students).

A book intended for all practicing physicians is much more challenging to write than one targeted at a specific group. We hope we have met this challenge successfully. If we have succeeded in providing a practical, easy to read source for all practicing physicians, we will have achieved our goals.

Gordon A. Irving, MB, BS, MSc(Med), M.Med, FFA(SA)
Mark S. Wallace, MD

Contents

SECTION III

Psychological Aspects of Pain Management and the Difficult Pain Patient

SECTION IV

Nonpharmacologic Pain Therapies

SECTION V

Future Therapies for Chronic Pain

Introduction

Most physicians are faced with the daily challenge of treating acute and chronic pain. This challenge can cause great frustration on the part of both physician and patient. With advances in knowledge and medication we have greatly improved our treatment of pain arising from surgery, childbirth, and trauma. Yet we have made little primary progress in the management of chronic nonmalignant and cancer pain. It has been estimated that in the United States almost $80 billion is spent annually on chronic pain. Approximately 80 million Americans (one-third of the population) suffer from chronic pain, and 433 million workdays are lost annually due to pain. Since pain management has a low priority in most medical school curricula the majority of these pain patients are treated by physicians without any special training.

The purpose of this book is to give the physician (1) a knowledge of pain principles, (2) a basic knowledge of the pharmacology of analgesics, and (3) guidelines for the management of acute and chronic nonmalignant pain and cancer pain. It provides guidelines as to when to refer the pain patient to a pain specialist. Because pain is an integral combination of an individual's physical and psychological background, it is impossible to provide a "cookbook" method of treating pain. However, we hope the algorithms of each syndrome will give a logical progression to rapid and effective therapy.

LEGAL ISSUES

Pain caused by unexpected trauma, including motor vehicle accidents, falls, industrial accidents, and medical malpractice, results in 80% of the cost of all litigation. Although difficult to quantify, noneconomic losses, such as pain and suffering, loss of consortium, and loss of pleasure, account for up to 80% of the award. These difficulties have led to a growing skepticism of the rising volume of chronic pain claims. The primary physician should prepare careful documentation of the nature of the injury and the patient's physical and emotional response to appropriate therapy so that the validity of these claims can be assessed. The physician must also encourage active modes of therapy and an early return to work to prevent patients from succumbing to a sickness role and chronic pain syndromes.

DEFINITIONS

A basic knowledge of pain language is necessary for the physician to adequately describe pain in discussing the pain syndrome with the pain specialist if referral is necessary. These specialized terms also provide clues to the possible etiology of the pain syndrome so that the physician can prescribe appropriate treatment. Most of these definitions are from the International Association for the Study of Pain Subcommittee on Taxonomy. Examples are given for each pain syndrome.

Acute Pain Pain that results from noxious stimulation produced by injury or disease of body tissues. Acute pain is self-limited and should not persist beyond 1 month of the usual course of the disease or injury. *Example:* A patient fractures the right index finger, resulting in pain that persists for 3 weeks and then slowly disappears.

Allodynia Pain due to a stimulus that does not normally provoke pain. *Example:* A wisp of cotton brushed over the painful area is perceived as painful by the patient.

Analgesia Absence of pain in response to stimulation that would normally be painful. This phenomenon occurs with local anesthetic blockade of nerves. We use this term to mean a decrease in pain or an increase in pain threshold, which results when analgesics such as opioids are used.

Analgesic An agent that produces analgesia. This may be a pharmacologic agent such as an opioid or a nonpharmacologic method such as transcutaneous electrical nerve stimulation (TENS).

Causalgia (Also called *complex regional pain syndrome type II*). A syndrome of sustained burning pain, allodynia, and hyperpathia after a traumatic nerve lesion, often combined with vasomotor and sudomotor dysfunction and, later, trophic changes. *Example:* A patient who sustains a gunshot wound to the wrist with damage to the median nerve, which results in burning pain.

Central Pain Pain resulting from a lesion to the central nervous system. *Example:* A paraplegic suffers from constant burning pain in an area below the level of the spinal cord injury.

Chronic Pain Although some clinicians use the arbitrary period of 6 months to designate pain as chronic, this interval may be too long, as the normal course of many acute pain problems is only 2 to 6 weeks. Bonica defines chronic pain as (1) persisting a month beyond the usual course of an acute disease or a reasonable time for an injury to heal; (2) associated with a chronic pathologic process that causes continuous pain; (3) recurring at intervals for months or years. *Example:* A patient has rheumatoid arthritis with flare-ups occurring once or twice a month. Between flare-ups, the patient is pain-free. These flare-ups have been occurring for 5 years.

Chronic Pain Syndrome A term used to describe patients who (1) present with persistent, intractable pain complaints, many of which are inappropriate to existing physical problems or illness; (2) have a history of multiple physician consultations and many nonproductive diagnostic procedures; (3) are excessively preoccupied with their complaints, which is supported by their family and friends. This term should be reserved for those pain patients who have had a total breakdown of social and coping skills as a result of their pain problem.

Deafferentation Pain Pain that results from the loss of sensory input into the central nervous system. *Example:* A patient sustains a complete avulsion of the brachial plexus with complete loss of sensation and loss of motor supply to the arm. A continuous sharp pain in the hand develops later.

Dysesthesia An unpleasant abnormal sensation, which can be spontaneous or evoked. *Example:* A wisp of cotton brushed over the painful area causes an unpleasant sensation. Note that dysesthesia is described as unpleasant, but allodynia is described as painful.

Hyperesthesia Increased sensitivity to stimulation, excluding the special senses. *Example:* Although a wisp of cotton brushed over the painful area does not cause pain or an unpleasant feeling, the patient does notice that the feeling is stronger than when performed over a normal area.

Hyperalgesia An increased response to a stimulus that is normally painful. *Example:* Pinching normal skin is painful but tolerable. Pinching a recent surgical incision is extremely painful and intolerable to the patient, that is, hyperalgesic.

Hyperpathia A painful syndrome, characterized by increased reaction to a stimulus, especially a painful stimulus. *Example:* A patient has chronic hand pain. When the hand is touched, the patient complains of both allodynia and dysesthesia and describes the pain as radiating up the arm and down the back like an explosion, persisting for minutes after the hand has been touched.

Hypalgesia Decreased sensitivity to a noxious stimulation. Although it is almost never used, this is a better term than analgesia when describing the effects of the commonly used analgesics. Perhaps hypalgesic would better describe opioid effects.

Hypesthesia Decreased sensitivity to stimulation, excluding the special senses. *Example:* A patient has decreased sensation to pinprick in any dermatome.

Neuralgia Pain in the distribution of a nerve or nerves. *Example:* A patient has acute herpes zoster with eruptions in many dermatomes. Although the lesions heal and disappear, the pain persists in these dermatomes (known as postherpetic neuralgia).

Neuritis Inflammation of a nerve or nerves. *Example:* A patient has a ruptured lumbar disc, and the contents of the disc spill onto the right second lumbar nerve root, which results in inflammation of the nerve root.

Neuropathic Pain Pain that results from injury to the nervous system. *Example:* A patient receives an intramuscular injection accidentally into the sciatic nerve. Years later the patient may still have persistent pain in the distribution of this nerve.

Neuropathy A disturbance of function or pathologic changes in a nerve: in one nerve, mononeuropathy; in several nerves, mononeuropathy multiplex; if symmetrical and bilateral, polyneuropathy. *Example:* A constant burning pain develops in both hands and both feet of a patient with acquired immunodeficiency syndrome.

Nociceptive Pain Pain that occurs with an intact or uninjured nervous system. Prolonged nociceptive pain may result in neuropathic pain because of pathologic changes that occur within the central nervous system as a result of persistent input of painful stimuli. *Example:* A patient strains the lower back after lifting a heavy object. Neurologic examination is normal. The patient suffers from paravertebral muscle tightness and pain. The pain resolves with 24 to 48 hours of bed rest and nonsteroidal anti-inflammatory drugs.

Paresthesia An abnormal sensation in the distribution of a nerve, whether spontaneous or evoked. *Example:* A patient presents with carpal tunnel syndrome. Lightly tapping the area over the median nerve at the level of the wrist produces electrical shocks into the hand (Tinel sign).

Radiculopathy A disturbance of function or pathologic changes in one or more nerve roots. *Example:* A patient suffers from a fractured lumbar vertebra, which results in a bone fragment that compresses the right second lumbar vertebra.

Sympathetically Maintained Pain Pain that is mediated or maintained by norepinephrine secreted by the sympathetic nervous system. If the sympathetic supply to the affected area is blocked, the pain subsides. *Example:* A patient sustains a crush injury to the hand, and 1 month later, a continuous burning pain develops in the hand. A stellate ganglion block is performed, and the pain subsides.

WHAT IS A PAIN CLINIC?

Some chronic pain patients will present management problems for the primary care physician. One of the goals of this book is to provide the primary care physician with guidelines to identify those patients who need referral to a pain clinic. We feel that most pain problems can be effectively managed by the primary physician, but if the need arises for a pain specialist referral, the primary physician should have a basic understanding of the role and function of the pain clinic. Most patients will be returned to the primary physician once the pain problem is stabilized.

In the 1950s, Dr. John Bonica recognized the undertreatment of chronic pain. He also recognized that pain is both a physical and psychological experience and felt the need for a multidisciplinary approach to chronic pain management. The first multidisciplinary pain clinic was established in Seattle, Washington. Since then, many pain clinics have opened around the world.

The International Association for the Study of Pain recognizes four types of pain treatment facilities. It is important that the referring physician understand the type of facility to which the patient is being referred. The four types of pain treatment facilities are as follows.

Multidisciplinary Pain Center An organization of health care professionals and basic scientists, which includes research, teaching, and patient care related to acute and chronic pain. It is the most comprehensive of the pain treatment facilities and usually coexists with a medical school or teaching hospital. The center employs a wide array of health care professionals, which may include physicians, psychologists, nurses, physical therapists, occupational therapists, and other specialized health care professionals. The medical specialties represented on the staff may include anesthesiology, neurology, and neurosurgery (but the center is not limited to these specialties). All of the health care professionals communicate on a regular basis.

Multidisciplinary Pain Clinic An organization identical to the multidisciplinary pain center but does not include research and teaching activities. The services are very similar to those provided by the multidisciplinary pain center.

Pain Clinic A health care facility that focuses on the diagnosis and management of patients with chronic pain. These clinics may specialize in certain pain syndromes or pains related to a specific region of the body (e.g., headache clinic). They usually exist in a health care institution that offers appropriate consultative services. The absence of interdisciplinary assessment and management distinguishes this type of facility from a multidisciplinary pain center or clinic.

Modality-Oriented Clinic A health care facility that offers a specific type of pain treatment. Examples are nerve block clinics, acupuncture clinics, and biofeedback clinics. They do not provide comprehensive assessment and management and therefore do not qualify for the term multidisciplinary.

TYPES OF PATIENTS TO REFER TO A PAIN CENTER

Patients with a persistent pain that may or may not be consistent with their physical findings may (1) have progressive deterioration in function at work, home, or in social activities, (2) increase use of pain medication or persistently request invasive medical or surgical procedures as a "physical fix," or (3) may show deteriorating coping abilities, as seen by emotional lability, depression, anger, or hostility.

CHOOSING A PAIN CENTER

Types of Pain Centers or Clinics to Avoid

- Pain clinics that claim to cure pain.
- Pain clinics that routinely perform a series of injections or blocks when the first injection was unsuccessful, or the subsequent second or third injection did not give any significantly increasing duration of pain relief.
- Pain clinics that are solely procedure-oriented and rarely use psychological services.
- Pain clinics that place emphasis on high technology procedures, such as spinal cord stimulators or intrathecal pumps, without adequate trials of conservative treatment or an initial psychological evaluation.
- Pain clinics in which the passive physical modalities, such as ultrasound, massage, and heat, are emphasized, as opposed to more active manual therapies.

Referring Pain Clinics

- Pain clinics that have outcome data on their results, which are available on request.
- Clinics that are staffed with physicians who are easily accessible for discussions about patients.
- Clinics that maintain good lines of communication between referring physicians, primary care physicians, and the patient. Dictated history and physical and treatment guidelines should be expeditiously sent to both referring physicians and primary care physicians.
- Clinics that have physicians who are adequately trained and experienced in pain management. There is still nothing to prevent any physician from claiming he is a pain medicine specialist, although he may have minimum or no postgraduate training. While postgraduate training and certification does not establish the physician as a good practitioner of pain medicine, it demonstrates a commitment and presumably a reasonable basic knowledge of the complexity of chronic pain management.
- The Commission for Accreditation of Rehabilitation Facilities (CARF) is an independent national organization. It sets guidelines and evaluates the clinical and administrative site reviews of pain centers that request accreditation. While CARF accreditation of a pain management program does not prevent poor practices, it ensures that the facility has fulfilled certain criteria for a quality-based pain center.
- Clinics that offer rehabilitation pain management programs eventually show a decrease in the use of health care services (physician's visits, surgery, and emergency room visits) for alleviation of pain, and improved function of the pain patient. Return to work may be a major aim of some programs. The reduction in pain intensity is of less importance than the improvement of the patient's ability to perform adequately in daily activities.
- If a multidisciplinary approach is claimed by the pain center, clear evidence from subsequent referrals should demonstrate interdisciplinary communication between the pain physician, psychologist or psychiatrist, physical therapist, and any other members of the pain team, for example, occupational therapist and vocational counselor. Unfortunately, at present, many clinics pay lip service to multidisciplinary rehabilitation while promoting continued dependency on medical interventions that are of questionable long-term efficacy.

HOW TO USE THIS BOOK

The first half of this book contains a basic science foundation for the management of pain. It is not our intention to provide an in-depth basic science foundation for pain management. However, the treating physician should have a basic understanding of the principles behind the treatments outlined in this book. Therefore, it is suggested that when a treatment plan is instituted from our clinical section, the physician should refer to the appropriate section in the first half of the book to gain an understanding of the principles behind the treatment.

SUGGESTED READINGS

Bonica JJ: Definitions and taxonomy of pain. pp. 18–27. In Bonica JJ (ed): The Management of Pain. Lea & Febiger, Philadelphia, 1990

Bonica JJ: Multidisciplinary/interdisciplinary pain programs. In Bonica JJ (ed): The Management of Pain. Lea & Febiger, Philadelphia, 1990

Merskey H, Bogduk N: Classification of Chronic Pain: Descriptions of Chronic Pain Syndromes and Definitions of Pain Terms. 2nd Ed. IASP Press, 1994

Pain, anatomy, physiology, and pharmacology

Pain, Anatomy, and Physiology

ANATOMY OF PAIN PATHWAYS

Primary Afferent Neurons

The peripheral sensory system is classified into three groups of neurons—A, B, and C—based on their cross-sectional area (Table 2-1). The myelinated A fibers are the largest in size and the fastest in nerve impulse conduction. The A group is subdivided into α, β, δ, and Δ fibers (i.e., 1–20 μm). The A-delta fibers are the smallest and least myelinated of the A fibers and are the only A fibers that transmit pain impulses, for example, the initial sharp, easily localized, pain experienced by a person who has just been injured. The A-beta fibers, larger and more myelinated than the A-delta fibers, transmit pressure, touch, and vibration—but not pain impulses, although they can modulate pain impulses that enter the spinal cord. The unmyelinated C fibers slowly conduct pain impulses, transmitting the dull, poorly localized, and prolonged pain experienced after injury (Fig. 2-1). Although the A-alpha and A-gamma neurons are efferent, and do not transmit sensory impulses, they are secondarily involved in pain because of their role in activating muscle fibers and causing muscle spasms. The B fibers are involved in pain by means of the sympathetic nervous system, which is discussed later.

Table 2-1. Classification of Peripheral Nerve Fibers

Fiber Group	Innervation	Mean Diameter (μm)	Mean Conduction Velocity (m/sec)
A-alpha	Primary muscle spindle; motor to skeletal muscle	12–20	70–120
A-beta	Cutaneous touch and pressure	5–15	30–70
A-gamma	Motor to muscle spindle	6–8	15–30
A-delta	Cold sensation; mechanical pain; ? heat pain	1–4	12–30
B	Sympathetic preganglionic	1–3	3–15
C	Heat sensation; mechanical and chemical pain; heat and cold pain	0.5–1.5	0.5–2

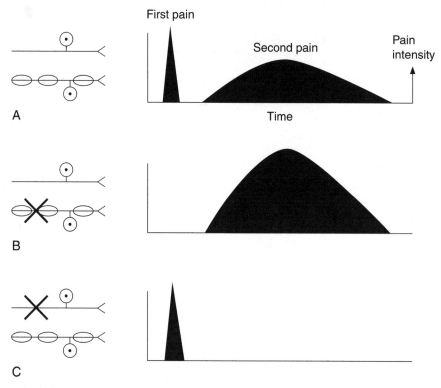

Fig. 2-1. A, The first and second pains are carried by two different pain fibers. The first pain occurs immediately after tissue injury and is transmitted by the A-delta fibers. This first pain is described as sharp and localized and lasts for 3–5 minutes, followed by a pain-free interval of 5–10 minutes. At about 10 minutes, the second pain begins, which is described as dull, aching, and burning. The second pain is transmitted by the C fibers. **B and C,** The first and second pain can be abolished by blocking the respective fibers that transmit the pain. By blocking the A-delta fibers, the first pain is abolished and the second pain is intensified. This phenomenon is explained by the gate control theory of pain (see Fig. 2-5). When the C fibers are blocked, the first pain is unchanged and the second pain is abolished.

Dorsal Horn

The neurons discussed in the preceding section terminate on second-order neurons in the dorsal horn, which ascend the spinal cord to synapse on third-order neurons in the brain. The second-order neurons in the spinal cord are grouped into layers called Rexed laminae. There are 10 Rexed laminae: 6 in the dorsal horn, 3 in the ventral horn, and 1 in the central canal of the spinal cord. The A-beta, A-delta, and C fibers terminate in various laminae of the dorsal horn. The A-delta fibers terminate primarily in laminae I and V, the C fibers primarily in lamina II, and the A-beta fibers primarily in laminae III and IV. The dorsal horn is rich in neurotransmitters and serves as a gate through which all pain impulses must travel; it also plays a prominent role in pain processing. Dysfunction of the dorsal horn can result in chronic pain (Fig. 2-2).

Spinothalamic Tract

Neurons originating in laminae I, II, and V cross the midline of the spinal cord and ascend in the anterolateral portion, called the spinothalamic tract (STT), which ascends the spinal cord to synapse on thalamic nuclei. The STT is divided into a medial and a

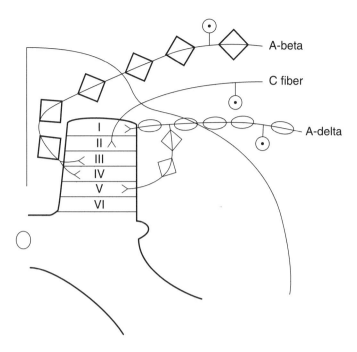

Fig. 2-2. Demonstration of the three nerve fibers terminating on dorsal horn cells. A-beta fibers synapse on cells located in laminae III and IV, which ascend ipsilaterally to reach the brain stem through the dorsal column tract. When they reach the brain stem, they cross the midline to ascend to the thalamus. A-delta fibers synapse on cells located in laminae I and V, and the C fibers synapse on cells located in lamina II. Projections from these cells cross the midline and ascend contralaterally via the spinothalamic tract to reach the thalamus.

lateral system. The lateral system is called the *neospinothalamic tract* and has a direct connection between the dorsal horn and the thalamus. It is a fast conducting system that transmits the initial sharp, localized pain experienced on injury. The medial system is called the *paleospinothalamic tract* and has connections to the brain stem and midbrain structures, such as the reticular formation, periaqueductal gray, limbic system, and hypothalamus before it reaches the thalamic nuclei. It is a slow conducting system that transmits the prolonged dull and poorly localized pain experienced after injury. This medial system also activates the brain stem and midbrain structures that arouse the organism and activate sympathetic responses and suffering (Fig. 2-3).

Thalamic Projections

The ventralis posterolateralis (VPL) nucleus receives input from the dorsal column tract (which consists of neurons originating in laminae III and IV, transmitting pressure, touch, and vibration) and the neospinothalamic tract. This nucleus projects to the sensory cortex and serves as a sensory discriminative function in pain perception. This system localizes and describes the painful area. The medial and posterior thalamic nuclei receive input from the paleospinothalamic tract and project to the association areas of the cortex. This system serves an affective function in pain perception and regulates the emotional or unpleasant aspects of pain. The paleospinothalamic tract also activates the limbic system, which may explain why different individuals respond differently to the same pain stimulus (Fig. 2-4).

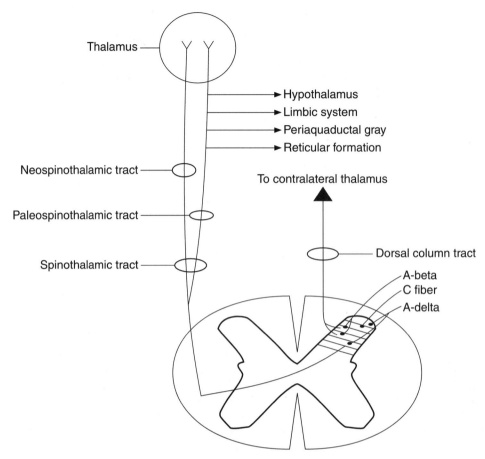

Fig. 2-3. Demonstration of the ascending pathways that originate in the dorsal horn. Cells that receive input from the A-beta fibers project ipsilaterally through the dorsal column tract to reach the brain stem. The tract then crosses the midline and ascends to the thalamus. Cells that receive input from the A-delta and C fibers cross the midline and ascend contralaterally by way of the spinothalamic tract to reach the thalamus. The spinothalamic tract is divided into the paleospinothalamic tract (medial tract) and the neospinothalamic tract (lateral tract). The neospinothalamic tract makes a direct connection between the dorsal horn cells and the thalamus, and the paleospinothalamic tract sends fibers to the deep brain structures before reaching the thalamus.

Descending Pain Modulating and Suppression Pathways

Three pathways exist between midbrain structures and the dorsal horn, which serve to modulate pain impulses arising from the peripheral nervous system: *pathway one* originates in the raphe magnus nucleus, *pathway two* arises from the nucleus locus ceruleus of the pons, and *pathway three* issues from the Edinger-Westphal nucleus. These three pathways descend to terminate on and inhibit pain-responsive neurons in the dorsal horn. When activated, pathways one, two, and three release serotonin, norepinephrine, and cholecystokinin, respectively. The periaqueductal gray (PAG) makes connections to these three pathways. The PAG is rich in opiate receptors, and when these receptors are activated, the PAG activates the three pathways to modulate pain impulses entering the dorsal horn. These PAG opiate receptors can be activated by endogenous release of endorphins and exogenous administration of opioids. The endogenous release of endorphins can be triggered by pain and stress. The dorsal horn of the

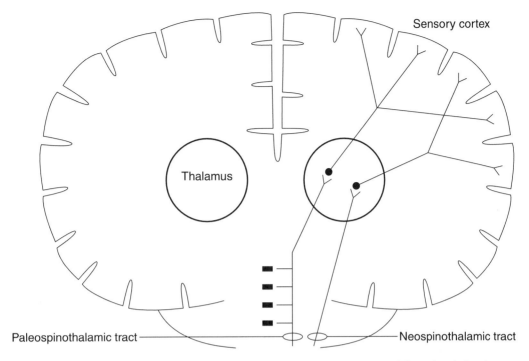

Fig. 2-4. Demonstration of the thalamic projections to the sensory cortex. The spinothalamic tract ascends to synapse on nuclei of the thalamus. Cells of the thalamus that receive input from the spinothalamic tract and dorsal column tract project to cells of the sensory cortex.

spinal cord is also rich in opiate receptors, which are located in lamina II and, when stimulated, produce powerful suppression of incoming C-fiber activity.

PHARMACOLOGY OF PAIN PATHWAYS

Primary Afferent Neurons

C fibers are the only primary afferent neurons responsive to chemical stimuli. Since local tissue damage results in the release of endogenous chemicals, C fibers are susceptible to both activation and sensitization by these chemicals. Stimulation of the C fibers result in an afferent axon reflex, which causes the release of substance P (sP) and calcitonin gene-related peptide (cGRP) from the peripheral terminals. These two peptides sensitize the C fibers to sensory input. Mast cells and platelets release histamine and serotonin, respectively, which directly activate C fibers. A variety of kinins are released by local tissue damage, especially bradykinin, which is a potent activator of the C fibers. Other substances released locally by the damaged cells include the prostaglandins, leukotrienes, and potassium. The prostaglandins and leukotrienes are derived from arachidonic acid, which is released from the cell membranes by phospholipase A, and are synthesized by cyclo-oxygenase and lipo-oxygenase, respectively. Prostaglandins and leukotrienes sensitize the C-fiber terminals, and potassium directly activates the terminals. Cytokines, such as the interleukins, result from the inflammatory reaction involving macrophages and have a powerful sensitizing effect on C fibers. The net result of the release of these various substances is a C-fiber activation and sensitization, which causes hyperalgesia of the affected area. Many of the drugs we use for acute pain inhibit this C-fiber activation and sensitization. Table 2-2 summarizes the primary afferent pharmacology.

Table 2-2. Chemical Mediators That Activate C Fibers

Chemical	Source	Effect on C Fiber
Potassium	Damaged cells	Activates
Serotonin	Platelets	Activates
Bradykinin	Plasma kininogen	Activates
Histamine	Mast cells	Activates
Prostaglandins	Arachidonic acid—damaged cells	Sensitizes
Leukotrienes	Arachidonic acid—damaged cells	Sensitizes
Substance P	C-fiber terminals	Sensitizes

Dorsal Horn

The dorsal horn is rich in neurotransmitters. Activation of C fibers results in the release of many amino acids and peptides that excite the cells of the dorsal horn. These substances include glutamate, substance P, neurokinins, and calcitonin gene-related peptide. Glutamate is interesting because it excites wide-dynamic range (WDR) neurons located in lamina V of the dorsal horn. Repetitive stimulation of C fibers will result in a progressively facilitated discharge of these WDR neurons. The WDR neurons respond only to high-threshold stimuli under normal conditions, but they may respond to low-threshold stimuli after C-fiber activation. This phenomenon is called "wind-up" and is mediated by glutamate. Wind-up can be prevented by pretreatment with opioids (which inhibit C-fiber input into the dorsal horn) and glutamate receptor antagonists.

Glycine is an inhibitory amino acid released by activation of large afferents. Large afferents have a powerful excitatory influence on dorsal horn cells but fail to have noxious effects because of the activation of the glycinergic interneurons. This phenomenon exemplifies the widely known "gate control theory" of pain. The activation of large myelinated fibers inhibits the incoming C-fiber activity, thereby triggering the mechanism of pain relief by transcutaneous electrical nerve stimulation, which has an excitatory effect on the large myelinated fibers responsible for pressure and touch. It is common for patients to report that rubbing the area decreases the pain; this also closes the gate to incoming C-fiber activity in the dorsal horn (Fig.2-5). Injury to peripheral nerves (e.g., trauma, postherpetic neuralgia, diabetic neuropathy) results in an imbalance of neural input into the spinal cord. As can be seen from the above discussion, this imbalance can lead to chronic pain.

Supraspinal System

The pharmacology of supraspinal pain pathways are poorly understood and beyond the scope of this text. However, supraspinal systems have a strong modulatory effect on the dorsal horn through serotonergic, noradrenergic, and endogenous opioid systems.

SUMMARY

Nerve fiber size is classified as A-beta, A-delta, and C fibers. A-beta fibers are large and myelinated, with high conduction velocities, and respond to low-threshold mechanical stimuli. They synapse on second-order neurons in laminae III and IV of the dorsal horn, which ascend ipsilaterally to the brain stem in the dorsal columns. A-delta fibers are small and myelinated, with slow conduction velocities, and respond to high-threshold mechanical and noxious stimuli and cold sensation. They synapse on second-order neurons in laminae I and V of the dorsal horn, which ascend to the brain stem contralaterally via the spinothalamic tract. C fibers are small and unmyelinated, with slow conduction velocities, and

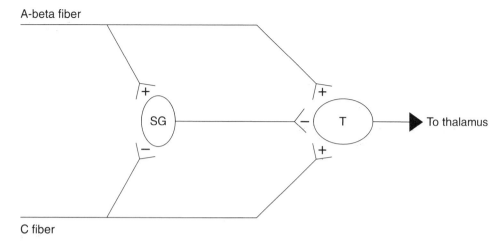

Fig. 2-5. The Gate Control Theory of Pain. There are cells within the dorsal horn that inibit and facilitate pain transmission. T cells (*T*) are located in lamina V and transmit pain impulses to the contralateral thalamus. The T cells are activated by input from the A-beta, A-delta, and C fibers. The substantia gelatinosa cells (*SG*) located in lamina II of the dorsal horn inhibit the T cells. The A-beta and A-delta fibers also activate the inhibitory SC cells and, therefore may "close the gate" to painful impulses from the C fibers. The C fibers inhibit the SC inhibitory cells to the T cells and, therefore, "open the gate" to painful impulses from the C fibers. This phenomenon helps to explains why rubbing a painful area, thus activating A-beta fibers, "closes the gate" and results in a decrease in pain.

respond to high-threshold mechanical and chemical noxious stimuli, hot and cold pain, and heat sensation; therefore, they are termed *polymodal*. They synapse on second-order neurons mainly in lamina II of the dorsal horn, which ascends contralaterally to the brain through the spinothalamic tract.

The functional specialization of primary sensory neurons enables, under normal circumstances, the response to low- and high-intensity peripheral stimuli to be differentiated. Low-intensity peripheral stimuli activate low-threshold receptors generating innocuous sensations, and high-intensity stimuli activate high-threshold nociceptors, which can lead to the sensation of pain. This pain is a physiologic sensation acting as a warning of potentially harmful stimuli. Clinical pain (or chronic pain) results from abnormal excitability in the nervous system and does not serve a physiologic function. Clinical pain involves both central and peripheral changes, and the net result is that a low-intensity stimulus can elicit pain. The transduction sensitivity of high-threshold nociceptors can be modified in the periphery by a combination of chemicals produced by damaged tissue, sensory terminals, and sympathetic terminals. Central sensitization represents a modification in sensory processing within the central nervous system, such that the sensations elicited by low-threshold primary sensory neurons, instead of being innocuous, can become painful. Nociceptor input not only has the capacity to produce pain directly, but, in producing hyperexcitability in the spinal cord, it can produce pain indirectly by changing the response to inputs that never normally produce pain. Finally, nerve growth factors, which normally regulate phenotypic expression of neural tissue, may be increased in chronic inflammation and nerve damage. This abnormal increase may stimulate abnormal phenotypic expression of neural tissue resulting in abnormal processing of sensory input, resulting in the perception of pain. Therefore, chronic pain may be genetic.

SUGGESTED READINGS

Fields HL: Pain. pp. 1–170. McGraw-Hill, New York, 1987

Yaksh TL: Neurologic mechanisms of pain. pp. 791–844. In Cousing MJ, Bridenbaugh PD (eds): Neural Blockade. Lippincott-Raven, Philadelphia, 1988

Opioid Pharmacology

The opiates come from the seed capsule of the opium poppy (*Papaver somniferum*). Opioids (which means opiatelike) are derivatives of opium and include naturally occurring opium derivatives, partially synthetic derivatives of morphine, and synthetic compounds (Table 3-1). The term *narcotic* means any drug that produces narcosis and therefore is a misnomer for opioids. "Narcotics," as used by the Drug Enforcement Agency, includes drugs other than the opioids, such as cocaine.

The opioids are the most powerful pain relievers. Unfortunately, there are many misconceptions about opioid use that hinder proper prescribing by the physician.

OPIOID PHARMACODYNAMICS

Opioid Receptors

Pharmacodynamics is defined as the effect of drugs on the body, and it is also the study of this effect at the receptor level. There are five groups of opiate receptors, which are widely located in the body (Table 3-2). Opiate receptors are located in the brain, spinal cord, peripheral nerves, ganglia, adrenal medulla, and gut. The different receptors produce different pharmacologic actions depending on their location. Most of the receptors in the brain are located in the periaqueductal gray. Stimulation of these receptors activate descending fibers, which modulate C-fiber input into lamina II of the spinal cord (see Chapter 2). The modulating neurotransmitters released in the spinal cord are norepinephrine and serotonin. Spinal cord opiate receptors are located in lamina II (substantia gelatinosa), and when stimulated, they inhibit the release of substance P from the presynaptic terminal and increase potassium conductance in the postsynaptic terminal. The role of peripheral opiate receptors is controversial; however, stimulation of the receptors on peripheral nerve terminals results in inhibition of substance P release.

Side Effects

The most common side effects seen with opioid therapy are respiratory depression, nausea, vomiting, constipation, and pruritus. Fortunately, the blood level of the opioid required to cause side effects is usually much higher than that required for analgesia. Also, these side effects are usually easily treated.

Table 3-1. The Opioids

Naturally Occurring Opium Derivatives	Partially Synthetic Derivatives of Morphine	Synthetic Compounds
Morphine	Heroin	Alfentanil
Codeine	Hydromorphone	Fentanyl
	Oxycodone	Levorphanol
	Oxymorphone	Meperidine
		Methadone
		Propoxyphene

Respiratory depression is the most serious side effect but is rarely seen with the most common doses used in daily practice. It is produced by stimulation of the opiate receptors located in the brain stem. It is more likely to occur in opioid-naive patients and in very high doses. Pain stimulates respiration, and this tends to counteract any respiratory depression caused by the opioid. Respiratory depression is rarely seen if the opioid is titrated slowly upward to achieve the analgesic effect.

Nausea and vomiting (N/V) is a less serious side effect of the opioids but can be a great hindrance to the effective use of these drugs. To properly treat N/V, the physician must have an understanding of the physiology of N/V. The vomiting center is located in the brain stem and is activated by three areas: the chemoreceptor trigger zone (CRTZ), the vestibular system (VS), and the gastrointestinal tract (GI). The CRTZ is directly activated by the opioids. It is also activated by dopamine and serotonin; therefore, the antidopaminergics (prochlorperazine, metoclopromide) and the antiserotonergics (ondansetron) prevent activation. The opioids sensitize the vestibular apparatus to movement, which can result in N/V. The VS is also sensitized by the cholinergics and histamine; therefore, the anticholinergics (scopolamine) and the antihistaminergics (diphenhydramine) prevent sensitization. Patients who complain of dizziness and N/V with movement would most likely benefit from drugs that prevent VS sensitization. Opioids also decrease GI motility, which may exacerbate N/V. Metoclopramide is a good treatment choice for opioid-induced N/V because of its antidopaminergic activity, as well as increasing GI motility.

Table 3-2. Opioid Receptors and Actions

Mu	Kappa	Sigma	Delta	Epsilon
Analgesia	Analgesia		Analgesia	Unknown
Euphoria	Dysphoria	Dysphoria		
Respiratory depression	Respiratory depression	Increased respiration	Respiratory depression	
Sedation	Sedation			
Miosis	Miosis	Mydriasis		
Nausea			Nausea	
Pruritus			Pruritus	
Urinary retention				
Dependence				
Tolerance				
Temperature increase		Temperature increase		
Bradycardia				
	Diuresis			

Constipation and *pruritus* are side effects of the opioids that are usually easily managed. Constipation results from the activation of the mu receptor in the GI tract. A prophylactic laxative and a high roughage diet with increased fluid intake is the most effective way to manage opioid-induced constipation. Some patients manage on diet changes alone. A bowel movement should occur daily. Pruritus results from activation of the mu receptor in the spinal cord. It is more commonly seen with the intraspinal administration of opioids, which is discussed later. A summary of the management of opioid-induced side effects are found in Table 3-3.

Tolerance and Dependence

Tolerance is defined as a decreased effect of a drug following repeated administration. Increasingly greater doses are required to achieve the desired effect. Both the physician and patient must understand this phenomenon to avoid escalating the dose of the opioid to unacceptable levels in an attempt to maintain pain relief. It is common to develop tolerance to the supraspinal effects of the opioids, such as analgesia, respiratory depression, euphoria, dysphoria, sedation, and N/V. Tolerance does not occur for constipation or miosis. Tolerance is more common with rapidly increasing doses, or large doses with short dosing intervals and usually occurs after 2 to 3 weeks of continuous administration. Tolerance may be reversed after a 2- to 3-week drug-free interval. This procedure is called a "drug holiday" and is accomplished by slowly tapering the opioid over 10 to 14 days and maintaining a drug-free interval of 2 to 3 weeks. The opioid can then be restarted at a lower dose with better pain relief achieved. It is very common for chronic pain patients to maintain a stable

Table 3-3. Management of Opioid Side Effects

Side Effect	Treatment
Respiratory depression	1. Dilute on ampule of naloxone (0.4 mg/cc) in 10 cc normal saline. Administer 1 cc (0.04 mg) every minute until respiration are >8/min. This technique prevents the reversal of the pain relief.
Nausea	1. Scopolamine patch every 72 hours. (Use $\frac{1}{2}$ of a patch if age >60). 2. If above fails, add metoclopramide 10 mg every 6 hours. 3. If above fails, add ondansetron 2–4 mg every 8 hours. 4. If step 3 fails, replace with prochlorperazine 5–10 mg every 6 hours or trimethobenzamide 100–250 mg every 6 hours or hydroxyzine 50–100 mg every 6 hours. 5. If step 4 fails, replace with diphenhydramine 25–50 mg every 6 hours. 6. If step 5 fails, decrease opioid. If this fails, discontinue opioid and refer to pain specialist.
Constipation	Prophylactic bowel maintenance program 1. Metamucil, 1 tablespoon each morning in juice. 2. Prune juice twice daily. 3. Senokot-S, 2 tablets at bedtime. 4. Encourage fluids. 5. If no BM in any 48-hour period: —Milk of Magnesia, 30 cc po —Dulcolax, 10 mg po at bedtime —Fleet enema 6. If patient requires antacids, choose Mylanta or Maalox.
Pruritus	1. Diphenhydramine 25–50 mg every 6 hours.

opioid dose for years without developing tolerance. However, if the dose escalation becomes a problem, a drug holiday should be considered.

Two types of dependence are recognized: physical and psychological. *Physical dependence* is a pharmacologic property of all opioids and means that withdrawal symptoms will occur if the opioid is abruptly discontinued, or if an antagonist is administered. Withdrawal occurs because the exogenous administration of opioids suppresses the normal endogenous production of opioids. If the exogenous source is abruptly stopped, the body lacks the normal blood levels of endogenous opioids, and withdrawal will occur. Table 3-4 summarizes the signs and symptoms of opioid withdrawal. Withdrawal can be prevented with a slow taper over 10 to 14 days to allow the body to restart endogenous opioid production. Unlike benzodiazepine and barbiturate withdrawal, opioid withdrawal is not life-threatening to the patient. The physician must keep this in mind when managing the noncompliant patient. If the patient is noncompliant with the treatment plan, a taper regime should be prescribed. If the patient remains noncompliant, it is acceptable to abruptly withhold the opioid. These patients may be managed best in a detoxification program (see Chapter 30 on the difficult pain patient).

Psychological dependence is commonly referred to as addiction, which is defined as a psychological and behavioral syndrome characterized by compulsive drug use, overwhelming interest in securing a supply, and return to drug use after drug detoxification. Addicted persons may exhibit drug hoarding, acquisition of drugs from multiple sources, increasing drug dosage on their own, and drug sales. Unfortunately, chronic pain patients on chronic opioid therapy are all too often labeled as addicts. There is considerable evidence that addiction is a rare outcome of opioid use by pain patients, at least among those with no prior history of drug abuse. Causes of addiction lie more in the psychology of the patient and in the environment than in the qualities of the medically administered drugs. Chapter 30 addresses these issues in more detail.

OPIOID PHARMACOKINETICS

An understanding of opioid pharmacokinetics is essential to proper prescribing of this class of analgesics. Pharmacokinetics is the effect of the body on the drug and will influence how the drug is administered. This section briefly discusses the pharmacokinetics of the opioids to give a better understanding of prescribing practices.

Absorption

Most of the opioids administered to outpatients are through the oral route. All opioids are readily absorbed in the GI tract. Due to the first pass effect through the liver, the bioavailability of the various opioids will differ. Methadone has a very low hepatic clearance and,

Table 3-4. Signs and Symptoms of Opioid Withdrawal

Hours After Last Dose	Signs and Symptoms
8–12	Lacrimation, rhinorrhea, yawning, sweating
18–20	Dilated pupils, anorexia, gooseflesh, tremors, restlessness, irritability, anxiety
48–72	Increased irritability; insomnia; marked anorexia; violent yawning; severe sneezing; muscle spasms; generalized body aches; nausea and vomiting; diarrhea; abdominal cramping; increased heart rate; increased blood pressure; chills and hyperthermia; flushing; low back pain; hyperpnea

therefore, the intravenous dose is just slightly lower than the oral dose. Morphine has a high hepatic clearance, therefore, the oral dose is three times the intravenous dose. These principles become important when trying to convert from an intravenous opioid regimen to an oral regimen. Table 3-5 gives the equianalgesic dose and parenteral: oral dose ratios for the most commonly used opioids. It is possible to administer opioids rectally, which bypasses the first pass effect but results in erratic absorption.

A new method of delivering opioids is transdermally. Drugs delivered by this route must have a high lipid solubility, high potency, and low molecular weight. The only opioid available for this route is fentanyl, which meets all the requirements. The fentanyl patch is a system composed of four functional layers: (1) an occlusive backing that prevents loss of drug and entry of water into the drug system; (2) a drug reservoir mixed with alcohol that increases the permeability of the skin to fentanyl and enhances the rate of drug flow; (3) release membrane adhesive that controls the rate of drug release from the reservoir (a fentanyl-saturated silicone layer holds the system in place and effectively administers a bolus of fentanyl after application; (4) protective peel strip. The penetration of the fentanyl through the skin varies from 46% to 66% and variations in drug penetration between skin regions can vary 20% to 40%. The onset of analgesia does not occur for about 2 hours due to the formation of a skin depot. Once the skin becomes saturated, the fentanyl is absorbed into the vasculature. Because of this skin depot, appreciable plasma levels remain 8 to 12 hours after removal of the patch. Factors that increase fentanyl absorption include vigorous exercise, excessive hydration, occlusion of the skin surface, skin damage, hyperfunction of the sweat glands, and hyperthermia.

Distribution/Metabolism/Elimination

The volume of distribution of a drug is the apparent volume a drug must be distributed if the concentration everywhere is equal to that in the plasma. This volume is dependent on the lipid solubility, protein binding, and ionization of the drug. Because of differences in lipid solubility, protein binding, and ionization, all of the commonly used opioids have similar volumes of distribution and therefore will not be discussed further.

All of the opioids are hepatically metabolized. Opioid metabolism depends more on plasma concentration and hepatic blood flow than on the intrinsic microsomal activity.

Table 3-5. Equianalgesic Doses of Commonly Used Opioids

	Equianalgesic Dose (mg)		Parenteral: Oral Dose Ratio
DRUG	*IV*	*PO*	
Morphine	10	30–60	0.17–0.33
Codeine	120	200	0.6
Fentanyl	0.1	—	—
Hydrocodone	—	30	—
Hydromorphone	1.5	7.5	0.2
Levorphanol	2	4	0.5
Meperidine	75	300	0.25
Methadone	10	20	0.5
Oxycodone	—	30	—
Oxymorphone	—	10	—
Propoxyphene	—	130	—
Butorphanol	2	—	—
Pentazocine	30	150	0.20

Liver dysfunction has little effect on opioid metabolism, unless it is severe. Therefore, it is rarely required to decrease the dose in liver dysfunction. All of the opioids are metabolized into inactive metabolites except morphine and meperidine. Morphine glucuronide, a metabolite of morphine, is 200 times more potent as an analgesic than morphine, but because of poor penetration of the blood-brain barrier, this analgesia is not appreciated. Meperidine is metabolized to normeperidine, which has half the potency of meperidine. However, normeperidine may induce seizures if plasma levels are high enough.

The kidneys excrete the metabolites of the opioids; therefore, in renal disease the metabolites may accumulate. This problem becomes significant in the use of meperidine because of the toxicity of the metabolite normeperidine to the central nervous system (CNS). The maximum recommended daily dose of meperidine is 800 mg. Morphine-6-glucuronide may serve as a reservoir of morphine, which is released by means of plasma hydrolysis. This morphine is then made available to cross the blood-brain barrier.

OPIOID MONOGRAMS

There are many opioids available for the management of acute and chronic pain. Some opioids have very different pharmacologic properties that affect the administration. They also come in different preparations, which will also affect administration. Opioids are divided into agonists, agonist-antagonists, and antagonists. The agonists bind to one or more of the opiate receptors and activate. The agonist-antagonists bind to the receptors without activation; therefore, they block agonist activity. The antagonists, as well as the agonist-antagonists, may induce withdrawal symptoms in opioid-dependent patients because of mu antagonism. Antagonists are frequently used to reverse life-threatening side effects of opioids, such as respiratory depression from opioid overdose. They are rarely used on a chronic basis. Table 3-6 lists opioids in common use. Table 3-7 lists the opioid preparations and recommended dosing schedule.

Agonists

Morphine. Morphine sulfate is the reference standard for all opioids. Its oral bioavailability is approximately one-third the intravenous dose; therefore, when converting from intravenous to oral morphine, the dose must be tripled. It is supplied in both immediate release and controlled release preparations. The immediate release preparation has an onset of 15 to 20 minutes and a duration of 3 to 4 hours. The controlled release preparation has a slow

Table 3-6. Commonly Used Opioids

Agonists	Agonist-Antagonists	Antagonists
Morphine	Butorphanol	Naloxone
Codeine	Buprenorphine	Naltrexone
Fentanyl	Nalbuphine	
Hydrocodone	Pentazocine	
Hydromorphone		
Levorphanol		
Meperidine		
Methadone		
Oxycodone		
Oxymorphone		
Propoxyphene		

Table 3-7. Opioid Preparations and Recommended Dosing

Generic Name	Trade Name	Dosage Form	Recommended Starting Dosage
Butorphanol	Stadol NS (V)	Nasal spray	1–2 puffs nasally q 6 hrs
Codeine	Codeine (II)	*Tab:* 15, 30, 60 mg	15–60 mg q 4–6 hrs
	Tylenol with codiene (IV)	*Tab:* acetominophen 300 mg with 7.5, 15, 30, 60 mg codeine	1–2 tabs QID (do not exceed 8/day)
		Sol: each 5 ml of sol. contains 12 mg codeine, 120 mg acetominophen	
Fentanyl	Duragesic (II)	*Transdermal:* rates of 25, 50, 75, 100 µg/hr	25µg/hr patch
Hydrocodone	Vicodin (IV)	*Tab:* acetominophen 500 mg with 5, 7.5 mg	1–2 tabs QID (do not exceed 8/day)
	Lortab (IV)	*Tab:* acetominophen hydrocodone 500 mg with 2.5, 5, 7.5, 10mg hydrocodone	1–2 tabs QID (do not exceed 8/day)
		Sol: each 5 ml of sol. contains 120 mg acetominophen and 2.5 mg hydrocodone	
	Lortab ASA (IV)	*Tab:* aspirin 500 mg with 5 mg hydrocodone	1–2 tabs QID (do not exceed 8/day)
	Lorcet-HD (IV)	*Tab:* acetominophen 500 mg with hydrocodone 5 mg	1–2tabs QID (do not exceed 8/day)
	Lorcet-Plus (IV)	*Tab:* acetominophen 650 mg with hydrocodone 7.5 mg	1–2 tabs QID (do not exceed 8/day)
Hydromorphone	Dilaudid (II)	*Tab:* 1, 2, 3, 4 mg	2 mg q 3–4 hrs
		Suppos: 3 mg	3 mg PR q 3–4 hrs
		Inj: 1, 2, 4 mg/ml	1–2 mg q 3–4 hrs SQ or IM; 0.2–1.0 mg q 1–2 hrs IV
	Dilaudid-HP (II)	*Inj:* 10 mg/ml	1–2 mg q 3–4 hrs SQ or IM; 0.2–1.0 mg q 1–2 hrs IV
Levorphanol	Levo-Dromoran (II)	*Tab:* 2 mg	2 mg q 6–8 hrs
		Inj: 2 mg/ml	2 mg q 6–8 hrs SQ
Meperidine	Demerol (II)	*Tab:* 50, 100 mg	50–100 mg q 3–4 hrs
		Syrup: 50 mg/5 ml	
		Inj: 25, 50, 75, 100 mg/ml	50–100 mg q 3–4 hrs SQ or IM; 12.5–25 mg q 1–2 hrs IV
Methadone	Dolophine (II)	*Tab:* 5, 10 mg	2.5–10 mg q 6 hrs
		Sol: 5, 10 mg/5 ml	

(Continues)

Table 3-7. *(Continued)*

Generic Name	Trade Name	Dosage Form	Recommended Starting Dosage
Morphine	Morphine (II)	*Tab:* 10, 15, 30 mg	5–30 mg q 3–4 hrs
		Inj: 10 mg/ml	2–4 mg q 1–2 hrs
	MS Contin (II)	*Tab:* 15, 30, 60, 100, 200mg	15–30 mg q 8–12 hrs
	MSIR (II)	*Tab:* 15, 30 mg	15–30 mg q 3–4 hrs
		Sol: 10, 20 mg/5 ml	
	RMS (II)	*Suppos:* 5, 10, 20, 30 mg	10–30 mg PR q 3–4 hrs
	Roxanol (II)	*Sol:* 20, 100 mg/5 ml	10–30 mg q 3–4 hrs
	Roxanol SR (II)	*Tab:* 30 mg	30 mg q 8–12 hrs
Oxycodone	Roxicodone (II)	*Tab:* 5 mg	5–10 mg q 3–4 hrs
		Sol: 5 mg/5 ml	
	Percocet (II)	*Tab:* acetaminophen 325mg with oxycodone 5mg	1–2 tabs QID (do not exceed 8/day)
	Percodan (II)	*Tab:* aspirin 325mg with oxycodone 5 mg	1–2 tabs QID (do not exceed 8/day)
	Oxycontin (II)	*Tab:* 10, 20, 40 mg	1 tab q 8–12 hrs
	OxyIR (II)	*Cpsl:* 5 mg	5–10 mg q 3–4 hrs
Oxymorphone	Numorphan (II)	*Suppos:* 5 mg	5 mg q 3–4 hrs
Pentazocine	Talwin (IV)	*Tab:* 50 mg	50 mg q 3–4 hrs
Propoxyphene Hydrochloride	Darvon (IV)	*Cpsl:* 32, 65	32–65 mg q 3–4 hrs
Napaylate	Darvon-N (IV)	*Tab:* 100	100 mg q 3–4 hrs
		Sol: 50 mg/5 ml	

Abbreviations: (II), Schedule II, Controlled Substance Act; (IV), Schedule IV, Controlled Substance Act; (V), Schedule V, Controlled Substance Act; Tab, tablet; Sol, solution; Suppos, suppository; Inj, injection; Cpsl, capsule; IM, intramuscularly; IV, intravenously.

onset, but a prolonged duration of 8 to 12 hours. Controlled release morphine is embedded in a wax base, which slowly releases the morphine. The analgesia peaks in 90 to 120 minutes (compared to 30–39 minutes for the immediate release). The tablet cannot be broken, as this will release a large quantity of the morphine. Immediate release morphine should be given every 3 to 4 hours, and controlled release morphine every 8 to 12 hours. Usually, controlled release morphine is administered on a time-contingent basis (every 8–12 hours) and immediate release morphine is given on an as-needed basis for breakthrough pain (every 3 to 4 hours prn). This method allows for more stable blood levels of morphine without peaks and valleys commonly seen with as-needed dosing. Morphine is also available in an elixir, which is more readily absorbed than tablets.

Methadone. Methadone is slightly more potent than morphine. It is less psychological dependence-producing than morphine because there is less euphoria and less sedation with methadone. It has an oral bioavailability of almost 90%, therefore, the intravenous and oral doses are almost equivalent. Methadone is poorly metabolized by the liver, which results in an extremely long half-life. This makes the drug valuable in the prevention of withdrawal in drug addicts because it only requires once-per-day dosing. However, the analgesia half-life is much shorter; therefore methadone is usually given every 6 to 12 hours for pain control. This dosing schedule makes it very popular for chronic narcotic therapy. Methadone is also available in an elixir, which is more readily absorbed than tablets.

Meperidine. Meperidine is less potent than morphine. It has a faster onset than morphine, so the patient may experience more euphoria. Because of the metabolite normeperidine and the potential for seizures, it is not the opioid of choice. This effect of normeperidine may be significant at doses greater than 1 g per day, or in renal failure. In addition to analgesic effects, meperidine also has atropinelike effects and local anesthetic effects. The atropinelike effects may lead to tachycardia. Neuropathic pain syndromes that are resistant to opioids may respond to meperidine, perhaps due to the local anesthetic action it possesses. Meperidine has been known to induce a syndrome characterized by tachycardia, increased blood pressure, arrhythmias, and hyperthermia in patients taking monoamine oxidase (MAO) inhibitors.

Hydromorphone. Hydromorphone is 6 to 8 times more potent than morphine. It is easily absorbed from the GI tract and has fewer side effects than morphine. It has a fast onset and a short half-life, requiring frequent doses (every 2–3 hours). It is more commonly used on an as-needed basis (to treat breakthrough pain), rather than a time-contingent basis.

Codeine. Codeine is a weak opioid with less intense side effects. It has a higher oral bioavailability than morphine and a quicker onset, but the duration is short. It is usually given with acetaminophen. In clinical usage its dosage is limited by the dose of acetaminophen it is combined with because of the risk of acetaminophen toxicity (see a discussion of acetaminophen toxicity in Chapter 4). Codeine is frequently used as an antitussive.

Hydrocodone. Hydrocodone has pharmacologic activity similar to codeine. It was previously used as an antitussive only, but now is a commonly used analgesic. It is only available in an acetaminophen preparation, therefore, the total daily dose is limited.

Oxycodone. Oxycodone is qualitatively similar to morphine in all respects. It is available in three preparations: oxycodone alone, oxycodone with acetaminophen, and oxycodone with aspirin. It is also available in a sustained release preparation with similar properties of controlled release morphine (every 8–12 hour dosing schedule).

Oxymorphone. Oxymorphone is 7 to 10 times more potent than morphine. It is a derivative of hydromorphone and comes in a 5-mg rectal suppository.

Levorphanol. Levorphanol is 4 times more potent than morphine. The incidence of nausea and vomiting, and constipation is less than with other agents. The duration is somewhat longer than morphine.

Propoxyphene. Propoxyphene is a derivative of methadone. It is a less effective analgesic than codeine: 60 mg is no more effective than 600 mg of aspirin, and 32 mg is no more effective than placebo. It has an alleged lower dependence potential, but this is disputed. The oral bioavailability is 50%, and it has a large volume of distribution, which accounts for its long half-life of approximately 10 hours; however, its analgesic action is short.

Fentanyl. Fentanyl is 100 times more potent than morphine. It is available in a transdermal patch only, for use in chronic pain (see the section Pharmacokinetics above).

Summary of Guidelines for Prescribing Opioids

- Watch for and treat all side effects.
- Be cautious in starting chronic opioid therapy in
    Young patients.
    Severe psychological pathology (personality disorders, schizophrenia, depression; chaotic family or social environment).
    Prior history of chemical dependency.
- If one opioid is ineffective, or significant side effects prevent further escalation of the dose, another opioid may prove to be effective. For example: changing morphine to trial methadone or a fentanyl match. When changing from one opioid to another a lower equivalent dose of the second opioid should be used as the starting dose.
- Patients with a low risk of abuse potential are
    Middle-aged or older with no prior drug or alcohol abuse with a stable family and social history.

Agonists-Antagonists

Butorphanol. Butorphanol is a kappa and sigma agonist with weak mu antagonism. Because of the kappa agonism, significant sedation may result. It causes 50% less nausea/vomiting than morphine, and other side effects are less common. Dysphoria is seen with this opioid. It is available in a nasal spray preparation. The success of this drug as a chronic analgesic has been limited, and it is not the opioid of choice.

Pentazocine. Pentazocine is a kappa and sigma agonist and mu antagonist. High doses may cause an increase in heart rate and blood pressure. There is a high incidence of psychomimetic effects (anxiety, dysphoria, nightmares, and hallucinations), which greatly limit the use of this drug. It is not the opioid of choice for chronic use.

Antagonist

Naloxone. Naloxone is a potent mu antagonist, which is short-acting (30–45 minutes). It is available in an intravenous form (0.4 mg/ml). The proper method of administration is to dilute the drug in 10 ml saline and titrate 1 ml every 1 to 2 minutes until the desired effect is reached. Bolus dosing of naloxone has been associated with tachycardia, hypertension, pulmonary edema, and cardiac dysrhythmia—thought to be the result of a sudden increase in sympathetic nervous system activity.

GUIDELINES FOR PRESCRIBING OPIOIDS FOR CHRONIC PAIN

Because of the many problems with opioids, such as side effects, tolerance, dependence, potential misuse, and legal issues, the chronic administration of opioids must be done with caution. Unfortunately, many patients are denied the potential benefits of opioids because of many misconceptions. In general, terminally ill patients experiencing pain should never be denied opioids if it is determined they will benefit. The treatment of chronic nonmalignant pain with opioids is somewhat controversial but many patients can benefit from long-term opioid therapy. General guidelines for chronic opioid therapy in chronic nonmalignant pain can be found in the following boxed list.

Guidelines for the Management of Opioid Therapy for Nonmalignant Pain

- A trial of opioids should be considered after all other reasonable attempts at analgesia have failed.
- A comprehensive medical history and physical examination should be documented.
- A trial of opioids does not imply a "last resort" or giving up on the patient. This should be communicated to the patient.
- A history of substance abuse (including alcohol abuse), severe character pathology, or a chaotic home environment are relative contraindications. If opioids are initiated in this group, it should be undertaken cautiously with careful monitoring. Evaluation and advice by a pain specialist should be considered in this population of patients.
- A single practitioner should assume primary responsibility for treatment.
- A verbal or written "contract" should be established with the patient. This agreement should include the possibility of the practitioner weaning the opioid if addictive behavior develops such as non-compliance, dose-escalation, social breakdown, etc.
- The patient should be provided an informed, verbal or written consent before starting therapy. Points to be covered include recognition of the low risk of true addiction, potential cognitive impairment, and likelihood of physical dependence.
- After drug selection, doses should be given on an around-the-clock basis and titrated to effect.
- Failure to achieve at least partial analgesia at relatively low initial doses in the non-tolerant patient raises questions about the potential treatability of the pain syndrome with opioids.
- Emphasis should be given to capitalize on improved analgesia by gains in physical and social function.
- The physician may permit additional doses of the opioid on top of the daily dose in times of increased pain only if tightly controlled and limited.
- Initially, patients must be seen and drugs should be prescribed at least monthly. Progress must be documented. When stable, less frequent visits may be acceptable.
- At each visit, assessment and documentation should specifically address:
  Comfort (degree of analgesia)
  Opioid-related side effects
  Functional status (physical and psychosocial)
  Existence of aberrant drug-related behaviors
  Mood

It must be remembered that opioids are not appropriate for all pain syndromes. They are very effective in nociceptive pain, which is pain without coexisting nervous system pathology. Opioids, in general, are much less effective in neuropathic pain, which is pain secondary to nervous system pathology (such as peripheral nerve injury or spinal cord injury). This is a generalization and does not apply to all patients, as some patients with neuropathic pain respond to opioids but usually at a much larger dose.

INTRAVENOUS AND SUBCUTANEOUS OPIOID THERAPY

It is not uncommon for end-stage cancer patients to require the intravenous administration of opioids. This can be accomplished with an intravenous patient-controlled analgesia pump (IVPCA), which can easily be managed in the comfort of the patient's home. The decision to change from oral opioids to intravenous opioids depends on many factors but, in general, if the patient is requiring large doses of opioids with frequent episodes of breakthrough pain, an IVPCA may be beneficial. It is easier to titrate the opioid to effect with the IVPCA than with oral opioids. However, IVPCA therapy requires intravenous access. This can be accomplished with a central line or a peripheral line with a subcutaneous port; most home health care nurses can easily access these systems. The following boxed list gives guidelines for IVPCA therapy.

Guidelines for Intravenous Patient Controlled Analgesia

- Request consult for intravenous line placement, either central or peripheral with a subcutaneous access port.
- Convert the total daily opioid dose to an intravenous dose (refer to Table 3-5).
- Take two-thirds of this total dose and administer over 24 hours as a continuous infusion. The patient will titrate in the remaining one-third by using the IVPCA bolus dosing. The typical bolus dosing is as follows:

  Morphine: bolus dose = 1–5 mg   lockout = 8–12 minutes
  Hydromorphone: bolus dose = 0.2–1 mg   lockout = 8–12 minutes
- If the patient is requiring frequent bolus dosing, increase the basal infusion by 10%–20% per day and the bolus dosing by 10%–20% per day until comfortable.
- If the patient is experiencing unacceptable side effects, decrease the basal infusion and bolus dosing by 10%–20% per day until side effects resolve.

CASE SCENARIO:

Mr. X suffers from pain secondary to metastatic lung CA to his lumbar spine. He is requiring 900 mg per day of morphine and in spite of good pain relief, he is experiencing frequent breakthrough pain. The decision to start IVPCA is made and a peripheral intravenous line with a subcutaneous port is placed. The conversion is as follows:

1. 900 mg oral morphine/3 = 300 mg IV morphine
2. two-thirds of 300 mg = 200 mg morphine to be administered continously over 24 hours which = 8 mg per hour
3. the bolus dose is 2 mg with a 10 minute lockout

The dose is slowly titrated up to an infusion rate of 15 mg per hour and a 5 mg bolus dose for a total of 600 mg per day of morphine. However, the patient continues to suffer from pain. The decision is made to convert to the more potent opioid hydromorphone. The conversion is as follows:

1. 600 mg IV morphine/6 = 100 mg IV hydromorphone
2. two-thirds of 100 mg = 66 mg hydromorphone to be administered continuously over 24 hours which = 2.7 mg per hour
3. the bolus dose is 0.5 mg with a 10 minute lockout.

This regimen is slowly titrated up and pain relief is achieved.

It is also possible to administer opioids with a PCA subcutaneously (SCPCA). This has the advantage of not requiring intravenous access. However, the disadvantages include less predictable blood levels than with IV opioids. Injection pain is minimized by concentrating the opioid in order to decrease the volume of the injectate required to 1 cc per hour or less. The injection site should be moved to different parts of the body every 2 to 3 days to avoid cellulitis. As with IVPCA, this technique can easily be managed by a home health care nurse. The same guidelines that apply to the IVPCA apply to SCPCA, except the opioid should be in concentrated form (i.e., morphine 10 mg/ml).

If a PCA device is not available, less expensive continuous syringe drivers can be used to provide a constant basal rate of analgesia intravenously or subcutaneously. Ideally, the volume of subcutaneous injectate should be not more than 1 ml per hour.

INTRASPINAL OPIOID THERAPY

Intraspinal opioid therapy is a technique used by pain specialists to provide potent analgesia. As you recall from Chapter 2, pain impulses travel to the central nervous system by means of the slow conducting A-delta and C fibers. The C fibers synapse on neurons in lamina II of the spinal cord. This lamina is called the substantia gelatinosa and is rich in opioid receptors. This is the site of intraspinal opioid action. By delivering the opioid into the epidural or the intrathecal space, much smaller doses are required, therefore, systemic side effects are less likely. However, since many of the systemic side effects of opioids are mediated through the spinal cord and brain stem receptors, these side effects may still occur with intraspinal opioids.

Acute intraspinal opioid infusions are accomplished by the epidural administration of the opioid, but chronic administration usually requires the drug to be delivered intrathecally. This is because much smaller volumes are required for intrathecal administration. Chronic delivery of intraspinal opioid is accomplished with an implantable pump that has a drug reservoir that is accessed percutaneously. This drug reservoir is approximately 18 ml, and the infusion rates are approximately 0.1–0.5 ml per day. Thus the pump will only require refilling every 1 to 3 months. These pumps are very expensive to place and are not recommended for patients with a short life expectancy. An alternative, and a much more cost-effective, technique in patients with a limited life expectancy is the placement of an epidural catheter with a percutaneous access port. This port can be accessed and connected to an external patient-controlled analgesic pump. With this technique the patient can self-administer the intraspinal opioids for pain relief. The principle risk of infection occurs with the changing of the reservoir bag containing the opioid. This can be decreased by having trained personnel only handling the bag changes; reducing the number of changes by increasing the volume of the reservoir bag and increasing the concentration of the opioid; and maintaining strict asepsis during the change process.

SUGGESTED READINGS

Butler SH: Systemic Analgesics. pp. 1640–1675. In Bonica JJ (ed): The Management of Pain. Lea & Febiger, Philadelphia, 1990

Mather LE: Clinical pharmacokinetics of analgesic drugs. pp. 620–635. In Raj PP (ed): Practical Management of Pain. Mosby Year Book, St. Louis, 1992

Portenoy RK: Chronic opioid therapy in nonmalignant pain. J Pain Sympt Manage 5:546–562, 1990

Zenz M, Strumpf M, Tryba M:. Long-term oral opioid therapy in patients with chronic nonmalignant pain. J Pain Sympt Manage 7:69–77, 1992

CHAPTER 4

Nonopioid Pharmacology

NONSTEROIDAL ANTI-INFLAMMATORY DRUGS

The nonsteroidal anti-inflammatory drugs (NSAIDs) are a class of nonopioid analgesics that have anti-inflammatory, antipyretic, and analgesic properties. They are recommended for the relief of mild to moderate pain. Depending on the mechanism underlying the pain, the NSAIDs can be quite effective. If there is a strong inflammatory component to the pain (i.e., bone pain) NSAIDs can provide potent pain relief. The analgesic actions of the NSAIDs are very similar across different classes of drugs but can differ greatly in duration of action. For moderate to severe pain, the NSAIDs are commonly combined with opioids. The NSAIDs are classified according to the parent compound from which they are derived (Table 4-1). If the patient fails to obtain pain relief from an NSAID trial of 2 weeks, an NSAID from a different class should be tried rather than one from the same class. If an NSAID from each class has failed, it is unlikely that the patient will obtain pain relief from further trials.

Mechanism of Action

The mechanism of action of NSAIDs is mainly through the inhibition of the enzyme cyclo-oxygenase, which prevents the breakdown of arachidonic acid to form prostaglandins. The prostaglandins induce inflammation and directly sensitize the peripheral terminals of C fibers to thermal, mechanical, and chemical stimuli. Because of this sensitization, the chemical mediators such as bradykinin, histamine, and substance P exert a greater effect on the pain receptors.

Side Effects

Unfortunately, the NSAIDs have side effects that may greatly limit their use. These side effects are divided into gastrointestinal, hematologic, and renal (Table 4-2). All are directly related to the inhibition of prostaglandin synthesis. As a group, the nonacetylated salicylates (Table 4-1) are less likely to cause these side effects.

NSAIDs cause a localized irritation of the gastric mucosa from a direct and indirect effect. Higher doses may cause erosive gastritis and gastric hemorrhage secondary to a decrease in PGE_2 and PGI_2. These prostaglandins inhibit gastric secretion and stimulate the formation of cytoprotective intestinal mucus. A history of peptic ulcer disease and/or gastric

Table 4-1. Classification of the Nonsteroidal Anti-inflammatory Drugs

Drug	Half-life (hours)
Carboxylic Acid	
Salicylic acids	
Acetylsalicylic acid (aspirin)	4–15
Nonacetylated salicylates	
Choline magnesium trisalicylate	4–15
Salicyl salicylate	4–15
Diflunisal	7–15
Acetic acids	
Indoles	
Indomethacin	3–11
Sulindac	16
Pyrole acetic acids	
Tolmentin	1–2
Ketorolac	3–8
Phenyl acetic acids	
Diclofenac	2
Propionic acids	
Phenylpropionic acids	
Ibuprofen	2
Fenoprofen	2
Flurbiproen	3–4
Ketoprofen	2
Naphthylpropionic acids	
Naproxen	13
Anthranilic acids	
Fenamates	
Meclofenamate	2–3
Pyrazoles	
Phenylbutazone	40–80
Oxicams	
Piroxicam	30–86

bleeding, continued use of alcohol, increasing age, and high doses of NSAIDs are risk factors to developing gastropathy from NSAID use. The use of prophylaxis for NSAID-induced gastropathy is controversial. The H_2 antagonists and prostaglandin analogues (misoprostol) have been used with varying success. The physician must weigh the risk/benefits and the cost. If the patient is obtaining good pain relief in the presence of gastropathy, it may be wise to continue the NSAIDs, but also to add a prophylaxis.

With the exception of aspirin, all of the NSAIDs reversibly inhibit platelet aggregation, therefore, normal hemostasis will be restored after five half-lives, which is the time required for the body to clear all of the drug. Aspirin irreversibly inhibits platelet aggregation and thus lasts for the life of the platelets (6–10 days). The varying effect of the NSAIDs on platelet function depends on the balance between the inhibition and synthesis of thromboxane A2 within the platelets and inhibition of prostacyclin synthesis within the endothelial cells. Thromboxane A2 stimulates and prostacyclin inhibits platelet aggregation. As NSAIDs will inhibit the synthesis of both these prostaglandins, the net balance determines the effect of each NSAID on platelet function. For instance, the nonacetylated salicylates have less of an effect on platelet function than the other NSAIDs in different classes.

Because of their antiplatelet effect, the NSAIDs should be used with caution in patients with underlying bleeding problems (e.g., those receiving anticoagulant therapy). If an NSAID must be used in patients with a bleeding disorder, a short-acting drug should be used (Table 4-1).

Nephrotoxicity from NSAIDs is rare in the healthy patient because renal blood flow and glomerular filtration are not prostaglandin-dependent. However, in patients who are volume-depleted or have congestive heart failure or hepatic cirrhosis, the risk of nephrotoxicity from the NSAIDs increases. This increased risk occurs because these conditions activate the renin-angiotensin system and sympathetic nervous system, which in turn promote local secretion of vasodilator prostaglandins. These vasodilator prostaglandins minimize the renal ischemia produced by these syndromes. As NSAIDs inhibit these prostaglandins this may lead to decreased renal perfusion and glomerular filtration. The nephrotoxicity is manifested by hematuria, proteinuria, and nephrotic syndrome. Prostaglandin inhibition produced by the NSAIDs may lead to fluid retention, impaired responsiveness to diuretic therapy, and hyperkalemia.

There are rare idiosyncratic reactions to NSAIDs that are not related to prostaglandin inhibition. These reactions are reviewed in Table 4-2. Although they may be serious, they are very rare.

Pharmacology

All the NSAIDs have a high oral bioavailability (80–100%) and are rapidly absorbed from the gastrointestinal tract. Ketorolac is the only NSAID approved for intramuscular (IM) or intravenous (IV) use in the United States. The NSAIDs have a low volume of distribution due to their high protein binding (80–99%). One would assume that the half-life of the NSAIDs is short because of the low volume of distribution; however, some can be quite long (Table 4-1). This is because the enzymes involved in the biotransformation of the NSAIDs are saturable and the elimination half-life will increase with increased dose. The NSAIDs are metabolized by the liver by oxidation and conjugation. The conjugated and oxidized products are then eliminated by the kidney.

Table 4-2. Side Effects of Nonsteroidal Anti-inflammatory Drugs

Gastrointestinal/Idiosyncratic	Hematologic	Renal
GI upset	Platelet inhibition	Nephrotoxicity
Bone marrow toxicity (phenylbutazone)		
Gastritis		Water retention
CNS symptoms (indomethacin)		
Aseptic meningitis (ibuprofen, sulindac, tolmentin)		
Dermatologic reactions (all NSAIDs)		
Asymptomatic transaminasemia (all NSAIDs)		
Bilateral pulmonary infiltrates (naproxen)		
Exacerbation of bronchospasm (all NSAIDs)		

ACETAMINOPHEN

Acetaminophen is a *p*-aminophenol derivative that differs from the NSAIDs because of its lack of anti-inflammatory properties. It is appropriate for mild to moderate pain relief when an anti-inflammatory effect is not necessary. It is commonly combined with narcotics.

Mechanism of Action

The mechanism of action of acetaminophen is unknown. It may produce analgesia by nitric oxide synthase inhibition in the spinal cord. Nitric oxide is a neurotransmitter that is released in the spinal cord dorsal horn when C fibers are activated. The presence of nitric oxide in the synaptic cleft can activate postsynaptic spinothalamic tract neurons. Acetaminophen also inhibits brain cyclo-oxygenase, which may account for its antipyretic activity.

Side Effects

The side effects of acetaminophen are minimal. It does not produce GI irritation or the platelet inhibition of the NSAIDs. The major serious side effect is hepatic necrosis, which can occur with large doses of acetaminophen (10–15 g). However, with chronic acetaminophen use, the total daily dose required for hepatic toxicity may be lower than the acute dose. The hepatic necrosis results from the formation of *N*-acetylbenzoquinoneimine, which reacts with glutathione and sulfhydryl groups of proteins. The treatment of this toxicity is acetylcysteine, which binds to *N*-acetylbenzoquinoneimine and inactivates it. There are many opioid-acetaminophen combinations that are developed for acute pain management and not for chronic use. Because of the triplicate system of prescriptions required for opioids in many states, and the fact that most opioid-acetaminophen combinations can be written or called in as normal prescriptions, there has been an inappropriate excessive prescription. This has resulted in many cases of liver toxicity. If the chronic pain syndrome cannot be managed with less than 4 g per day of the acetominophen in the opioid/acetaminophen combinations, other opioids without acetaminophen should be considered.

Pharmacology

The pharmacology of acetaminophen is very similar to the NSAIDs, with the exception of a larger volume of distribution due to its low protein binding (20%). Acetaminophen is metabolized by the liver and eliminated by the kidney.

TRAMADOL

Tramadol hydrochloride is a drug that has been in use in Germany to provide pain relief since the late 1970s. This drug is now available in 70 countries throughout the world. This drug became available in the United States in early 1995. Tramadol hydrochloride is a transisomeric form of a phenyl-substituted aminomethylcyclohexanol. It is produced as a racemic mixture of two optically active enantiomers designated (+) and (–) tramadol.

Mechanism of Action

Tramadol produces analgesia through two mechanisms. One mechanism relates to its weak affinity for mu opioid receptors (about 6,000-fold less than morphine, about 100-fold less than *d*-propoxyphene, and about the same as dextromethorphan [antitussive found in cough syrups]) (see Chapter 3 on opioid pharmacology). Therefore, it is an extremely weak opioid agonist. An active metabolite (*O*-desmethyltramadol) binds to opioid receptors with a greater affinity than the parent compound and might contribute to this component. However, clinical trials suggest that the primary analgesic action of tramadol is mediated through nonopioid mechanism(s). This nonopioid mechanism appears related to the ability of tramadol to enhance the release or inhibit the neuronal reuptake of the central monoamine neurotransmitters 5-hydroxytryptamine (serotonin) and norepinephrine. Several lines of evidence suggest that the two mechanisms of action of tramadol combine synergistically to produce analgesia (see Chapter 5 on co-analgesics and antidepressants).

Side Effects

The most common side effects of tramadol are nausea, somnolence, dizziness, vomiting, and headache. In long-term trials, nausea has been the most common side effect. Side effects are reduced if lower doses are used upon initiating the drug. The side effects of tramadol are similar in type, but not in frequency, to the weak opioids and antidepressants. There are no serious side effects. There is no evidence of euphoria, abuse, dose escalation, spontaneous withdrawal, or naloxone-induced withdrawal.

Pharmacology

Tramadol is readily absorbed from the gastrointestinal tract with only 20% protein bound; it is metabolized by the liver, and the metabolites are excreted by the kidney. The onset of analgesia is slightly longer than weak opioids, but the duration of actions is longer.

Recommended Dosage

The proposed recommended dose of tramadol in adults is 50–100 mg every 4 to 6 hours. The total dose should not exceed 400 mg in persons with normal renal and hepatic function. In otherwise healthy elderly patients up to age 75, dose adjustments are not needed. In individuals older than 75, the total daily dose should be decreased to 300 mg. In renally impaired patients, the dose of tramadol should be 50–100 mg every 12 hours. In patients with advanced cirrhosis, the recommended dose is 50 mg every 12 hours.

SUGGESTED READINGS

Denson DD, Katz J: Nonsteroidal antiinflammatory agents. pp. 606–619. In Raj PP (ed): Practical Management of Pain. Mosby Year Book, St. Louis, 1992
Denson DD, Katz J: Nonsteroidal antiinflammatory agents. pp. 112–123. In Sinatra RS, Hord AH, Ginsberg B, Preble LM (eds): Acute Pain. Mosby Year Book, St. Louis, 1992

CHAPTER	
5	

Co-Analgesics

The co-analgesics are drugs used in pain management that may or may not have intrinsic analgesic properties. However, they provide pain relief in certain pain syndromes or potentiate the common analgesics such as opioids. All of the co-analgesics used in pain management were originally developed for treatment of diseases other than pain. As we have gained a greater understanding of the physiology underlying pain syndromes, there has been increasing use of these co-analgesics for pain. In many circumstances, the co-analgesics are the treatment of choice instead of the opioids and nonopioid analgesics. When administering these co-analgesics, the practitioner must make it clear to the patient why these drugs are being used. Often there is confusion among the patients and pharmacists because the use of these drugs for pain therapy is not in the master drug file. This chapter presents the commonly used co-analgesics.

ANTIDEPRESSANTS

The antidepressants are commonly used in certain chronic pain syndromes for pain relief. The analgesic doses are lower than the antidepressant doses. Whether the antidepressants actually treat underlying depression (which is known to exacerbate chronic pain) with a corresponding decrease in pain is unknown. However, it appears that these drugs have a direct effect on certain painful conditions. Pain syndromes that have been shown to respond to antidepressants are postherpetic neuralgia, diabetic neuropathy, tension headache, migraine headache, and atypical facial pain. However, most neuropathic pain syndromes (see the section Definitions in Chapter 1) may respond to the antidepressants. The antidepressants are most effective for diffuse, burning, and dysesthetic pain. Most patients can be managed at or below antidepressant doses. However, some patients may require antidepressant levels, in which case blood levels should be monitored.

Mechanism of Action

The antidepressants inhibit the reuptake of biogenic amines (norepinephrine and serotonin) into the nerve terminals, which results in an increase in the concentration and duration of action of the neurotransmitters at the synapse. Both serotonergic and noradrenergic neurons in the brain stem project to and inhibit C-fiber input into the spinal cord. The antidepressants are thought to activate these descending inhibitory neurons. As discussed in Chapter 3 on

Table 5-1. Side Effects of the Antidepressants

Anticholinergic	Antihistiminic	Alpha-1 Blockade	Antidopaminergic	Cardiac
Dry mouth	Sedation	Orthostatic hypotension	Dystonia	Conduction defects
Constipation				
Urinary retention				
Sedation				

opioid pharmacology, the opioids also activate these brain-stem inhibitory neurons, and the antidepressants potentiate the action of the serotonin and norepinephrine released by the opioids. The antidepressants also have alpha-1 blocking activity, which may account for some of the pain relief in neuropathic pain (see the section Alpha-1 Blockers and Alpha-2 Agonists below). It has recently been shown that the antidepressants have intrinsic NMDA antagonist activity (see Chapter 2 on anatomy and physiology of pain pathways and Chapter 34 on the future in pain management), which may account for their action on neuropathic pain.

Side Effects

The antidepressants have anticholinergic, antihistaminic, antidopaminergic, and alpha-1 blocking activity (Table 5-1). Because of this activity, the following side effects may occur:

1. Anticholinergic: dry mouth, constipation, urinary retention, sedation
2. Antihistaminic: sedation
3. Alpha-1 blockade: orthostatic hypotension
4. Antidopaminergic: dystonia

The sedation seen with the antidepressants may be advantageous, as many chronic pain patients suffer from insomnia. Because of this side effect, the drug is usually administered at bedtime. If a pain patient suffers from insomnia, it is best to use an antidepressant with more sedating properties, such as amitriptyline or doxepin. The antidepressants with fewer anticholinergic effects (e.g., trazadone and nortriptyline) are less sedating and therefore useful in patients who do not suffer from insomnia. The antidepressants also cause depression of cardiac excitability, which may result in cardiac conduction defects.

Pharmacology

The antidepressants are well absorbed from the gastrointestinal tract and have very long half-lives; therefore single daily doses can be effective. The antidepressants are metabolized by the liver, and the tertiary amines, imipramine and amitriptyline, are demethylated to desipramine and nortriptyline, respectively.

Drug Monograms

The antidepressants are divided into the tricyclics, serotonin-specific reuptake inhibitors, and the atypical antidepressants. Table 5-2 gives a summary of the antidepressants commonly used in pain management.

Tricyclics

The tricyclics are the oldest of the antidepressants. Unfortunately, they have the highest side effect profile. Because of this, they are generally administered as a single bedtime dose. In general, for patients over 65, the initial starting dose is 10 mg at bedtime and increased by 10 mg as tolerated. For patients under 65, the initial starting dose is 25 mg and increased by 25 mg as tolerated. Most of the tricyclics are available in elixir form.

Table 5-2. The Antidepressants Used in Pain Management

Drug	Sedating Quality	Dosage
Tricyclics		
Amitriptyline	++++	Over 65 y/o: 10 mg q hs, increase
Nortriptyline	++	up to 100 mg q hs, as tolerated.
Imipramine	++	Under 65 y/o: 25 mg q hs, increase
Desipramine	+	up to 100 mg q hs as tolerated.
Doxepin	+++	
Amoxapine	++	
Serotonin-specific reuptake inhibitors		
Fluoxetine	±	Initial dose: 20 mg q AM, increase to 60 mg q AM, as tolerated.
Paroxetine	+	Initial dose: 20 mg q AM, increase to 60 mg q AM, as tolerated.
Sertraline	+	Initial dose: 50 mg q AM, increase to 200 mg q AM, as tolerated.
Atypical antidepressants		
Trazadone	+	Initial dose: 50 mg q AM, increase to 200 mg q AM, as tolerated.
Maprotiline	+	Initial dose: 50 mg q AM, increase to 200 mg q AM, as tolerated.
Venlafaxine	±	Initial dose: 75 mg q AM, increase to 150 mg q AM, as tolerated.

Amitriptyline. Amitriptyline is the most commonly used antidepressant for pain management. The efficacy of this drug has been proven in many clinical studies. It is a tricyclic that inhibits the reuptake of both serotonin and norepinephrine. Unfortunately, it has a potent side effect profile because of the anticholinergic, antihistaminic, and alpha-adrenergic blockade. It may also cause considerable weight gain, which is difficult to reverse even when the drug is discontinued.

Nortriptyline. Nortriptyline is a major metabolite of amitriptyline and is therefore classified as a secondary amine. Although the antidepressant effect occurs within a therapeutic window, the pain-relieving properties do not. It primarily inhibits the reuptake of norepinephrine. It has a lower side effect profile than amitriptyline.

Imipramine. Imipramine blocks the reuptake of both serotonin and norepinephrine (norepinephrine more than serotonin). Its side effect profile falls between amitriptyline and nortriptyline. It is used in psychiatry to treat anxiety disorders and thus may be helpful in pain patients who suffer from anxiety.

Desipramine. Desipramine is the active metabolite of imipramine. It blocks the reuptake of serotonin and norepinephrine (norepinephrine more than serotonin). It has a low side effect profile. It may actually stimulate some patients.

Doxepin. Doxepin has a side effect profile slightly less than amitriptyline. It has antihistaminic effects comparable to cimetidine.

Amoxapine. In addition to inhibiting norepinephrine and serotonin reuptake, amoxapine is antidopaminergic. This is explained by its close structural relationship to the neuroleptic drugs. It has a high incidence of producing seizures in the overdose situation. It has also been associated with neuroleptic malignant syndrome.

Serotonin-Specific Reuptake Inhibitors

The serotonin-specific reuptake inhibitors (SSRIs) are a new class of antidepressant that selectively inhibits the reuptake of serotonin. These agents have minimal side effects when compared to other antidepressants. They have not been in use long enough to demonstrate absolute effectiveness in pain management, but they appear to have a role in this area. Because they are generally stimulating, the dose is given in the morning. It is not uncommon to administer an SSRI in the morning and a low-dose tricyclic in the evening.

Fluoxetine. Fluoxetine has been inappropriately attacked by the lay press. Except for occasional anxiety and nausea, the side effects are minimal. This drug may lessen the frequency of migraine headache attacks.

Paroxetine. Both sedation and insomnia have been reported with paroxetine. Nausea, sweating, dizziness, weakness, diarrhea, constipation, and ejaculatory disturbances have also been reported.

Sertraline. Sertraline is a new antidepressant that lacks many of the side effects of the tricyclics. The efficacy of Sertraline in chronic pain management is unknown.

Atypical Antidepressants

Atypical antidepressants are nontricyclic drugs that are chemically unrelated to the classic tricyclic structure.

Trazadone. Trazadone has a relative lack of antidepressant side effects. It is mildly sedating and is given in doses twice that of the tricyclics. It has been associated with priapism.

Maprotiline. Maprotiline has relatively few anticholinergic side effects and a lower incidence of cardiovascular side effects. It has been reported to cause seizures in normal doses.

Venlafaxine. The efficacy of venlafaxine in chronic pain management is unknown.

Guidelines for the Antidepressants

Because of the side effects of the antidepressants (especially the tricyclics), patient compliance may be poor. The most common cause of noncompliance with the tricyclics is an initial dose that is too high. It is best to start at the smallest dose possible and gradually increase slowly over 2 to 4 weeks. The choice of the tricyclic will depend on the patient's sleep disturbance. If the patient suffers from a sleep disturbance, a more sedating tricyclic will be necessary. If there is no sleep disturbance, a less sedating tricyclic will be the drug of choice (Table 5-2). Some patients may benefit from the stimulating effect of the SSRIs in the morning and the sedative effect of the tricyclics in the evening, therefore, these drugs may be given together.

Therapeutic serum levels of the antidepressants that apply for depression do not apply for pain management, therefore serum levels are usually not necessary.

ANTICONVULSANTS

The anticonvulsant drugs have been demonstrated to be effective in pain syndromes with an intermittent lancinating quality. They have also been used successfully in neuropathic, continuous burning pain syndromes. The anticonvulsants used in chronic pain management

Table 5-3. Anticonvulsants Used in Pain Management

Drug	Dosage
Carbamazepine	100 mg bid, increase by 100 mg every other day up to 300 mg qid if tolerated
Phenytoin	100 mg bid, increase by 100 mg every other day up to 200 mg tid if tolerated
Valproic acid	15 mg/kg/day, increase by 5–10 mg/kg/day every other day up to 60 mg/kg/day if tolerated
Clonazepam	0.5 mg tid, increase by 0.5 mg/day every third day up to 10 mg/day if tolerated
Gabapentin	300 mg tid, increase by 300 mg every week up to 600 mg tid if tolerated

include carbamazepine (drug of choice), gabapentin (may replace carbamazepine as drug of choice due to low side effect profile), phenytoin, and valproic acid. Conditions that have been shown to be responsive to the anticonvulsants include trigeminal neuralgia, glossopharyngeal neuralgia, paroxysmal pains of multiple sclerosis, diabetic neuropathy, and miscellaneous lancinating pains (postlaminectomy, postamputation, and postherpetic neuralgia). They are generally started at low doses and gradually increased until the emergence of toxicity or intolerable side effects. The "therapeutic" serum levels that apply for the treatment of epilepsy do not apply for pain management. Therefore the drugs should be titrated to pain relief and side effects. Table 5-3 lists the commonly used anticonvulsants that are used in pain management.

Mechanism of Action

The mechanism of action is unclear; however, the anticonvulsants appear to affect the peripheral nerves much the same way they affect the brain. The anticonvulsants suppress ectopic foci in the brain, thereby preventing seizures, and they also reduce the discharge from sites of ectopic foci in damaged peripheral nerves, which are thought to be responsible for intermittent lancinating pain. They most likely suppress this abnormal activity by blocking the sodium channel.

Side Effects

Unlike the tricyclic antidepressants, the anticonvulsants are chemically unrelated and therefore have different side effects (Table 5-4).

All of the anticonvulsants, with the exception of gabapentin, possess the potential for liver toxicity. Valproic acid and tegretol have the highest incidence. When starting valproic acid and tegretol, baseline liver function tests should be performed and repeated every 2 to 3 months. If the liver functions become abnormal, the drug should be discontinued.

Table 5-4. Side Effects of the Anticonvulsants

Side Effect	Causative Drug
Liver toxicity	All anticonvulsants (except gabapentin and clonazepam)
Aplastic anemia	Carbamazepine
Gingival hyperplasia	Phenytoin
Withdrawal seizures	All anticonvulsants

Carbamazepine is the only anticonvulsant with the potential for causing aplastic anemia. Blood counts should be monitored when using this drug. Phenytoin may cause gingival hyperplasia; good oral hygiene must be stressed. If hyperplasia occurs, the drug should be discontinued. The most common side effect of gabapentin is sedation and ataxia, which subside within 2 weeks of therapy in most cases.

Patients with a seizure disorder will have an increase in seizures if the anticonvulsants are abruptly stopped. Therefore the anticonvulsants should be weaned slowly in these patients. In patients without a history of seizures, withdrawal rarely occurs. However, if these patients are receiving high doses, it is wise to taper the drug.

Guidelines for the Anticonvulsants

With the exception of gabapentin and clonazepam, baseline liver function tests (LFTs) and a full blood count is necessary before starting the anticonvulsants. If the LFTs are elevated, it is wise to try gabapentin only. Start the drug at the lowest dose and slowly increase over 2 to 4 weeks. If side effects occur, decrease the dose. Therapeutic levels that apply for the anti-seizure activity do not apply for pain relief. However, because of the seriousness of the toxicity associated with these drugs, it is wise to monitor serum levels. LFTs and a full blood count should be monitored monthly for the first few months. If these studies remain stable, they may be checked every 3 to 6 months; if, however, they become abnormal, it is suggested that the medication be discontinued.

Gabapentin is unique in that it is not necessary to monitor blood levels or liver functions during therapy. It is not metabolized in the liver and therefore has fewer drug interactions. Gabapentin has no known systemic toxicities nor have therapeutic blood levels been established. Side effects that may occur include sedation and ataxia, which, in most cases, will subside within 2 weeks. The recommended starting dose is 300 mg tid and may be increased up to 1,800 mg per day. Doses as high as 3,600 mg per day have been reported in seizure therapy with no serious side effects.

ANTIARRHYTHMICS

Some of the antiarrhythmics have been shown to affect certain chronic pain syndromes (Table 5-5). These drugs work much the same way as the anticonvulsants in that they are most effective in treating pain that is intermittent and lancinating. However, they are also effective in pain that has an allodynic and dysesthetic component. Bretylium and guanethidine are used in the treatment of sympathetically maintained pain. These two drugs should be reserved for physicians experienced in pain management as they are used in intravenous regional blockade. Guanethidine is not approved for use in the United States. Lidocaine is used for diagnostic and therapeutic purposes. Intravenous lidocaine infusions are com-

Table 5-5. Antiarrhythmics Used in Pain Management

Drug	Route of Administration	Dosage
Mexiletine	Oral	150 mg bid, increase by 150 mg every other day up to a maximum of 10 mg/kg/day divided tid if tolerated
Tocanide	Oral	400 mg tid, increase by 400 mg every other day up to 1800 mg/day
Lidocaine	Intravenous	
Bretylium	Intravenous regional	
Guanethidine	Intravenous regional	

monly performed in pain clinics to determine if the pain syndrome is responsive to the sodium channel blockers, such as the anticonvulsants and antiarrhythmics. Because of the severe toxicities that can result from intravenous lidocaine, this procedure should be reserved for specially trained physicians. The only two antiarrhythmics used orally for chronic pain are mexiletine and tocanide. Mexiletine, tocanide, and lidocaine are used to treat the same syndromes that are responsive to the anticonvulsants.

Mechanism of Action

Mexiletine, tocanide, and lidocaine. The antiarrhythmics mexiletine, tocanide, and lidocaine appear to act on ectopic foci in damaged nerves much the same way as the anticonvulsants. They suppress the abnormal activity in peripheral nerves through sodium channel blockade. The concentrations required to suppress ectopic foci and abnormal activity is far below that required for nerve conduction blockade.

Bretylium and guanethidine. Bretylium and guanethidine act by inhibiting the release of norepinephrine from the postganglionic adrenergic neurons. Because of this action, they produce a chemical sympathectomy. Bretylium lasts from 12 to 24 hours, and guanethidine lasts from 24 to 72 hours. The chemical sympathectomy produced by these drugs decreases the pain associated with sympathetically maintained pain (see the section Definitions and the discussion of clinics in Chapter 1). These drugs are also diagnostic for this syndrome.

Side Effects

The side effects differ between the antiarrhythmics because they are chemically unrelated (Table 5-6).

Nausea and vomiting may occur with all of the antiarrhythmics. It is commonly seen in intravenous regional blockade with bretylium after the tourniquet is deflated. It is also common with mexiletine if the dose of this drug is increased too rapidly. A slow increase over a couple of weeks up to a maximum of 10 mg/kg per day may prevent this side effect.

Tremors and irritability may occur with mexiletine, especially in older patients. This side effect usually disappears if the dose is decreased.

Seizures may occur with lidocaine, mexiletine, and tocanide if given in high doses. However, this is extremely rare in the dosage range used for chronic pain management.

Guidelines for the Antiarrhythmics

The most commonly used antiarrhythmic for pain is mexiletine. This drug should be started at the lowest dose possible twice a day. Slowly increase the drug over 2 to 4 weeks to three times a day up to a maximum of 10 mg/kg per day. If side effects occur, decrease the dose. Therapeutic serum levels that apply to the antiarrhythmic effect of this drug do not apply to pain relief, therefore serum levels are usually not necessary.

If the patient is on other cardiac drugs or has a history of congestive heart failure, a consultation with a cardiologist should be sought before starting this drug.

Table 5-6. Side Effects of the Antiarrhythmics

Side Effect	Causative Drug
Nausea/vomiting	All antiarrhythmics
Tremors/irritability	Mexiletine
Seizures	Lidocaine, mexiletine, tocainide

ALPHA-1 ANTAGONISTS AND ALPHA-2 AGONISTS

The sympathetic nervous system (SNS) is involved in many chronic pain syndromes. If it is determined that the SNS is involved in the pain problem, then medications can be administered to alter the SNS. The alpha-1 blockers and alpha-2 agonists are used for this purpose. The commonly used alpha receptor agonists and antagonists are given in Table 5-7.

A phentolamine infusion is commonly performed by pain specialists before starting oral prazosin, or phenoxybenzamine. Routinely, 0.5–1 mg/kg of phentolamine is infused intravenously over 30 minutes until pain relief occurs or unacceptable tachycardia or hypotension occurs. If this infusion is successful, a trial of this class of drugs may be beneficial. Another method of determining if the pain syndrome is sympathetically mediated is by blocking the sympathetic nerve supply to the painful area. This can be accomplished by blocking the stellate ganglion for upper extremity pain or the lumbar sympathetic chain for lower extremity pain.

Mechanism of Action

Peripheral nerve terminals possess alpha receptors that may become active in neuropathic pain conditions. The SNS releases norepinephrine, which stimulates these receptors and leads to pain. The alpha blockers block the action of norepinephrine on these receptors. The alpha-2 agonists inhibit the release of norepinephrine from the postganglionic sympathetic nerve terminals. In this way, these drugs produce a chemical sympathectomy.

Side Effects

Orthostatic hypotension is the most common side effect of both alpha-1 antagonists and alpha-2 agonists. The alpha receptors are also located on blood vessels where they increase vascular tone, therefore, if this response is inhibited, orthostasis results. As the body fluids shift to compensate for the change in vascular tone, this side effect usually disappears with time.

Due to its central effect of stimulating the pain inhibitory pathways, clonidine may result in sedation. This sedation usually disappears with time (Table 5-8).

Guidelines for the Alpha-1 Antagonists and Alpha-2 Agonists

Alpha-1 antagonists and alpha-2 agonists are well tolerated with few side effects. These drugs must be titrated to blood pressure rather than pain relief. If unacceptable low blood

Table 5-7. Alpha-1 Antagonists and Alpha-2 Antagonists Used in Pain Management

Drug	Route of Administration	Dosage
Alpha-1 antagonists		
Prazosin	Oral	1 mg tid, increase by 1 mg every other day up to 5 mg tid
Phenoxybenzamine	Oral	10 mg tid, increase by 10 mg every other day up to 40 mg tid
Terazosin	Oral	1 mg every day, increase by 1 mg every other day up to 5 mg q day
Phentolamine	Intravenous	
Alpha-2 agonist		
Clonidine	Oral and transdermal	0.1 mg bid, increase by 0.1 mg every other day up to 0.3 mg bid

Table 5-8. Side Effects of the Alpha-1 Antagonists and Alpha-2 Agonists

Side Effect	Causative Drug
Cardiac	
Orthostatic hypotension	All drugs
Tachycardia	Prazosin, phenoxybenzamine, and terazosin
CNS	
Sedation	Clonidine

pressure occurs before pain relief, then these drugs must be discontinued. If the patient will tolerate it, a combination of an alpha-1 antagonist and an alpha-2-agonist may be tried. All of these drugs should be started at the lowest dose twice a day (once a day for terazosin) and increased slowly over 2 to 4 weeks. The maximum doses are prazosin 20 mg per day, terazosin 5 mg per day, phenoxybenzamine 40 mg per day, and clonidine 0.6 mg per day. Blood pressure should be monitored closely while initially titrating these drugs.

MISCELLANEOUS DRUGS

There are a few miscellaneous drugs that can be utilized for chronic pain management. These drugs are less frequently used than those mentioned above; however, in resistant cases, these drugs may be considered. Table 5-9 lists these drugs.

Baclofen. Baclofen is a GABA-B (γ-aminobutyric acid) agonist that has antispasmodic acitivity. It is most commonly used for spasms that result from spinal cord injury. It has been shown to provide relief of pain that has a shooting or lancinating component. It also provides muscle relaxation. Baclofen has been recently approved for intrathecal use for the management of spasticity of spinal origin.

Antihistamines. As discussed in Chapter 2, histamine can activate C fibers. Therefore, it seems reasonable to administer an antihistamine to block this C-fiber activation. Hydroxyzine is the only antihistamine that has been proven to have intrinsic analgesic activity of its own. Hydroxyzine potentiates the effects of narcotics, and because of this, it is commonly used in conjunction with these agents. Phenyltoloxamine and orphenadrine have also been used in chronic pain management.

Skeletal muscle relaxants. The use of muscle relaxants are usually a part of a therapeutic regimen and are rarely given alone. In conjunction with narcotics, NSAIDs, and physical therapy, they can be quite effective in pain management. However, the long-term use of the muscle relaxants is controversial and not recommended at this time. The skeletal muscle relaxants are divided into the antispasmodics and centrally acting muscle relaxants.

The antispasmodics include baclofen and dantrolene. Baclofen is a muscle relaxant and antispasmodic, which is mainly used for spasticity after spinal cord injury. It is now approved for intrathecal use in these patients. The antispasmodic effect of this drug is thought to be secondary to GABA-B activity at the spinal cord level. Baclofen may prove efficacious in pain secondary to muscle spasms and may also be used in intermittent lancinating pain.

Dantrolene is a potent antispasmodic that dissociates the excitation-contraction coupling mechanism of skeletal muscle by interfering with the release of calcium from the sarcoplasmic reticulum. Fatal and nonfatal liver disorders may occur with dantrolene, therefore, this drug should be used in selected cases only, and therapy should be stopped if benefit is not evident by 45 days. The main indication for this drug is spasticity secondary to spinal cord injury.

Table 5-9. Miscellaneous Drugs Used in Pain Management

Drug	Dosage
Antihistamines	
Hydroxyzine	50–100 mg q hs
Skeletal muscle relaxants	
Antispasmodics	
Baclofen	5 mg tid, increase by 5 mg every third day up to 20 mg tid
Dantrolene	25 mg q day, increase gradually up to a maximum of 400 mg/day
Centrally acting agents	
Carisoprodol	350 mg tid
Chlorphenesin carbamate	400–800 mg qid
Chlorzoxazone	250–500 mg tid
Cyclobenzaprine hydrochloride	10 mg tid
Methocarbamol	1000–1500 mg tid
Orphenadrine citrate	100 mg bid
Antipsychotics	
Pluphenazine	1–2.5 mg qid
Haloperidol	0.5–5 mg tid
Corticosteriods	
Methylprednisolone	Individualize dose
Dexamethasone	
Prednisone	
Stimulants	
Dextroamphetamine	5–30 mg q AM
Methylphenidate	5–30 mg q AM
Caffeine	65–130 mg q AM
Creams	
Capsaicin 0.025% or 0.075%	Apply to painful area 3–4 times per day
EMLA cream	Apply to painful area 3–4 times per day (occlusive dressing will increase dermal penetration); leave on area for up to 4 hours

The centrally acting muscle relaxants include carisoprodol, chlorphenesin carbamate, chlorzoxazone, cyclobenzaprine hydrochloride, methocarbamol, and orphenadrine citrate. Many of these are available in combination with certain other drugs.

Capsaicin cream. Capsaicin is a derivative of red chili pepper that depletes substance P from C fiber terminals by blocking transport and synthesis. Initially, the cream may burn after application; however, this will disappear with continued use. As significant depletion of substance P from the peripheral terminals takes up to 3 weeks, treatment must be continued for this minimum period of time before efficacy can be gauged. The patient must use this cream 3 to 4 times per day for it to be effective. It is available in a 0.025% and 0.075% cream.

EMLA cream. EMLA (eutectic mixture of local anesthetic) is an emulsion of lidocaine 2.5% and prilocaine 2.5%. It was developed as a topical local anesthetic to allow painless intravenous cannulation in children. The efficacy of EMLA cream in pain management has not been studied, although there are reports of effective treatment of superficial painful syndromes such as postherpetic neuralgia and superficial neuromas.

Sedatives, hypnotics, and tranquilizers. The use of sedatives, hypnotics, and tranquilizers for chronic pain management is controversial. Despite this, their use in combination with opioids and antidepressants is not uncommon. In certain pain conditions where psychosis and anxiety are major symptoms, these drugs may prove useful. However, consultation with a psychiatrist may be indicated. Benzodiazepines often cause significant disturbances of REM sleep, tolerance and habituation can be a problem, and these drugs can be extremely difficult to withdraw. It is still unclear whether these drugs have intrinsic analgesic activity. Because their use remains controversial, they should be used in selected cases only.

Corticosteroids. The corticosteroids have been proven efficacious in advanced cancer. They appear to provide short-term analgesia by both a direct analgesic effect and secondary to tumor size reduction. Methylprednisolone and dexamethasone are the drugs of choice, but other corticosteriods may be used. The corticosteriods may be useful in pain resulting from diffuse bony metastasis and tumor infiltration of neural structures such as the brachial plexus or lumbosacral plexus. Pain resulting from spinal cord compression has also been reported to be responsive to the corticosteroids. Another advantage of the corticosteroids is improvement of appetite and mood. The dosing of corticosteroids is empirical and should be individualized.

Stimulants. Cancer patients often obtain pain relief from high-dose opioid therapy with sedation as the only side effect. The addition of a stimulant to their regimen can be very beneficial. Dextroamphetamine, caffeine, and methylphenidate are the most commonly used stimulants; if these drugs are taken in the morning, daytime sedation induced by the opioids can be prevented.

SUGGESTED READINGS

Fields HL: Anticonvulsants, psychotropics, and antihistaminergic drugs in pain management. pp. 285–306. In Fields HL (ed): Pain. McGraw-Hill, New York, 1987
Haddox JD: Neuropsychiatric drug use in pain management. pp. 636–659. In Raj PP (ed): Practical Management of Pain. Mosby Year Book, St. Louis, 1992

Medical management of pain syndromes

Chronic Pain Management

GENERAL PRINCIPLES

Chronic pain can be defined as pain that is present on a daily or almost-daily basis for 6 months or more. Once pain has been present for this length of time, it is difficult to eradicate, and some continuing pain will often have to be accepted by the patient.

Accurate figures on the incidence of chronic pain are not available. However, data from various surveys suggest that, in 1989, at least one-third of the American population suffered from chronic pain syndromes.

When assessing patients in chronic pain and the response to treatment, the primary physician should document various aspects that can assist in both diagnosis and response to therapy.

DIAGNOSTIC TECHNIQUES

Spatial Distribution of Pain

Getting the patient to mark or shade in painful areas on a line drawing of the body can indicate possible anatomic problems. Shading of the whole of an extremity, or several body areas, makes identification of a single physical pain pathology less likely and psychological and environmental issues should be explored.

The Visual or Verbal Analogue Pain Score

The patient is asked to score his or her pain from 0 to 10, where 0 is no pain and 10 is the worst pain imaginable. Having a subjective number allows treatment to be assessed. If the individual persistently complains of pain 10/10 "or higher," significant, real or perceived, environmental stressors are often present.

Pressure Algometers

Some forms of chronic pain have myofacial trigger and tender points. A spring-leaded algometer placed over these areas allows the pressure that causes pain to be documented. This is moderately reliable in measuring pain thresholds and can be used for both fulfilling diagnostic criteria in primary fibromyalgia and for following the effects of treatment.

Disability

Disability can be measured by a number of different methods. The Sickness Inventory Profile (SIP) is reliable and valid, providing useful clinical information in physical function, communication, and cognitive and social activity. Von Korff and colleagues (1992) have proposed a graded classification of pain and disability. The level of disability due to pain is graded from low, where the pain does not interfere with usual activities, to high, where the pain significantly interferes. These gradings are as follows:

I	Low disability	Low intensity pain
II	Low disability	High intensity pain
III	High disability	Moderately limiting
IV	High disability	Severely limiting

In III and IV, pain is rarely less than 5/10 on a scale where 0 is no pain and 10 is the worst pain imaginable.

Verbal Pain Descriptions

Verbal pain descriptions are usually measured using the McGill Pain Questionnaire (MPQ). This is a patient checklist of 20 groups of adjectives describing pain.

Back Pain Function

The disability caused by back pain and the improvement with therapy can be assessed by a number of measures. The Quebec Back Pain Disability Scale, devised by Kopec and colleagues (1995), is easy to complete and can give indications of both the dysfunction and the response to therapy (Fig. 6-1).

Sleep Disturbance

Difficulty in falling asleep, number of awakenings because of pain, and duration of sleep during a 24-hour period are all self-report measures that should be asked. Improvements in sleep often correspond with improvements in pain and dysfunction. Early morning awakening may indicate significant depression.

Ambulation

Getting the patient to do a timed 50-yard walk can act as a guide for physical therapy success. As they cope more effectively with pain, the patients tend to decrease both their time and the number of their pain behaviors.

Sit/Stand

Sit/stand is another useful method of monitoring physical improvement, especially in patients with low back pain. The number of times the patient can stand from a sitting position, preferably from a chair without arms, in 2 minutes is recorded. As physical function improves, the number of repetitions the patient is able to perform increases, and the number of pain behaviors decreases.

Pain Diaries

Pain diaries can serve an important function in identifying food allergies, diurnal rhythms, external stressors, and effectiveness of medication. Unfortunately, they are seldom kept

THE QUEBEC BACK PAIN DISABILITY SCALE

Today, do you find it difficult to perform the following activities because of your back?

Response options (0–5):
0, not difficult at all
1, minimally difficult
2, somewhat difficult
3, fairly difficult
4, very difficult
5, unable to do

	Not difficult				Unable to	
1. Get out of bed.	0	1	2	3	4	5
2. Sleep for at least 6 hours.	0	1	2	3	4	5
3. Turn over in bed.	0	1	2	3	4	5
4. Travel 1 hour in car.	0	1	2	3	4	5
5. Stand up for 20–30 minutes.	0	1	2	3	4	5
6. Sit for 4 hours.	0	1	2	3	4	5
7. Climb one flight of stairs	0	1	2	3	4	5
8. Walk a few blocks (300–400 yds.)	0	1	2	3	4	5
9. Walk several miles.	0	1	2	3	4	5
10. Reach up to high shelves.	0	1	2	3	4	5
11. Throw a ball.	0	1	2	3	4	5
12. Run two blocks.	0	1	2	3	4	5
13. Take food out of the refrigerator.	0	1	2	3	4	5
14. Make your bed.	0	1	2	3	4	5
15. Put on socks (pantyhose).	0	1	2	3	4	5
16. Bend over a sink for 10 minutes.	0	1	2	3	4	5
17. Move a table.	0	1	2	3	4	5
18. Pull or push heavy doors.	0	1	2	3	4	5
19. Carry two bags of groceries.	0	1	2	3	4	5
20. Lift 40 lbs.	0	1	2	3	4	5

Fig. 6-1. The Quebec Back Pain Disability Scale.

conscientiously and should probably be used only for a few days at a time for most patients. Most patients do not fill in pain diaries at the time but later by recall. Asking the patient to fill in their pain ratings at a regular time, such as wake up/breakfast, lunch, evening meal, and bedtime, improves compliance. All medications taken and the time when they are taken should also be noted.

For intermittent chronic pain syndromes such as headaches, the onset and offset of the pain and its maximum pain score should be recorded. (See Fig. 15-1.)

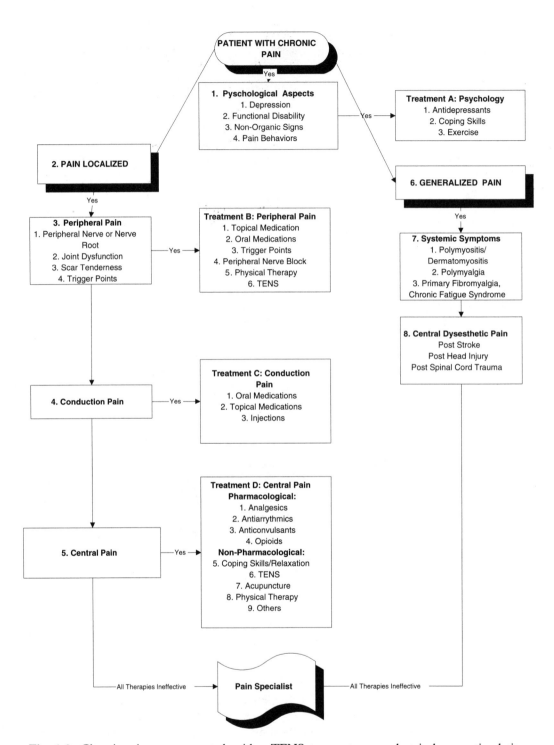

Fig. 6-2. Chronic pain management algorithm. TENS, transcutaneous electrical nerve stimulation.

Figure 6-2 presents an algorithm for the management of chronic pain.

TREATMENT PLANS

Psychological Aspects

Depression

The patient presenting with pain must be closely observed for a flat affect, early morning wakening, and emotional lability. Suicidal ideation must be asked about. If severe depression or suicidal ideation is present, referral to a psychiatrist must be sought immediately. Depression can mimic chronic pain or can be present secondarily to chronic pain. The difference is often difficult to determine, even for a psychiatrist or psychologist.

Functional Disability

Questions regarding how the pain has affected the individual's function, both socially and at work, should be asked. A person who is not working because of pain, or is socially withdrawn because of pain, will often exhibit marked pain behaviors (see below) indicating poor coping skills. It is not the pain that disables a person but how he or she decides to function with it.

Nonorganic Signs

Waddell (a Scottish orthopaedic surgeon) developed his "nonorganic signs for low back pain" to identify those patients in whom physical treatment, such as surgery or physical therapy, was likely to have poor results. He identified axial rotation and axial pressure, distraction causing an alteration in physical signs, a nonanatomic distribution of the pain, and exaggerated signs or pain behaviors as being indicative of a "psychogenic cry for help." Surgery, even when "technically successful," in this group was often unsuccessful in decreasing pain. These signs should always be looked for when examining the low back. There are other nonorganic signs that have been described for other body areas.

Pain Behaviors

Pain behaviors include frequent grimacing, sighing, verbalizing, visibly guarding muscles, and rubbing of the painful area. While this is understandable in the acute pain context, for the chronic pain individual it often indicates poor coping skills and, if not a conscious, it may be an unconscious request for compassion and perhaps secondary gain.

TREATMENT A

Antidepressants. The role of tricyclic antidepressants (amitriptyline, nortriptyline, imipramine) in chronic pain is well documented. By their action on the serotonin, norepinephrine, dopamine, and alpha-1 receptors, they appear to have a more marked analgesic effect than the newer serotonin-specific reuptake inhibitors. Amitriptyline is useful as a sedative medication if the patient has sleep difficulty. It is initially given at 10 or 25 mg q hs, depending on the age of the individual. It can be titrated up every 3 days until adequate sleep is achieved. This often coincides with patient complaints of a dry mouth. If the dry mouth is a significant problem, methylcellulose mouth sprays can be prescribed, or the patient can be instructed to chew gum. Once a level of 100 to 150 mg has been reached, without sleep or pain improvement, a drug blood level should be taken. Based on this level, the dose should be increased to antidepressant range and kept there for 1 month. If, after this time, there is no improvement in the patient's pain, the medication should be stopped.

Amitriptyline may reset the brain center that governs body size. If the patient starts putting on weight on amitriptyline, the medication should probably be changed or a permanent weight gain may occur. Nortriptyline appears less likely to cause this problem. The patient should be closely monitored while being treated for depression and a referral to a psychiatrist made if the patient has an adverse alteration or no improvement in mental status.

Coping skills. There are many tapes of relaxation and stress management techniques available. If the individual can relax his or her muscles effectively, the pain is often reduced. A psychologist trained in pain management is a very effective professional to whom the patient should be referred for coping skills training in dealing with environmental stressors. Biofeedback is useful in teaching the individual to relax if this is a problem.

Exercise. General exercise should always be encouraged. This can be walking, swimming, or bicycling. Aerobic exercise will improve the patient's function and health, give the individual an important coping mechanism for dealing with pain. Specific stretching exercises for the individual's pain problem can be given by a physical therapist or athletic trainer. Advice on exercise can be as simple as parking at one end of the car park and walking further to the shop, or walking up two to three flights of stairs before taking the elevator higher. Taking on the responsibility of aerobic exercising regularly is of great benefit in improving self-esteem.

Localized Pain

If pain is localized, a careful history should be taken of the probable mechanism of injury. This can indicate the forces involved and the potential structures that may have been damaged.

Peripheral Pain

Although chronic pain is a combination of peripheral sensitization and central hyperexcitation within the spinal cord, there are some syndromes that are predominantly peripheral in origin:

1. *Peripheral nerve or nerve root.* A careful examination should establish whether the pain is within the distribution of a nerve root or peripheral nerve.
2. *Joint dysfunction.* Pushing on an individual joint such as a cervical zygapophyseal (facet) joint may reproduce the individual's pain. This indicates that the joint, or structures surrounding it, may be involved in the pain process.
3. *Scar tenderness.* Neuromas may be present in any scar. Gently "rolling" the scar or pressure over it may cause severe pain.
4. *Trigger points.* Trigger points are localized areas of muscle spasm, which, when pressure is exerted on them, cause pain referral into the painful site. Stretching the muscle may also recreate the pain.

TREATMENT B

Topical medication. Acute sensitivity of the skin or allodynia (which means "light touch" not normally perceived as painful is felt as being exquisitely painful), over a small area, may be effectively decreased by capsaicin cream. Capsaicin works by depleting substance P and needs to be rubbed on 3 to 4 times a day. It takes 3 to 6 weeks to effectively deplete substance P stores peripherally and centrally. The cream, made from red peppers, causes an intense burning sensation that patients might find intolerable. However, the burning usually lessens after a few days of use. The patients should be warned to wash their hands carefully afterward and to avoid rubbing their eyes during application of the cream or a severe irritation of the eyes will occur. EMLA cream, a mixture of lidocaine and prilocaine can be placed on small spots of acute tenderness. The cream should be placed as a thick layer with a transparent dressing placed over it. The cream should be left in place for 4 hours, after which time it can be removed. The area will remain anesthetic for a further 4 hours. This may be effective in desensitizing small painful areas. There are many other over-the-counter preparations, as well as those prepared by herbalists and others, which, when rubbed onto areas of pain, are said to diminish the pain sensation. If the over-the-counter creams, lotions, or sprays do not financially embarrass the individual and are found to be effective, with minimal side effects, their use should not be discouraged.

Oral medications. In the acute phase of pain, nonsteroidal anti-inflammatory drugs are very useful. In chronic pain, the nonsteroidal drugs probably have more effect centrally than peripherally and tend to be less effective. In areas of inflammation, opioids may work peripherally. However, in chronic pain their site of action is probably central. Some medications such as the alpha-1 blockers (prazocin) are useful in sympathetically maintained pain syndromes. Mexiletine, an oral analogue of lidocaine, and a sodium channel blocker may be effective in chronic pain associated with diabetic neuropathy.

Trigger points. When trigger points (localized areas of muscle tenderness referring pain) are present, ischemic massage, cold spray and stretch techniques, ice massage and stretch, dry needling, and local anesthetic injections all have a role. Any trigger point treatment should be accompanied by a home stretching and range of movement exercise program. If trigger points are a factor, the patient can be taught to deactivate latent trigger points that may become active in the future.

Peripheral nerve block. At certain sites peripheral nerves are easily accessible to an injection of local anesthetic. Good knowledge of the anatomic location of the nerve, use of a nerve stimulator, and careful injection can deaden the nerve going to a painful area. If pain relief is nearly total, this may indicate the pain is being initiated peripherally. For confirmation, a second successful block should be performed at a later date. If the pain is centralized, although the peripheral skin area will be numb, the patient's pain will be unrelieved. Care must be taken not to inject within a nerve. This causes extreme pain during the injection and may subsequently form a neuroma within the substance of the nerve. A joint or inflamed bursa can also be injected with local anesthetic to gauge their contribution to the pain syndrome. Joint injection can be done under fluoroscopy with contrast confirmation.

Physical therapy. In chronic pain, a physical therapist should use hands-on techniques. Joints that are stiff due to disuse or muscle spasm must be mobilized and stretched manually. Heat and ultrasound can be used to relax muscles to allow more effective mobilization. Mobilization of the joints and surrounding connective tissue is the key factor. The physical therapist should also be skilled at giving the patient specific exercises for home use and encouraging a general home exercise program.

TENS. Transcutaneous electrical nerve stimulation (TENS) is a useful modality and should be trialed in most patients with chronic pain. The patient should be instructed on the placement of the electrodes and the frequencies to be trialed. When placed correctly, a stimulation pattern should be felt over the painful region. If TENS does not help after 1 week, it is unlikely it will be of value. Of those patients in whom TENS was initially successful, 50% claim that the effect appears to wear off over the next year. Initially TENS is useful in approximately 60% of patients with chronic pain.

Conduction Pain

Conduction pain usually occurs when a nerve has been damaged due to trauma, entrapment, or demyelination. The regenerating nerve is often extremely sensitive to norepinephrine, which increases the afferent input to the spinal cord.

TREATMENT C

Oral medications. Most medications are ineffective for this type of pain. Anticonvulsants such as gabapentin or sodium channel blockers such as mexiletine can be trialed.

Topical medications. EMLA or capsaicin cream may be useful in desensitizing the regenerating nerves.

Injections. Injection into a presumed neuroma, which removes the pain, may indicate that the site of the neuroma is accessible to either neurolytic therapy or surgical removal. The neuroma should be injected on at least two occasions, with similar satisfactory results, before neurolytic therapy is undertaken.

Central Pain

Once pain has been present for a period of time, the dorsal horn of the spinal cord is thought to be altered, perhaps permanently. Wide dynamic range nociceptors are "wound up" and stimulate other nociceptor cells within the spinal cord dorsal horn, thereby increasing the receptive field and increasing the area over which pain is felt. This explains the glove and stocking distribution of pain felt in some neuropathic pain syndromes, e.g., diabetic neuropathy, or sympathetically maintained pain. This "pain memory" is thought to explain why pain remains chronic. We have no medication, as yet, to turn off this "wind-up" of the central nociceptors.

TREATMENT D

Pharmacologic. *Analgesics.* Simple analgesics such as tramadol, maximum dose 100 mg qid, acetaminophen-opioid combinations up to a maximum of 4 g acetaminophen a day, and acetaminophen maximum 4 g per day are all useful and can be trialed in patients with chronic pain. Any improvement of reported pain should be accompanied by an improvement in function. In chronic pain, unlike malignant pain, the analgesic requirements should remain fairly constant with time. A rapid escalation in pain requirements usually signifies either progression of the disease or an environmental stressor that has worsened the pain perception.

Antiarrhythmics. Certain antiarrhythmics, such as the sodium channel blocker mexiletine, which is converted to a lidocaine-like substance in the liver, calcium channel blockers, and beta blockers, have been used for treatment of various pain disorders. Mexiletine has been used for centralized neuropathic pain and is often effective in treatment of diabetic neuropathic pain. Calcium channel blockers and beta blockers have been used in prophylaxis against headaches.

Anticonvulsants. Chronic pain, especially that associated with shooting, "lancinating" pains, has been likened to epilepsy of the spinal cord. Thus, drugs such as carbamazepine, phenytoin, and valproic acid can be trialed. The new anticonvulsants, such as gabapentin (maximum 1,800 mg per day), appear to be far less toxic and anecdotally are proving effective in several forms of neuropathic and central dysesthetic pains.

Opioids. There is much evidence that opioids can be extremely effective in the management of chronic pain. The risk of addiction is low, and organ toxicity is minimal. The side effect of constipation is, however, unavoidable in most patients, and, when giving opioids, a second prescription should routinely be given for laxatives. It is worthwhile to have a "drug contract" with the patient (Fig. 6-3). This stipulates that the patient will (1) only get drugs from one physician, (2) ask permission before increasing the opioids for exacerbation of pain, (3) take care not to lose the prescription, and (4) consent to random drug testing should this be

OPIOID CONTRACT

I, _____ , understand that in order to receive care for the treatment of pain in the University Center for Pain Medicine and Rehabilitation I must comply with the following rules:

1) I will take medications at the dose and frequency prescribed. Any changes in the dose or frequency will be discussed with my attending physician, Dr. _____ , or with another designated attending physician in my physician's absence.

2) I will receive prescriptions at the following interval:

_____

3) I will not receive controlled substances for the treatment of pain from any source other than the University Center for Pain Medicine and Rehabilitation.

4) I will communicate with my primary physician that I am on contract with the University Center for Pain Medicine and Rehabilitation for the controlled prescribing of pain medications.

5) I will consent to random drug testing.

6) I will safeguard my prescribed medications.

7) I will comply with my scheduled appointments.

8) I will comply with all guidelines printed on the reverse side of this contract.

_____   _____
Patient   Date

_____   _____
Pain Center Physician   Date

_____   _____
Pain Center Nurse   Date

_____
Renewal Date

_____ Copy given to patient.

Fig. 6-3. Opioid contract. *(Figure continues.)*

PAIN CENTER GUIDELINES FOR CONTROLLED SUBSTANCES

1) Dr. _____ is available for pain clinic appointments on:

_____

2) Check the time and date of your next Pain Center appointment before leaving. If you must leave, call the receptionist within three days to verify your appointment.

3) Contact the Center at least three days in advance if you need to cancel or reschedule your appointment.

4) Requests for medication refills will be taken before noon Monday through Friday. Call your request for refill at least three days prior to your last dose of medication. Do not wait until the day you will run out of medications. Prescriptions for controlled substances will not be sent by mail or courier service, nor will any Schedule II prescriptions be called in by telephone. Written prescription must be picked up at the Pain Center.

5) It is our policy not to replace damaged, lost or stolen medications. It is your responsibility to keep your medications in a secure place.

6) You must discuss any changes in the way you take your pain medications with your attending physician before making changes. Do not suddenly stop taking your medications.

7) If you are having problems such as intractable, unrelieved pain and/or your condition becomes unstable, i.e., signs and symptoms unacceptable to you, or if you have questions or concerns, please contact the pain service.

Important Phone Number: Pain Center (713) 704-7246

Your Attending Physician: _____

Your Case Manager: _____

Fig. 6-3. *(Continued)*.

considered necessary. Many pain physicians also require the patient to have a drug-free holiday for 2 to 3 weeks after a year on chronic opioid therapy. This may increase the sensitivity of the individual to opioids once they are restarted, or it may allow the individual to come off opioids once they have been withdrawn. In either event, it enhances the feeling of trust between patient and doctor, which is extremely important for most physicians signing ongoing triplicate prescriptions. If one type of opioid is unsuccessful, a second class of opioid can be tried. Thus, if morphine is not successful, methadone, a fentanyl patch, or hydromorphone (Dilaudid) could be trialed. If aberrant behavior or prescription loss occurs, the physician retains the right to wean the patient and discharge him or her from his care. To effectively wean a patient without withdrawal symptoms means withdrawing the medication at a rate between 20% and 50% of the dose per day. After 1 week, most patients can be successffully withdrawn from even large doses of opioids.

Nonpharmacologic. *Coping skills and relaxation.* By releasing various neuropeptides, relaxation and improving coping skills can dampen the pain response. They allow the patient to have a good quality of life despite pain.

TENS. TENS should be trialed on an organized basis for 1 week. If pain relief does not occur after this time, TENS will probably be ineffective.

Acupuncture. If acupuncture is going to be successful, 50% of patients respond within three treatments and probably 90% within six treatments. If no improvement occurs after six treatments, given initially biweekly, and then weekly, therapy should be discontinued. Acupuncture may be with needles only, or with needles and electrical stimulation. If the patient responds well to acupuncture, the duration of pain relief varies. Periodic booster treatments are usually required.

Physical therapy. Specific stretching and mobility exercises, as well as an aerobic program, should be given.

Other treatments. There are many other treatments for pain. For example, there is some evidence that magnets placed over trigger point areas, or over the nerve serving the area, may diminish the pain response. This is probably by central neuromodulation.

Generalized Pain

The individual who presents with generalized pain will not usually respond to specific blocks or surgery. Some diseases, such as polymyositis, dermatomyositis, and polymyalgia rheumatica, can present with diffuse aching pain and need to be excluded by careful examination and perhaps laboratory studies.

Polymyositis and Dermatomyositis

Polymyositis and dermatomyositis are usually associated with weakness in the proximal limb muscles, especially the hips and thighs, as well as shoulder girdles. A deep aching pain in calves and buttocks occur in up to 50% of these patients, with tenderness on palpation of the thighs. Muscle enzyme levels are raised. Treatment is with high-dose steroids. Referral to a rheumatologist is mandatory.

Polymyalgia Rheumatica

Polymyalgia rheumatica usually presents as a diffuse aching pain and stiffness in the neck, hip, and shoulder girdles. The patient has a raised ESR and chronic anemia. Referral to a rheumatologist is important. Treatment is with steroids, which should be started immediately if the patient's vision is affected, or tenderness of the temporal arteries or a decrease in temporal arterial pulsation is present. A delay in treatment of temporal arteritis may lead to permanent blindness.

Primary Fibromyalgia/Chronic Fatigue Syndrome

Generalized pain without ESR or enzyme changes may be due to primary fibromyalgia or chronic fatigue syndrome. These terms have been used interchangeably and may be a part of a continuum of the same disease. Clinically, fibromyalgia appears to be a musculoskeletal system response to stress. There is generalized body aching and pains with stiffness involving three or more anatomic sites. The symptoms tend to get worse with physical activity, and sleep disturbance is almost universal. The subject often complains of swelling of the hands and feet with exercise, and many have irritable bowel-type symptoms. These patients also complain of anxiety attacks and chronic headaches, and they often complain of nonradicular and nondermatomal numbness. Treatment is with low-dose tricyclic antidepressants, such as doxepin hydrochloride, initially at night, or with larger dose serotoninergic reuptake inhibitors in the morning. Flexeril in small doses of 10 mg bid–tid has been reported to be useful. Nonsteroidals are usually not effective unless an acute inflammatory component is present. Vitamin D in large doses and the antioxidants, vitamin E and selenium, have been said to improve muscle pain. Calcium and magnesium tablets 400–600 mg taken 45 minutes before sleep appear to improve the sleep pattern by decreasing muscle aching. The main form of treatment of these individuals is with aerobic exercise, stress management techniques, and deep relaxation. Trigger point therapy with dry needling or cold and stretch techniques may be useful. TENS is often disappointing. However, localized areas of tenderness may respond favorably to TENS, and, with its low side effect profile, it should be trialed. These syndromes remain extremely difficult to treat successfully.

Central Dysesthetic Pain

Patients who have had a stroke, closed head injury, or spinal cord trauma may present with intractable pains. These pains may be resistant to most forms of therapy. TENS should be trialed, as should anticonvulsants such as gabapentin. Occasionally, nerve blocks may help localize the pain. Opioids should be tried; however, they are usually ineffective. Pains that occur in response to muscle spasm may respond to neurolytic injections into the motor points of the affected muscles, or intrathecally. Intrathecal baclofen has proven very effective in reducing painful spasms.

PAIN SPECIALIST

If the various treatments for chronic pain prove to be ineffective, referral to a pain specialist should be made. The pain specialist should reevaluate the patient, preferably in consultation with a psychologist who is trained in pain management. Treatment suggested by the "pain team" may include medication optimization, diagnostic pain blocks, diagnostic joint injections, infusions of lidocaine or phentolamine, differential spinal or epidural injection. Invasive procedures may include radiofrequency ablation, intrathecal pumps, spinal cord stimulators, or peripheral nerve stimulators. Together with a large battery of potential tests, both diagnostic and therapeutic, the pain specialist should have access to a multidisciplinary pain management program. The main object of such programs should be to increase the functionality of the individual and give him or her back a good quality of life despite the pain. Returning to work where possible should be a major goal.

CASE STUDY

Mr. R. was a 38-year-old firefighter who had been badly burned on both hands while fighting a fire some three years previously. His burns had healed without the need for skin grafting, but his right hand had continued to give him pain. He described the pain as 80/100 most of the time, increasing to 95/100 if he tried to use the hand. At best it was 70/100. He was sleeping badly. The pain made getting to sleep difficult, and he was awakened frequently with pain. He had tried numerous NSAIDs without effect. He took 12–16 codeine/acetaminophen combination tablets per day. This dose amounted to 6–8 g of acetaminophen per day and diazepam 10 mg three times a day. He was drinking heavily to "take his mind off the pain" but had no previous history of substance abuse. He described the pain as a continuous burning over his thumb and back of his right hand. Cold or hot packs did not make the pain worse, but barometric pressure changes, associated with weather fronts, aggravated his pain. He had had three emergency room admissions over the last 6 months because of his pain. On each occasion he was given Demerol 100 mg by intramuscular injection with marked relief of his pain (100/100 decreased to 50–60/100).

He was married with two children. He had attempted to return to work 6 months after his accident. His painful right hand (he was right-handed) prevented him from achieving much productive work, and he had stopped work after 1 month. He had been a firefighter for 12 years and had enjoyed it. He wanted to return to it in some capacity.

On examination he protected his right hand and wore an elasticized glove to decrease the swelling. Nail and hair growth appeared normal. There was normal skin temperature when compared to the left side. He had marked allodynia (light touch caused pain) over the dorsum of his hand and thumb as well as hyperpathia (mildly painful stimulus caused pain, which lasted significantly longer than the stimulus). He was unable to oppose his thumb, and movements of all fingers were decreased by pain and stiffness. The hand swelling was not marked.

Impression Central pain, possibly conduction pain (radial nerve).

Plan

1. Nortriptyline 25 mg at night, increasing every 3 nights until either 100 mg is reached or a good night's sleep occurs.
2. Capsaicin cream 0.025% to rub on four times a day.
3. Gabapentin (anticonvulsant) 300 mg, increasing by 300 mg a day until 600 mg tid.
4. Consider opioids.
5. Tell him to stop his alcohol intake.
6. Put him on slow taper schedule to withdraw the benzodiazepine.
7. See him in 10 days.

The patient returned stating he was feeling slightly improved. His pain score was 70/100. He was sleeping much better on 50 mg nortriptyline, but did not like the side effects of dry mouth and constipation. He had stopped his alcohol intake. The capsaicin cream had been too uncomfortable to use, as the intense burning had persisted for many hours after application. He was on gabapentin 300 mg tid. When he increased it further, he had felt very drowsy. He had decreased his analgesics to six per day.

Plan

1. Trial TENS.
2. Encourage him to increase the gabapentin dosage slowly by 300 mg every 2 days. If excessive drowsiness occurs, he should stay at a lower dosage until tolerance to this side effect occurs (usually 1–2 weeks).

3. Congratulate him on stopping his alcohol intake.
4. Encourage finger exercises.
5. Increase nortriptyline.
6. See him in 1 week.

He returned in 1 week stating he was sleeping much better on 75 mg nortriptyline at night. His dry mouth was not as troublesome if he chewed gum to relieve it. His constipation had been effectively treated by adding more roughage and prune juice to his diet.

The TENS worked well when it was on, decreasing the pain to 50/100, which was the best it had been since the accident. The pain relief only lasted a few minutes after turning the device off.

He was still off alcohol and taking 6 to 8 analgesics per day. He was taking gabapentin 300 mg morning and noon and 600 mg at night.

His average pain was 60–70/100.

Plan

1. He was instructed on other TENS settings. He was using TENS in a conventional with burst mode. An acupuncturelike mode (low frequency, high intensity) over the acupuncture or trigger points of the wrist and forearm might give him a longer duration of relief. He was concerned about wearing the TENS for too long a period. He was told he could use the TENS as long as he wanted; skin irritation was the only potential side effect.
2. As he had conformed to requests to come off alcohol and decrease his acetaminophen/codeine analgesics and had had no prior history of drug abuse or chaotic home environment, a trial of opioids was started. He was commenced on methadone 10 mg every 8 hours and told not to expect any major improvement for 2 to 4 days, as methadone has a slow onset of effect. He could continue his analgesics but slowly taper them over the next 3 to 4 days. Thereafter he was to take them on an "as-needed" basis but to take note of how many he was requiring. He was given a prescription for laxatives and a prepared instruction sheet about the treatment of constipation.
3. He was maintained on the nortriptyline and gabapentin.
4. See him in 1 week.

He returned in 1 week, delighted with his progress. His pain decreased to 30/100 at best and 50/100 on average. He was requiring 3 to 4 extra analgesics per day. Mentally he stated he was feeling alert and was taking 1 to 2 laxatives per day to maintain a daily bowel movement. He had started some simple carpentry, which had been his hobby before the accident, but which he had not attempted since because of pain. The acupuncture-type TENS was not as effective as the burst/conventional mode. He was wearing the TENS approximately 12 hours a day.

Plan

1. Refer to physical therapist for hand exercises and mobilization. This resulted in a marked improvement over the ensuing weeks.
2. Increase methadone to 15 mg in morning and afternoon and keep at 10 mg in evening. This helped his pain further and decreased his "rescue" medications to periods when he knew his pain would be worsened, for example, just before physical therapy.
3. Continue on the nortriptyline and gabapentin.
4. Encourage him to investigate prospects of returning to work in some administrative position.
5. See him at regular intervals to assess progress and give encouragement.

If the above regimen had not been successful, referral to a pain specialist would have been appropriate. In this patient a radial nerve block may have been indicated. If successfully reducing his pain by more than 50%, he may have been a candidate for a peripheral nerve stimulator. A lidocaine infusion to see the potential efficacy of sodium channel blockers would be another consideration. Sympathetic-maintained pain is unlikely, as cold did not make his pain worse; however, this could be ruled out or verified by a stellate ganglion block or a phentolamine infusion. Other opioids might be trialed if methadone was proving ineffective or if there were significant side effects.

SUGGESTED READINGS

Kopec JA, Esdaile JM, Abrahamowicz M et al: The Quebec Back Pain Disability Scale. Spine 3:3410–352, 1995

Van Korff M, Ormel J, Keege FJ, Dworkin SF: Grading the severity of chronic pain. Pain 50:133–149, 1992

Williams RC: Toward a set of reliable valid measures for chronic pain assessment and outcome research. Pain 35:239–251, 1988

Acute Pain

GENERAL PRINCIPLES

Acute pain is commonly mistreated both in the postoperative period, where surveys have indicated failure to relieve pain in up to 50% of patients, and in the acute medical or post-trauma settings.

Inadequately treated pain contributes to patient discomfort, longer recovery periods, and increased use of health care resources. There is also some evidence that if acute pain is not treated aggressively, there is an increased possibility of chronic pain developing.

The first 48 to 72 hours after any injury are usually the most painful. Both drug and nondrug methods, such as reassessment and reassurance, should be used during this period. Patients may have myths about pain and medication which should be addressed. Early mobilization should be a goal after any painful episode to prevent joint stiffness and muscle atrophy adding to the individual's discomfort and immobility.

If the analgesics give inadequate relief or unacceptable side effects, they should be changed or the side effects treated.

If pain persists for more than 4 weeks following the usual healing pattern of the injury, referral to a pain specialist or other specialists should be strongly considered for appropriate therapy.

Figure 7-1 presents an algorithm for the management of acute pain.

BONE INJURY

If the trauma is significant and there is a clinical suspicion of bone or joint damage, investigations such as x-ray, CT (computed tomography) scan, or MRI (magnetic resonance imaging) may be indicated. In the initial phase of the injury a plain x-ray is the most appropriate. If surgical intervention is warranted because of damage to underlying structures, a specific CT scan or MRI may be ordered by the specialist. Problems with no obvious signs of bone damage do not require an x-ray.

TREATMENT PLANS

Dirty Wounds

TREATMENT A

The dirty wound should be cleaned and dressed. A tetanus toxoid should be given if tetanus immunity is not recent. Obvious dead and nonviable tissue should be debrided, which may require local anesthesia or general anesthesia. Antibiotics should be given as indicated. Some wounds may require extensive debriding in the emergency room. Such wounds are usually best left open initially and not covered until the full nature of the damage and viability of the remaining tissue has been assessed some days later.

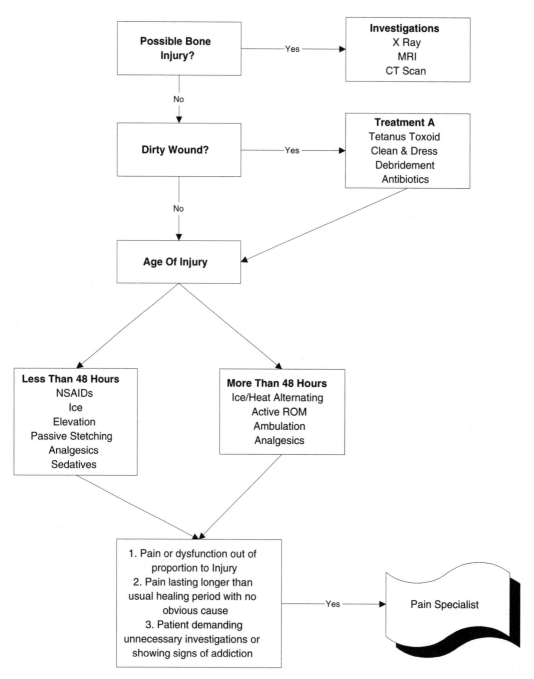

Fig. 7-1. Acute pain management algorithm. NSAIDS, nonsteroidal anti-inflammatory drugs; CT, computed tomography; MRI, magnetic resonance imaging.

Age of Injury Less Than 48 Hours

TREATMENT B

Nonsteroidal anti-inflammatory drugs. In any acute injury, tissue damage releases phospholipids from the tissue membranes leading to the formation of leukotrienes and prostaglandins, both of which sensitize the nociceptors. Nonsteroidal anti-inflammatory drugs (NSAIDs) block the formation of prostaglandins, decrease nociceptor sensitization, and decrease the swelling associated with acute injuries. Most NSAIDs have significant side effects, mainly involving the gastric mucosa, causing gastritis and hematemesis. Because of the potential for side effects and the physiology of the healing process, the use of NSAIDs should be limited to the first 48 to 72 hours. After this time, an analgesic such as acetaminophen or tramadol is probably safer.

Ice. Cooling the area by ice placed in a plastic bag, or a commercial polyglycol ice bag from the freezer, significantly decreases the swelling and diminishes the pain. To prevent frosbite, ice should be kept on an extremity for only 20 minutes every hour. The treatment can be repeated frequently over the first 48 hours of an injury. Putting a cream on the skin before icing and wrapping the ice bag in a paper towel will prevent damage to the skin.

Elevation. Swelling and edema prolong the healing process and cause more discomfort and pain. Elevation improves drainage from the area and decreases edema. If possible, the injured area should be elevated above the level of the heart. Elevation is most effective in the first 24 to 48 hours after injury.

Rest. Depending on the injury, rest allows tissues to heal without concurrent muscle spasms. Rest more than 48 hours, however, unless there has been significant trauma, can be counterproductive and can initiate a sickness role.

Stretching. Passive stretching of an injured joint is important even in the early stages of recovery. Collagen fibers are laid down and aligned according to the degree of stress and movement put on the tissues. Moving an injured joint early not only improves blood flow but encourages a faster recovery to full function. Most joints, unless they are fractured or have been operated on, can be gently stretched passively by the patient. Stretching should occur every 1 to 2 hours for a period of 5 to 10 minutes. If stretching causes a worsening of the pain or swelling, stretching should be stopped and recommenced after 24 to 48 hours.

Analgesics. Analgesics such as acetaminophen and opioid combinations, if prescribed, should be taken on a round-the-clock schedule for a limited period, probably 48 to 72 hours only, depending on the nature of the trauma. This can be followed by a prn (as necessary) schedule for 3 to 4 days further. Areas of inflammation have opioid receptors upregulated on the C-fiber terminals. This means the opioids act not only centrally but also peripherally, making them one of the most effective treatments in the acute pain of trauma.

Sedation. Sedation is usually not necessary for most acute trauma. Difficulty in sleeping because of enforced rest may be treated by chloral hydrate 500–1,000 mg at night. This is a safe medication with limited side effects and is nonaddictive. Sleeping tablets given on an as-necessary basis should be avoided because of the risk of addiction.

Age of Injury 48 to 72 Hours and Older

TREATMENT C

Alternating ice/heat. After the initial 48 hours, bleeding will have stopped and alternating heat and cold will allow the tissues to begin mobilizing any excessive fluid. It will also allow the individual to begin moving the injured part and joints. Any hot pack used must not be hotter than the face can tolerate. Ice/heat alternating can be done 2 to 3 times a day together with active range of movement exercises.

Active range of movement. After the initial rest period, active range of movement of the joints and ambulation of the patient should commence. While pain may persist, the ability to move and to mobilize the tissues is important in speeding up the healing process. It also encourages the patient to have self-reliance and not be dependent on passive modes of therapy.

Analgesics. Acetaminophen-opioid combinations can be continued for a few days longer but should probably be on a prn basis at this stage. After 5 to 7 days, analgesics such as acetaminophen alone can be used.

FURTHER TREATMENT

Strong opioids. If the initial therapy is not effective and the pain is still severe, strong opioids should be considered. When opioids are trialed the patient must be aware that they are on a temporary basis. Escalation of the drug without the physician's knowledge will be taken as indicating the drug is ineffective and it will be discontinued (see drug contract, Fig. 6-3). If strong opioids are given, they should be on a time-contingent basis and when stopped should be withdrawn at a rate of 20% to 50% per day. In this way withdrawal symptoms will be avoided.

Reevaluation. Pain causing significant dysfunction 1 week after the injury should be reevaluated. If the pain is significantly more than the initial diagnosis would suggest, further investigations may be relevant. These investigations may lead to a referral to a specialist. If there are indications that the pain has a strong affective component, environmental factors such as job and home environment should be taken into account.

Anxiolytics. If the patient remains extremely anxious and especially if sleep is affected, anxiolytics may be appropriate. The patient must be aware that the anxiolytics will be given on a time-contingent basis only and for a trial period. If poor coping skills are evident, once the acute phase has settled down, referral to a psychologist or psychiatrist may be appropriate. Most anxiolytics are contraindicated for chronic pain conditions. In acute pain, however, especially those associated with underlying anxieties, a short treatment period may be useful.

PAIN SPECIALIST

If, despite appropriate treatment, pain from the acute trauma lasts 4 weeks longer than it usually takes for a particular injury to heal, referral to a pain specialist should be considered. The pain specialist should evaluate the patient not only from a physical but also from an emotional standpoint. At this stage a psychological evaluation may be required, and environmental stresses carefully assessed. Early referral to a pain specialist should result in more appropriate care and less chronic disability, with less drain on society and the primary physician.

SUGGESTED READING

Acute Pain Management Guidelines: Agency for Health Care Policy and Research (HHCPR), P.O. Box 8547, Silver Spring, MD 20907, or call 1-800-358-9295 for free copy.

Abdominal Pain

Acute abdominal pain may be relatively straightforward to diagnose, requiring observation, medication, or even surgery for therapy. Abdominal pain lasting 3 to 6 months or longer is often much harder to diagnose. A careful history noting the periodicity of symptoms is of great importance. A rectal and vaginal examination should be always done, as well as a careful assessment of hernial orifices and external genitalia. Assessment of the other organ systems, for example, heart and lungs, should be done routinely as part of the general examination, especially if the history leads one to suspect an extra-abdominal cause of the pain— for example, cardiac failure causing right hypochondrium pain due to hepatic distention.

Pain in the abdomen is usually caused by visceral disorders. Somatic referred pain, however, must be looked for. The lower half of the thoracic parietal pleura, the periphery of the diaphragmatic pleura, and the upper 85% of the abdominal wall are supplied by the 6th or 7th thoracic spinal nerves. Lesions of any of these structures or surrounding connective tissues can cause similar pain.

The Nuprin Pain Report noted in 1985 that 46% of Americans had significant episodes of abdominal (stomach) pain. In 1986, the National Hospital Discharge Survey indicated that about 6.7 million operations were performed to diagnose and treat digestive and renal disorders each year.

Figure 8-1 presents an algorithm for chronic abdominal pain management.

SURGICAL CAUSE

To rule out any surgically amenable cause, various investigations may need to be carried out. These include computed tomography (CT) scan, magnetic resonance imaging (MRI), or ultrasound of the abdominal viscera. Blood work should be done to rule out pancreatitis, infections, and parasitic infestations. Markers for colon or prostatic cancer may indicate the need for further investigations. Barium studies or endoscopy may confirm suspicious lesions. Based on the results of these investigations, laparoscopy or other surgery may be indicated.

Visceral causes of pain that may require surgery include gallbladder disease, gastric or duodenal ulcer, carcinoma of the stomach and gastrointestinal tract, bowel diseases such as ulcerative colitis or Crohn's disease, and diseases of the ovaries and uterus, bladder and kidneys, liver, or pancreas.

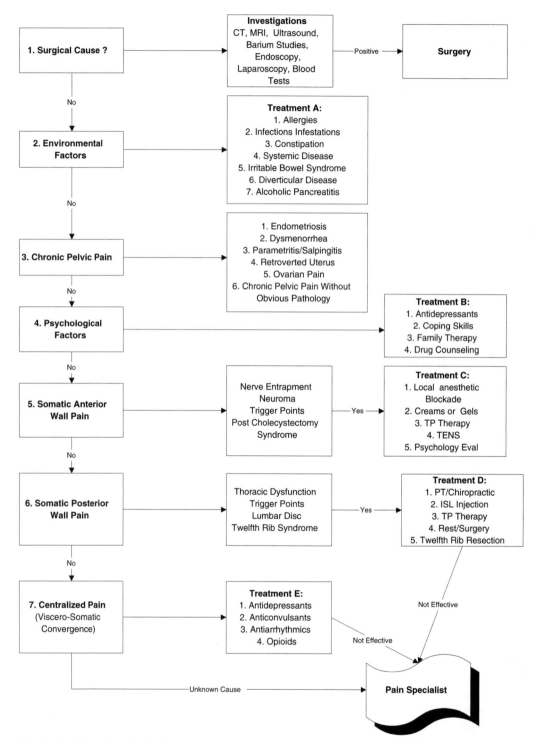

Fig. 8-1. Chronic abdominal pain management algorithm. ISL, interspinous ligament injection; TP, trigger point; TENS, transcutaneous electrical nerve stimulation.

TREATMENT PLANS

Environmental Factors

The environment, both physical and emotional, can cause abdominal pain. These include allergies, metabolic and environmental toxins, systemic disease, infestations or infection, irritable bowel syndrome, diverticular disease, and constipation.

TREATMENT A

Allergies. Where allergies are suspected, a food and pain diary (Fig. 8-2) should be given to the patient to look for periodicity of pain as well as precipitating factors. Food allergies may present with pain within 48 to 72 hours after digesting an allergen. Lactose intolerance should always be inquired about, especially in those racial groups such as the black and the Jewish populations in whom the gene for the lactase enzyme is often absent. If a food that is taken regularly is suspected, the patient should be instructed to avoid that food for 10 to 14 days. After this time they can "binge" on it. If they are "allergic" to the foodstuff, the period of abstinence will cause a hypersensitivity. Although the abdominal pain may not be improved by the 2-week avoidance trial, taking a large amount causes severe abdominal cramps and pain. This strategy can be followed for various suspect foodstuffs. A food diary (Fig. 8-2) can be valuable in documenting the allergy.

FOOD DIARY

Date _____   Name _____

Hour	Pre-Meal Pain Score	Food/Beverage Intake	Quantity	Time taken over meal/drink	One hour post-meal pain score

Fig. 8-2. Food diary.

Infections or infestations. Parasites and worms should be carefully investigated with stool analysis, careful history, and examination. Specific treatment for the infestation can then be instituted. Knowledge of the common infestations in the particular geographic area is important. A history of recent overseas or out-of-state trips should be part of the history. Some infestations may take several weeks to show clinical signs.

Constipation. Persistent constipation can result in anxiety, pain, decreased appetite, and intestinal pseudo-obstruction. The pain of constipation is usually felt over the left lower quadrant and upper abdomen, which may vary from constant and dull to sharp or severe. It does not awaken the patient. Defecation usually brings partial relief. Pain may be made worse by high-bulk foods or laxatives if they fail to cause defecation. The abdomen may be chronically distended, and colonic fecal contents can often be palpated in the transverse and descending colon. The rectum may be full of hard feces or empty, but with feces palpable on bimanual examination, in the sigmoid colon. Opioids taken concurrently for abdominal pain or for other unrelated ailments are a common cause of constipation.

Treatment of constipation depends on its severity. Mild constipation can be treated by increasing fluid intake, activity, and fiber (20–60 g per day). Mild to moderate constipation can be treated by adding bulking agents such as bran, methylcellulose, and psyllium. Bisacodyl 1 to 3 tablets or Senokot 1 to 4 tablets per day may be prescribed. Severe constipation with no bowel action for 3 days, where feces are felt in the rectum, can be treated with milk of magnesia 15 to 30 ml at night, or Lactulose 10 to 20 ml. The action of these agents usually produces a semifluid stool within 3 hours. If no bowel action has occurred for more than 3 days and no stool is felt in the rectum, in addition to milk of magnesia and Lactulose, a glycerine or Biscodyl suppository can be given. In refractory cases a sodium phosphate (Fleet) enema should be tried. Manual disimpaction, usually under a general anesthetic, may be necessary. The goal is to have one or more soft stool actions per day.

Systemic disease. The abdominal pain of uremia and diabetes is often nonspecific. Urinalysis and blood tests should provide the diagnosis. Treatment of the renal failure or diabetes will usually "cure" the abdominal pain.

Irritable bowel syndrome. Irritable bowel syndrome (IBS) is more common in females (up to 5:1 ratio) in the second, third, or fourth decades. It is associated with a disturbance in motility throughout the gut from esophagus to anus. It may be associated with increased sensitivity to gastrointestinal hormones and prostaglandins (in diarrheal patients).

Nausea and vomiting are common, but usually not anorexia or weight loss. Bowel habits are altered; morning diarrhea is often followed by constipation later in the day. Some patients are lactose-intolerant. A barium enema may show chronic spasm. Pain is often constant but does not awaken the patient. Tenderness is usually maximum over the descending colon.

Smokers should stop smoking, and a lactose-free diet should be tried. Bulk laxatives may help the morning diarrheal episodes. Psychological counseling for poor stress coping skills is often indicated.

Diverticular disease. Diverticula are mucosal and connective tissue sacs that penetrate the circular muscle bands of the colon. Pain is usually dull and worsened with constipation. Acute, severe pain may be associated with inflammation which lasts 1 to 2 weeks. Diverticula are usually seen on barium enema or at endoscopy.

Treatment is with a high-bulk diet, with laxatives if needed, to prevent constipation. Acute diverticulitis is treated with broad-spectrum antibiotics and correction of fluid and electrolyte losses. Abscess formation may necessitate surgery, as may strictures. Carcinoma may be difficult to rule out by endoscopic biopsies, and suspicious strictures should probably be resected.

Alcoholic pancreatitis. Recurrent abdominal pains should alert the practitioner to the possibility of alcoholic pancreatitis. Other stigmata of chronic alcohol use may be present, and a blood count may reveal macrocytosis. At this stage complete abstinence from drinking may be curative, or the patient may still progress to chronic pancreatitis (see the section Centralized Pain below).

Chronic Pelvic Pain/Diseases of the Uterus or Ovaries

Endometriosis

Endometriosis is ectopic endometrium outside the uterus. Up to 40% of lesions are asymptomatic. Pain, when present, may be continuous, or influenced by the menstrual cycle. Dysmenorrhea is often present, especially if the uterus is fixed in a retroverted position due to adhesions. Bladder endometriotic foci may cause pain on micturition and hematuria during menstruation. Adhesions in the pouch of Douglas may cause painful defecation. Pelvic examination usually shows a fixed retroversion of the uterus with tender, enlarged, adherent adnexa.

Treatment is with cyclical estrogen-progestogen preparations. It is successful in easing the pain in 50% of individuals. Continuous progesterones can also be used. Danazol, a potent antigonadotropin, may be indicated in resistant cases. Surgical opinion for laparoscopic laser ablation or surgical removal of endometriotic foci may be necessary. In resistant cases total hysterectomy and bilateral salpingo-oophorectomy may be performed. Sometimes, however, even with this radical surgery the pain continues.

Dysmenorrhea

Dysmenorrhea is recurrent pain occurring around the menstrual period. The pain is usually in the lower abdomen and often in the sacrum and upper buttocks. Secondary dysmenorrhea may be due to endometriosis, submucous fibroids, or obstruction to outflow of menstrual products. Primary dysmenorrhea starts a few months after menarche and may last for several years. The cause is unknown.

Treatment of primary dysmenorrhea is with reassurance, nonsteroidal anti-inflammatory drugs, and, if necessary, cyclic estroprogestogens. Treatment of secondary dysmenorrhea depends on the cause.

Parametritis/Salpingitis

Infection of the parametrial tissues, usually associated with a chronic cervicitis, or a salpingitis, often presents with pelvic and low back pain with dyspareunia but often no temperature. Night sweats and weight loss suggest tuberculous salpingitis. Pelvic examination reveals a tender, painful cervix, parametrium, or tubo-ovarian masses. Diagnosis can be determined by the presence of agglutinated leukocytes in the cervical mucus during the ovulation period (parametritis) or a positive tuberculin test with tubercle bacilli found in the menstrual blood or endometrial biopsy (tuberculous salpingitis). Laparoscopy may be necessary for diagnosis.

Retroverted Uterus

Retroversion may cause venous congestion of the uterus, giving rise to lower abdominal and sacrogluteal pain around the time of menstruation. Pain is often relieved by lying flat. A tender, retroverted, mobile uterus is usually found. Insertion of a vaginal pessary should relieve the pain within 2 to 3 days. Treatment is by insertion of a vaginal pessary for 6 to 8 weeks. If the pain returns on removal of the pessary, surgical correction should be considered.

Ovarian Pain

Recurrent ovarian cysts may cause pain. Diagnosis is by laparoscopy and treatment by oral contraceptives. After an oophorectomy, ovarian remnants may cause recurrent pains. Diagnosis is by suppressing adrenal production of estrogen by a short course of corticosteroids. Persisting estrogen levels indicate functioning ovarian tissues. Treatment is surgical removal of the remnants.

Chronic Pelvic Pain Without Obvious Pathology

In a situation where the pelvic pain is chronic, or recurrent, but no pathology can be found, venous pelvic congestion may play a role, as may psychosomatic disorders. The diagnosis should be one of exclusion. Cyclic estroprogesterones may help some patients, and continuous progesterones may help others. A referral for a psychological or psychiatric opinion is usually necessary.

Psychological Factors

Abdominal pain primarily caused by psychological or emotional factors varies in type, location, and other characteristics. There is usually no relation to meals. The pain is often worse during the evening, and nausea and vomiting are rarely observed. On examination no reflex abdominal spasm is felt, and signs and symptoms often vary from visit to visit. A careful history may indicate depression, secondary gain (often of an emotional nature), or drug-seeking behavior.

TREATMENT B

Antidepressants. If depression is thought to be a factor, antidepressants should be trialed. Nortriptyline should be the first choice, as it may improve any neuropathic pain component present. Tricyclics may cause constipation, which may worsen the patient's pain.

Coping skills. Emotional trauma and inadequate coping skills can maintain or worsen any chronic pain syndrome. A pain psychologist consultation is important in helping the patient cope emotionally with the various stressors of his or her daily life and learning mechanisms by which they can diminish the pain. There are now several books available for the public that give coping skill exercises and techniques.

Family therapy. Family therapy in dysfunctional households can be very effective. This is especially true in the adolescent age group.

Drug counseling. Abdominal pain is a common presentation for those seeking drugs for recreational purposes. Careful history and examination should help rule out these patients who require psychiatric and psychological help and not further narcotics.

Somatic Anterior Wall Pain

Pain felt in the anterior wall may be due to a neuroma or nerve entrapment due to previous surgery. Frequently this occurs at the lateral border of the rectus sheath. Trigger points in surrounding musculature may also refer pain to the anterior wall. The patient's pain is usually made worse by tensing the abdominal muscles. One way to identify muscular pain is to have the patient attempt a sit-up from lying. Preventing them from rising by pushing back against their chest recreates their pain.

The postcholecystectomy syndrome is poorly understood. It occurs as right hypochondrium pain soon after gallbladder surgery. It may be colicky in nature, usually occurring during the day and not at night. It varies in intensity from dull to severe and can continue for years.

TREATMENT C

Local anesthetic blockade. Local anesthetic injected around the intercostal nerve can differentiate somatic pain of the anterior wall. An injection of 2–5 ml lidocaine injected on the intercostal nerve posterior to the midaxillary line (before the anterior cutaneous branches of the intercostal nerves are given off) will block the somatic sensation to that area. It may be necessary to block two or three intercostal nerves for an accurate diagnosis. Adequate blockade is shown by a dermatomal loss of sensation to cold or light pinprick. Local anesthetic infiltration of a painful scar may stop the pain if a neuroma is present. Peripheral nerve blocks of the iliolumbar, ilioinguinal, or genitofemoral nerves may also block the pain if it is of somatic origin. The results of the local blocks are usually short-lived and should be considered as diagnostic, not therapeutic.

Creams or gels. If a neuroma is felt to be superficial, as shown by light touch recreating the pain and subcutaneous infiltration of local anesthetic stopping the pain, a local anesthetic cream or gel can be trialed. Emla cream is a mixture of lidocaine and prilocaine. A thick layer of Emla cream placed over the painful area with an occlusive dressing and left for four hours will create a numbness over the area for a further four hours. Thus one application can give pain relief for 8 hours or longer. It can be repeated 2 to 3 times a day if successful. After a period of time it is hoped the neuroma will be desensitized. This period will vary, and stopping the EMLA cream or local anesthetic gel every week for a period of 24 hours should be encouraged.

Trigger point therapy. If trigger points are found in the paravertebral muscles or abdominal musculature, they should be treated with either local anesthetic or dry needling. Care must be taken to inject the anesthetic, or place the acupuncture needle, within the band of the trigger point. This tender band is usually evidenced by a twitch response from the muscle and either a numbness or heaviness felt with dry needling, or reproduction of the pain felt when the needle enters it. Trigger point therapy should always be followed by specific stretching of the affected muscle. If the patient lies supine on the bed, by positioning the legs over the edge, and with cushions under the back, a good stretch should be felt in the anterior abdominal wall muscles.

TENS. Transcutaneous electrical nerve stimulation (TENS) should be trialed with electrodes placed just proximal to the painful area, as well as over the paravertebral muscles of the corresponding dermatome. A week's trial of TENS will show if it is effective (see Fig. 33-1).

Psychological evaluation. Syndromes such as postcholecystectomy syndrome need a psychologist to be involved in therapy, as the pathology of the pain generator is unknown, and the tendency for significant pain behaviors and drug addiction is high.

Somatic Posterior Wall Pain

Passive rotation of the patient's upper body while sitting stresses the thoracic spine. If abdominal pain is increased with, or triggered by, this maneuver, the amount of rotation that provokes pain should be recorded for comparison after treatment. Direct pressure over the thoracic spine may indicate tightness, or reproduce pain, if dysfunction of the zygapophyseal or costotransverse joints is present. An anterior protrusion of a lumbar disk or internal disk disruption may cause referred pain into the abdomen, usually in the groin and into the testicle or vulva (usually an L4–L5 disk). The lumbar spine will be painful on posterior/anterior mobilization. The 12th rib syndrome causes intermittent or continuous loin, and sometimes groin, pain. It is usually reproduced by alternating flexion and extension of the spine and by palpation of the 11th or 12th rib or both. Intercostal nerve blocks should confirm the diagnosis, which is thought to be due to irritation of the nerve by the rib.

TREATMENT D

Physical therapy/chiropractic. The thoracic spine should be mobilized by specific mobilization and manipulation techniques. A home exercise program should be given, which should include frequent thoracic rotations. Improvement is usually seen within 3 to 4 therapy sessions. If no improvement is evident after 3 weeks, other therapy should be tried.

Interspinous ligament injection. If pressure on the spinous process of a thoracic vertebra reproduces the abdominal pain, injection of 4 ml of local anesthetic into the interspinous ligament on either side of the spinous process may markedly diminish it. The injection is diagnostic, and may allow easier mobilization of the back for the physical therapist. Injection into the interspinous ligament should be done by a practitioner who is aware of the anatomy, and all injections should be done with a relatively short 1½-inch needle. Injection should be done during withdrawal of the needle to avoid epidural injection.

Trigger point therapy. Trigger points in the posterior paravertebral muscles, which refer pain to the abdominal wall, are often associated with zygapophyseal joint (facet joint) problems. Trigger points should be treated at the same time as the thoracic spine is being mobilized.

Rest/surgery. If an anterior wall disk rupture or disk degeneration is suspected, an MRI can be ordered. Unfortunately, a disk can be abnormal on MRI and not the cause of pain, or can be normal and the source of the patient's pain. A discogram, either provocative or analgesic, may respectively reproduce the pain or abolish the pain temporarily. Subsequent therapy depends on the result of the discogram.

Twelfth rib syndrome. If the pain in the 12th rib is interfering with the quality of life, and at least two intercostal blocks on separate occasions remove the pain, surgical excision of as much of the offending rib as possible is recommended. Neurolysis of the intercostal nerves may also give long-lasting relief.

Centralized Pain (Viscerosomatic Convergence)

Spinal input from the viscera projects onto the dorsal horn. Cross-connections can occur with the somatic afferent input to this same area. Thus, visceral pain can be perceived as a somatic type of pain. With chronic visceral pain a "wind-up" centralized pain is thought to be created, similar to chronic pain syndromes pains elsewhere. This may be the mechanism of action of syndromes such as irritable bowel syndrome, interstitial cystitis, or chronic pancreatitis.

The patient with chronic pancreatitis usually has a past history of alcohol abuse and presents with constant upper epigastric pain, often referred to the back. Exacerbations are usually so severe the patient paces up and down, unable to get into a position of comfort. Unless the pancreas is almost totally destroyed, chronic steatorrhea is not present initially; however, exocrine deficiency becomes apparent with time, leading to malabsorption and weight loss. About 15% of patients become insulin-dependent diabetics, and the remainder usually have abnormal glucose function tests. Narcotics are usually required to control their pain. Even though these patients may have addictive behavior patterns, narcotics should not be denied, but their use must be carefully controlled.

TREATMENT E

Antidepressants. Tricyclic antidepressants, such as nortriptyline, should be trialed starting at doses of 25 mg and increasing up to antidepressant levels.

Anticonvulsants. Anticonvulsants, including gabapentin, phenytoin, and carbamazepine (Tegretol), can be trialed.

Antiarrythmics. If a lidocaine infusion decreases the pain significantly, Mexitil may well be effective and should be trialed up to a dose of 10 mg/dg per day in three divided doses. A Mexitil trial on its own without lidocaine infusion can also be given. Unfortunately, Mexitil has a high incidence of nausea, which limits its use in clinical practice.

Opioids. Opioids should be the last resort in chronic abdominal pain. However, with centralized pain, opioids may be the most effective therapy. An opioid contract (see Fig. 6-3) should be discussed and signed: The patient is informed he or she will be taken off the opioid should it prove to be ineffective. A laxative should always be prescribed at the same time as the opioid. It is also useful to initially prescribe an antinauseant, such as metoclopramide, and an antipruritic medication, such as diphenhydramine. The patient is told to fill the latter prescriptions if nausea and itching are problematic. Both of these side effects usually settle down over the first few days of taking an opioid.

PAIN SPECIALIST

If the above therapies prove ineffective, referral to a pain specialist is indicated. The pain specialist should reevaluate the patient and look at medication optimization. A differential diagnosis between visceral and somatic pain may be attempted by intercostal blocks, interpleural blocks, celiac plexus blocks, or superior hypogastric blocks. In highly resistant cases, intrathecal trials with morphine or morphine-bupivacaine may be suggested. A multidisciplinary pain management program is important and should often be undertaken before more invasive procedures. During the diagnostic workup for chronic abdominal pain, a surgically amenable cause may be found.

CASE STUDY

Mr. A., aged 53, came in complaining of right hypochondrial and right scrotum pain of 5 years' duration. The pain had been present since a right inguinal hernia repair, but had been getting worse over the last few months. The pain was only slightly eased by over-the-counter nonsteroidal anti-inflammatory drugs and acetaminophen. Because of the pain, he stated he drank 6 to 8 beers a night plus a few large whiskeys to help him sleep. His bowel habits were erratic; he had a bowel movement, usually of hard feces' every 3 to 4 days. Occasionally, he took a laxative. He had noticed his pain was worse when he strained with defecation. He described the pain as, on average, being 80/100, at best 70/100, at worst "120/100." The only thing that helped his pain was lying with his knees bent and a warming blanket over his abdomen. His weight was steady. His sleep pattern was poor, with early morning awakening and difficulty getting to sleep. He was undergoing a divorce from his second wife after 12 years of marriage, and he was worried about his job. He worked in a paint factory. He had recently had several warnings because of absenteeism and poor work. He had attributed this to his pain but admitted that his drinking could have contributed to his recent poor work performance.

Other significant details of his history were a recent episode of hematemesis and a chronic cough, which he ascribed to his smoking 40 cigarettes a day.

On examination he had a flat affect. On standing, he was obese and in no obvious distress. Flexion, extension, and side bending showed full lumbar spinal movement. Thoracic rotations while sitting caused pain referred to the right groin. In the supine position, examination revealed a large soft abdomen with exquisite tenderness localized over the well-healed, right inguinal herniorrhaphy scar. Palpation of the scar did not refer his pain. He was also tender over the lateral edge of his rectus abdominis muscle. He was unable to perform a sit-up because of exacerbation of his pain. There was no guarding or rebound tenderness. The liver edge was felt 4 fingers below the right ribs and was slightly tender to palpation. In the prone position, examination revealed pain to palpation over the T10, T11, and T12 vertebrae. Gently mobilizing these vertebrae by repeatedly pushing the spinous processes to the side caused referral of pain to the right hypochondrium. There were trigger points in the paravertebral muscles at this level. The rest of the back examination was normal. In particular, pushing on his lumbar spine was not painful.

Rectal examination revealed a normal-size prostate with a well-demarcated central sulcus. Firm pellets of feces were felt in the rectum. Genital examination showed normal-size testes with no abnormal masses. Auscultation of his chest revealed scattered rhonchi throughout both lung fields, which decreased after a forced cough.

Impression

1. Possible environmental component: constipation.
2. Possible psychological component: drinking heavily, probably depressed (no suicidal ideation), family and work problems.
3. Possible anterior wall component: tender scar/neuroma, trigger points in the rectus abdominis.
4. Possible thoracic dysfunction: thoracic rotations and mobilizations cause referred pain.
5. Possible centralized pain: five-year history of pain.

Plan

1. Get a chest x-ray to exclude major pathology causing his cough.
2. Stop his NSAIDs, as they may have caused the hematemesis.
3. Prescribe lactulose 10–20 ml at night. Emphasize plenty of roughage in his diet. He had been eating erratically, usually junk food, since his wife had left him.
4. Referral to a psychiatrist for evaluation and possibly treatment of his depression and drinking problems.
5. Referral to Alcoholics Anonymous.
6. Administered 8 ml of 1% lidocaine into his scar. This numbed his skin but did not change his pain.
7. Referral to a physical therapist or chiropractor for mobilization of his thoracic vertebrae.
8. Draw blood for full blood count, ESR, and lead level. See him again in 1 week.

He missed his 1 week appointment and returned 2 weeks after the initial examination.

His pain was unchanged, although he was having almost a regular daily bowel action with a soft stool. This was achieved by a combination of a higher bulk diet, prune juice, one laxative in the morning if no bowel movement, and lactulose 10 ml in the evening if still no bowel action that day.

He had seen the psychiatrist who had started him on an antidepressant (nortriptyline 100 mg), which he took in the morning. He was finding it making him very drowsy as well as giving him a dry mouth, which he found uncomfortable.

He had been to a meeting of Alcoholics Anonymous, but didn't think it was "for him." He had tried to cut down his drinking but was finding it difficult. He still had a significant sleep disturbance.

The local anesthetic scar injection had caused a lot of discomfort and had increased his pain for 3 days. He did not want any more scar or other injections.

His chiropractor had "cracked his back" on three occasions, and his back felt "easier." He noticed he could turn around more comfortably when reversing, which, for a couple of months, had been very difficult for him to do.

His blood tests were all within normal limits.

On examination, his thoracic rotation was full and pain-free. He had only minimal discomfort on mobilizing T10, T11, and T12, with no pain referral. The paravertebral trigger points were only locally tender. He was still extremely tender in the scar and over the rectus abdominis.

Plan

1. Reassure him that there is still no evidence of anything "sinister."
2. Change the nortriptyline to an evening dose, as the side effect of drowsiness can be used to normalize the sleep pattern.
3. Prescribe a methylcellulose mouth spray or recommend chewing gum to decrease the unpleasant dry mouth effect of the nortriptyline.
4. Discuss with the psychiatrist the patient's drinking problem and his other stressors.
5. Refer to a physical therapist for myofascial treatment of his rectus and abdominal muscles and for a home stretching program. An aerobic exercise program was also suggested as a management modality.

The psychiatrist saw him frequently over the next 4 weeks and managed to get him into an alcohol rehabilitation outpatient program.

He returned for follow-up after 4 weeks. His pain was unchanged, but he scored it as 50/100 at best and 85/100 at worst; on average it was 70/100. He was sleeping well on nortriptyline 175 mg (which gave him antidepressant therapeutic blood levels) and lorazepam (Ativan) 2 mg at night. His bowel habit was becoming more regular with less frequent need for a laxative or lactulose. He had been off alcohol for 2 weeks and was attending Alcoholics Anonymous sessions regularly. His work had been very supportive, allowing him to attend the outpatient alcoholic rehabilitation clinic. The physical therapy had not helped, although his abdominal trigger points were less.

Plan

1. Encourage him and congratulate him on his achievement of stopping drinking.
2. Discuss with him his improvements so far, and again reassure him there is no evidence of his having cancer.
3. Trial TENS as the "paresthesia" is over the scar (see Fig. 33-1).
4. See him in 2 weeks.

He returned in 3 weeks looking like a different man. He had lost over 20 lb since stopping drinking. He had met a woman and was thinking of "going steady." He continued to attend the AA meetings and was seeing the psychiatrist on a biweekly schedule. He was reducing his smoking and had decided to quit in the near future. His bowel habits were regular, and, apart from his nortriptyline and lorazepam, he was on no other medication. The TENS reduced his pain from a 60/100 to a 30–40/100, which he found was tolerable. He was sleeping well. On examination he was still very tender over his scar.

At this stage it was decided not to treat him with any other therapy, as he was coping well, and he was unwilling to become a "pill popper." He would be seen at monthly follow-up initially to ensure that he continued to adhere to his new "resolutions." If his pain became worse or he started to become dysfunctional, a trial of anticonvulsants such as gabapentin could be started. In view of his recent alcohol and cigarette abuse, regular opioids were not advised. If gabapentin did not improve his pain, referral to a pain center for multidisciplinary evaluation, perhaps with intercostal diagnostic blocks, lidocaine infusion, or differential spinal, with follow-up treatment would be recommended.

Impression Probable centralized pain syndrome exacerbated by various environmental, psychological, and somatic components.

SUGGESTED READING

Abdominal pain. pp. 1146–1185. In Bonica JJ (ed): The Management of Pain. Lea & Febiger, Philadelphia, 1990

AIDS-Related Pain Syndromes

In the United States 1 in 250 inhabitants is HIV-positive. Acquired immunodeficiency syndrome is becoming a leading cause of death, with pain occurring in as many as 80% to 97% of the patients. As with cancer pain, it has many etiologies and is often undertreated. AIDS-related pain syndromes fall into the following categories: cancer-related pain, headache, herpes zoster-related pain, musculoskeletal pain, oropharyngeal pain, and peripheral neuropathy. Cancer-related pain, headache, and herpes zoster-related pain are discussed in other chapters and are not discussed here.

Musculoskeletal pain can occur secondary to both inflammatory and noninflammatory myopathies. Primary muscle wasting is common with AIDS and is frequently associated with a myopathy. This myopathy can present as slowly progressive muscle weakness and electromyographic changes consistent with myopathy. Secondary muscle wasting may result from toxic myopathies, which occur as a consequence of AZT therapy.

Oropharyngeal pain often occurs secondary to opportunistic infections, most commonly *Candida albicans* (oral thrush). This infection can cause severe pain.

AIDS peripheral neuropathy is a significant cause of pain. Sensory neuropathy occurs in 10% to 30% of AIDS patients. It can occur secondary to the antiviral therapy, which is usually reversible with cessation of the drug, or may be a direct result of the HIV infection. It is often indistinguishable from diabetic neuropathy. The patients often complain of bilateral dysesthesias and pain in the distal legs and arms, which may progress to frank numbness of the feet and hands. Although it is not known why AIDS patients develop peripheral neuropathy, it is well known that the human immunodeficiency virus (HIV) has a high predilection for the nervous system. HIV can be isolated from nerves early in the disease.

The AIDS patient can be overwhelming for the physician. Because of this, pain may become a secondary consideration. It is important to recognize the pain syndromes as the disease progresses and treat them accordingly.

TREATMENT PLANS

Musculoskeletal Pain

TREATMENT A

Discontinue antivirals. AIDS-related myopathy occurs both early and late in the disease. Early myopathy is usually secondary to the virus, and late myopathy is secondary to antiretroviral use. At this stage the decision should be made whether or not to discontinue the antiretroviral drugs.

TREATMENT B

Corticosteroids. Since AIDS-related myopathy may have an inflammatory component (polymyositis), a trial of corticosteroids may be beneficial. Studies have supported the use of corticosteroids in the management of AIDS. AIDS patients treated with corticosteriods had an improvement in appetite and weight gain with no significant adverse effect on the course of the disease.

The management of musculoskeletal pain is presented algorithmically in Figure 9-1.

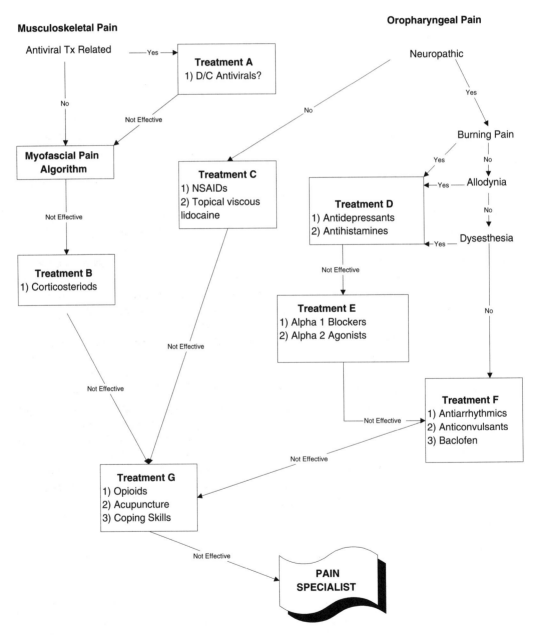

Fig. 9-1. Management of AIDS-related musculoskeletal and oropharyngeal pain. D/C, discontinue; NSAIDs, nonsteroidal anti-inflammatory drugs; Tx, treatment.

Oropharyngeal Pain

TREATMENT C

Nonsteroidal anti-inflammatory drugs. NSAIDs can be very helpful in nociceptive pain. The pain of oral candidiasis should be responsive to the NSAIDs and is a reasonable first-drug therapy.

Topical local anesthetics. Topical local anesthetics include 2% viscous lidocaine, benzocaine, or over-the-counter throat lozenges. They may be beneficial in oropharyngeal pain secondary to mucosal irritation.

TREATMENT D

Antidepressants. Antidepressants may be beneficial in neuropathic pain, with the TCAs the treatment of choice. The newer antidepressants may also prove to be beneficial. The choice of antidepressant will depend on the patient's sleep pattern and tolerance. If the patient has disturbed sleep, a more sedating antidepressant, such as amitriptyline, should be chosen. If no sleep disturbance is present, a less sedating antidepressant, such as nortriptyline, may be beneficial. Doses up to 150 mg per 24 hours have been reported effective. A combination of amitriptyline and fluphenazine may be tried if a TCA alone is ineffective. A 2- to 4-week trial of therapy should be attempted before the decision of efficacy is made.

Antihistamines. The addition of hydroxyzine at bedtime may improve the patient's symptoms and also improve sleep.

TREATMENT E

Alpha-1 blockers. AIDS-related oropharyngeal pain may result from sympathetic instability. Because of this, the alpha-1 blockers may be beneficial. The drugs of choice are prazosin, phenoxybenzamine, or terazosin titrated to effect. Significant improvement should be noticed within 1 to 2 weeks if effective.

Alpha-2 agonists. Clonidine may improve AIDS-related oropharyngeal pain by preventing the release of norepinephrine. Clonidine may be administered via the oral route or transdermal patch. Significant improvement should be noticed within 1 to 2 weeks if effective.

TREATMENT F

Antiarrhythmics. Mexiletine, an antiarrhythmic drug, may be effective in neuropathic pain. This drug can be titrated up to a maximum of 10 mg/kg per day. Another antiarrhythmic drug that may be effective is tocanide; significant improvement should be noticed within 1 to 2 weeks if effective.

Anticonvulsants. Carbamazepine is the current anticonvulsant of choice; however, gabapentin may be a worthwhile first-line drug, as it has a very low side effect profile. Others that may be effective include phenytoin and valproic acid. Clonazepam has also been used with some success. Significant improvement should be noticed within 1 to 2 weeks if effective.

Baclofen. Baclofen is an antispasmodic drug that may be beneficial in neuropathic pain. This drug can be titrated to effect. Significant improvement should be noticed within 1 to 2 weeks if it is effective.

TREATMENT G

Opioids. If all the foregoing treatment regimens fail, a trial of opioids may be of benefit. If a reasonable dose of opioids is not effective in pain treatment, referral to a pain specialist should be considered.

Acupuncture. By central neuromodulation and decreasing local muscle spasm, acupuncture should logically help in AIDS-related musculoskeletal pain. Unfortunately, there are no controlled studies published.

Coping skills. Inquiry should be made into mood and suicidal ideation. Patients with overt depression or active suicidal thoughts should be referred to a psychiatrist for therapy to run in conjunction with other therapies. Simple coping skills should be taught and family support encouraged in all instances where these are found to be lacking.

The management of oropharyngeal pain is presented in the algorithm in Figure 9-1.

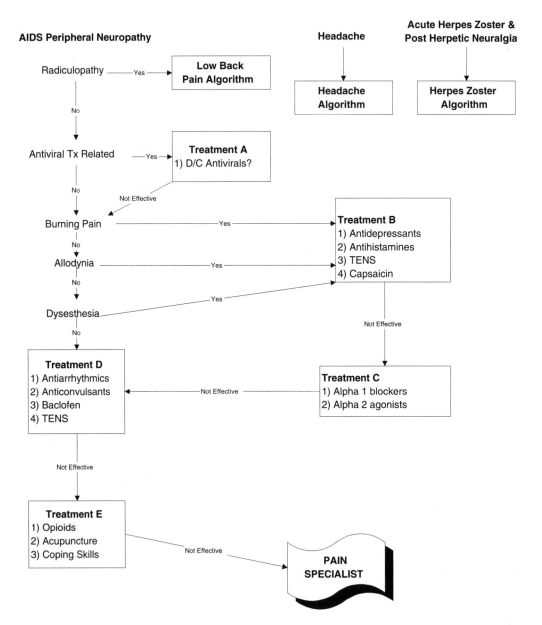

Fig. 9-2. Management of AIDS-related peripheral neuropathy, headache, and acute herpes zoster/postherpetic neuralgia. D/C, discontinue; TENS, transcutaneous electrical nerve stimulation; Tx, treatment.

Peripheral Neuropathy

TREATMENT A

Discontinue antivirals. AIDS-related peripheral neuropathy may be caused by anti-retroviral medications. The benefits of these drugs should be weighed against the pain of the peripheral neuropathy. A trial off of the anti-retrovirals should determine if the neuropathy is related to this drug. If the neuropathy does not improve, then it can be asssumed that the virus is the cause.

TREATMENT B

Antidepressants. Antidepressants may be beneficial in AIDS peripheral neuropathy with the TCAs the treatment of choice. The newer antidepressants may also prove to be beneficial. The choice of antidepressant will depend on the patient's sleep pattern and tolerance. If the patient has disturbed sleep, a more sedating antidepressant, such as amitriptyline, should be chosen. If no sleep disturbance is present, a less sedating antidepressant, such as nortriptyline, may be beneficial. Doses up to 150 mg per 24 hours have been reported effective. A combination of amitriptyline and fluphenazine may be tried if a TCA alone is ineffective. A 2- to 4-week trial of therapy should be attempted before the decision is made that it will be ineffective.

Antihistamines. The addition of hydroxyzine at bedtime may improve the patient's symptoms and also improve sleep.

TENS. A transcutaneous electrical nerve stimulator (TENS) may improve AIDS peripheral neuropathy pain. If no benefit is seen after a week of using different frequencies on a set regimen, it is doubtful that it will be of long-term benefit (see Fig. 33-1).

Capsaicin. Capsaicin cream may be helpful in AIDS peripheral neuropathy. It is suggested that initially 0.025% capsaicin be tried. If this is unsuccessful, then a 0.075% cream can be tried. Initially, this cream may burn after application; however, this will usually disappear with continued use. As significant depletion of substance P from the peripheral nerve terminals takes up to 3 weeks, treatment must be continued for this minimum period of time before efficacy can be gauged. The patient must use this cream 3 or 4 times per day in order to be effective.

TREATMENT C

Alpha-1 blockers. AIDS-related peripheral neuropathy may result from sympathetic instability. Because of this, the alpha-1 blockers may be beneficial. The drugs of choice are prazosin, phenoxybenzamine, or terazosin titrated to effect. Significant improvement should be noticed within 1 to 2 weeks if effective.

Alpha-2 agonists. Clonidine may improve AIDS-related peripheral neuropathy by preventing the release of norepinephrine. Clonidine may be administered via the oral route or transdermal patch. Significant improvement should be noticed within 1 to 2 weeks if effective.

TREATMENT D

Antiarrhythmics. Mexiletine, an antiarrhythmic drug, may be effective in neuropathic pain. This drug can be titrated up to a maximum of 10 mg/kg per day. Tocanide is another antiarrhythmic drug that may be effective. Significant improvement should be noticed within 1 to 2 weeks if these drugs are effective.

Anticonvulsants. Carbamazepine is the current anticonvulsant drug of choice; however, gabapentin may be a worthwhile first-line drug, as it has a very low side effect profile. Others that may be effective include phenytoin and valproic acid. Clonazepam has also been used with some success. Significant improvement should be noticed within 1 to 2 weeks if effective.

Baclofen. Baclofen is an antispasmodic drug that may be of benefit in neuropathic pain. This drug can be titrated to effect. Significant improvement should be noticed within 1 to 2 weeks if effective.

TENS. TENS may improve AIDS peripheral neuropathy pain. If no benefit is seen after a week of using different frequencies on a set regimen, it is doubtful that it will be of long-term benefit.

TREATMENT E

Opioids. If all the foregoing treatment regimens fail, a trial of opioids may be of benefit. If a reasonable dose of opioids is not effective in pain treatment, a referral to a pain specialist should be considered.

Acupuncture. By central neuromodulation and decreasing local muscle spasm, acupuncture should logically help in AIDS-related peripheral neuropathy. Unfortunately, there are no controlled studies published.

Coping skills. Inquiry should be made into mood and suicidal ideation. Patients with overt depression or active suicidal thoughts should be referred to a psychiatrist for therapy to run in conjunction with other therapies. Simple coping skills should be taught and family support encouraged in all instances where these are found to be lacking.

An algorithm for management of peripheral neuropathy is given in Figure 9-2.

PAIN SPECIALIST

If pain persists despite the above regimen, referral to a pain specialist is indicated. The pain specialist should evaluate the patient both physically and psychologically. Therapies may include the following.

Medication optimization or withdraw. Frequently, the pain specialist will optimize medications by adjusting doses or trying different combinations. In cases where the excessive or improper use of medications interferes with the patient's ability to function, the pain specialist may withdraw the medications.

Diagnostic nerve blocks to evaluate the pain mechanism. If the pain is localized to a specific area of the body, a local anesthetic block of the nerve that supplies this area will give information on the pain pathway taken. If the pain is significantly decreased with this procedure, neurolytic or stimulatory techniques may be tried.

Intravenous drug infusions. Pain specialists frequently use intravenous drug infusions to determine what type of drug the pain responds to. These infusions include lidocaine, phentolamine, or opioids. These infusions will give the pain specialist information on the physiologic aspects of the pain and will guide therapy.

Differential spinal or epidural block. If the patient suffers from pain in the trunk or lower extremity, a spinal or epidural injection of local anesthetic can provide information on the pain pathways. If a sensory and motor block occurs in the painful area but the patient continues to report pain, the pain is considered centralized.

Spinal cord stimulation. Patients who suffer from pain in the extremities may benefit from spinal cord stimulation, which can also be performed for trunk pain, although it is more difficult to achieve good stimulation.

Intraspinal drug therapy. Infusion of opioids, baclofen, or local anesthetics into the intrathecal or epidural space may provide excellent pain relief in selected cases. Oral trials of these drugs should have shown them to be at least partially effective, but side effects, such as somnolence or nausea, prevent further titration. Internalized systems can provide for long-term drug therapy.

A multidisciplinary pain management program. The multidisciplinary approach involves a group of specialists trained in pain management. Each member of the team addresses specific problems the patient faces. The team usually includes a pain physician, psychologist or psychiatrist, and physical therapist. Other members may include a social worker, vocational rehabilitation counselor, and others. The objectives are to rationalize medication, teach coping skills, educate, and give vocational guidance where appropriate. The long-term objective is to allow the individuals to control their pain and not let the pain control them.

CASE STUDY

Mr. X is a 35-year-old hemophiliac with AIDS. He first tested HIV-positive 6 years previously. He was started on AZT at the time of diagnosis but discontinued the drug 2 months later because of intolerable side effects. He was not on any antivirals at the time of the initial consult. He was diagnosed with AIDS 1 year ago. He had survived two episodes of *Pneumocystis carinii* infections and a cytomegalovirus (CMV) infection. He presented with pain mainly in his feet, which he had first noticed as numbness in the soles of his feet approximately 6 months previously. Although this was uncomfortable, it was not painful. The numbness became progressively worse to the point where he was having difficulty walking. Over the last month he developed pain in a stocking glove distribution on both legs. He described the pain as continuous and burning. His VAS score was 90/100 with no relief from ibuprofen or acetaminophen. His sleep pattern was disturbed due to the pain. He had no history of diabetes, and his blood sugar was normal.

Impression AIDS peripheral neuropathy.

Plan

1. Amitriptyline at bedtime.
2. TENS unit.
3. Capsaicin cream to feet.
4. See patient in 10 days.

The patient returned, stating that pain his pain score had decreased from 90/100 to 50/100. His sleep had improved, but he requested more pain relief.

Plan

1. Add an alpha-1 blocker (prazosin up to 6 mg per day).
2. See him in 10 days.

The patient returned with no change in his pain.

Plan

1. Discontinue the alpha-1 blocker.
2. Add gabapentin (up to 600 mg tid).

The patient returned, reporting that his pain was much improved with the gabapentin (VAS 30/100), but he occasionally suffered from exacerbations once or twice a week when the pain increased to 50–60/100.

Plan

1. Start tramadol prn for the exacerbations.
2. See him in 10 days.

The patient returned, reporting that, although his VAS is 30/100 most of the time, he still suffered from the exacerbations with no relief with the tramadol.

Plan

1. Discontinue the tramadol.
2. Start an opioid for mild to moderate pain such as codeine or hydrocodone with acetaminophen.

The patient did well on the above regimen for approximately 4 months. He returned with an increase in pain in spite of increasing the gabapentin to 3,600 mg per day. He was taking two codeine tablets with acetaminophen every 3 hours without any relief.

Plan

1. Continue gabapentin.
2. Discontinue the codeine with acetaminophen, as he is receiving an excessive dose of acetaminophen (more than 4 g per day).
3. Start an opioid such as methadone or morphine for moderate to severe pain.

The patient was placed on methadone every 6 hours. His baseline pain score had decreased to a tolerable level, but he continued to suffer occasional exacerbations.

Plan

1. Add immediate-release morphine for breakthrough pain.

The patient returned stating that the morphine had no effect on pain exacerbations.

Plan

1. Discontinue the morphine.
2. Add Dilaudid for breakthrough pain.

The above measures can and should be instituted on a primary care level. If they fail to produce relief, consultation with a pain specialist should be considered. Early referral is recommended when the usual treatment modalities, as outlined above, are proving inadequate.

SUGGESTED READINGS

Janisse T. Pain management of AIDS patients. pp. 546–578. In Raj PP (ed): Practical Management of Pain. Mosby Year Book, St Louis, 1992

Lebovits AH, Lefkowitz M, McCarthy D et al: The prevalence and management of pain in patients with AIDS: a review of 134 cases. Clin J Pain 5:245–248, 1989

Arthritis

The prevalence of osteoarthritis (OA) is approximately 9% of the population, with an increasing incidence relative to age and obesity. Joint injury and surgery increase the risk of OA. Most nonsteroidal and analgesic drug use is related to the treatment. OA may be radiographically positive, symptom-negative, or symptom-positive with normal radiographs. The pain is usually described as "deep and aching." Many symptoms can be eased by treating the painful soft tissues surrounding the arthritic joint. The actual cause of the pain experienced in OA is poorly understood. Night pain, which may be severe enough to interfere with sleep, may be caused in part by increased interosseus venous pressure. On weightbearing, the thickened synovial membrane of the joint may not distend to dissipate the joint fluid pressure. This increased intra-articular pressure may be a cause of the pain experienced with walking. No official diagnostic criteria exist for OA, although criteria have been proposed for OA of the hip.

There are two main variants of rheumatoid arthritis (RA), with significant prognostic differences. Epidemiologic RA is usually rheumatoid factor-negative and runs an intermittent course with long periods of remission. Clinical RA, usually rheumatoid factor-positive, remits in only 5% to 10% of cases. RA is three times more common in women, with a peak incidence between 40 and 60 years of age. Its prevalence is approximately 1% of the population. Although infectious etiologies have been investigated for many years, no one infection has been shown to cause RA. Recently it has been suggested a slow virus may be responsible, attacking people with a genetic susceptibility. Active RA is almost always associated with pain.

The estimated direct cost of RA in 1983 dollars in the USA was $777 million. The cost of OA was $2.06 billion.

Pain management algorithms for the arthritides are given in Figure 10-1.

OSTEOARTHRITIS

Location

Osteoarthritis (OA) is a disease of synovial joints. The main joints affected are the small joints of the hands, usually the distal interphalangeal joints and thumb base, which produce the swellings termed *Heberden's nodes*. The knees, hips, and zygapophyseal joints of the neck and lumbar spine may also be affected in a nonsymmetrical fashion.

Diagnostic Criteria for Rheumatoid Arthritis

- Morning stiffness in and around joints, lasting at least 1 hour before maximal improvement.
- Simultaneous soft tissue swelling or fluid in at least three joint areas, observed by a physician. The 14 common areas are right or left proximal interphalangeal (PIP) joints, metacarpophalangeal (MCP) joints, wrist, elbow, knee, ankle, and metatarsophalangeal (MTP) joints.
- At least one area of soft tissue swelling or effusion in a wrist, MCP, or PIP joint.
- Symmetrical arthritis. Simultaneous involvement of the same joint areas in both sides of the body. Absolute symmetry is not necessary with involvement of MCP, PIP, or MTP joints.
- Rheumatoid nodules.
- Positive test for rheumatoid factor.
- Radiographic changes typical of RA on posteroanterior views of the hand or wrist, including erosions and periarticular bone decalcification.

Four of these seven criteria must be present; one to four of these must have been present for more than 6 weeks.

Radiographic Appearance

The pathologic changes of OA cause local areas of destruction of the articular cartilage and remodeling. This is controlled by chondrocytes, which both synthesize and degrade the cartilage matrix. Radiographs may show sclerosis or cyst formation in the underlying bone due to the increased chondrocytic activity. Fibrillation, and thinning of the articular cartilage joint space narrowing is also seen. The laying down of cartilage and bone is shown as osteophytes at the joint margins.

Generalized Osteoarthritis

Primary generalized OA usually occurs in middle-aged women and affects the distal and proximal interphalangeal joints, first metatarsal phalangeal joint, base of the thumb, knees, and hips. These joints intermittently become swollen and inflamed.

RHEUMATOID ARTHRITIS

Symmetrical Peripheral Polyarteritis

Typically, RA causes a symmetrical peripheral polyarteritis. The hips are usually spared, as are the shoulders and elbows. The most commonly involved joints are the small joints of the feet and hands, ankles, knees, and neck.

Extra-articular Signs

Vasculitis. This is an uncommon, but potentially fatal, complication. All sizes of blood vessels may be involved, causing nail bed hemorrhages, gangrene in the fingers, small bowel infarction, or pulmonary hypertension. Small vessel infarction may be the cause of peripheral neuropathy and nodule formation. If severe vasculitis is present, admission to a hospital is necessary, with treatment by corticosteroids and immunosuppressives.

Lung disease. Pleural effusions and pleuritic pain are the most common form of lung involvement. Severe interstitial fibrosis occasionally occurs, usually in those who have been exposed to industrial dusts, such as coal.

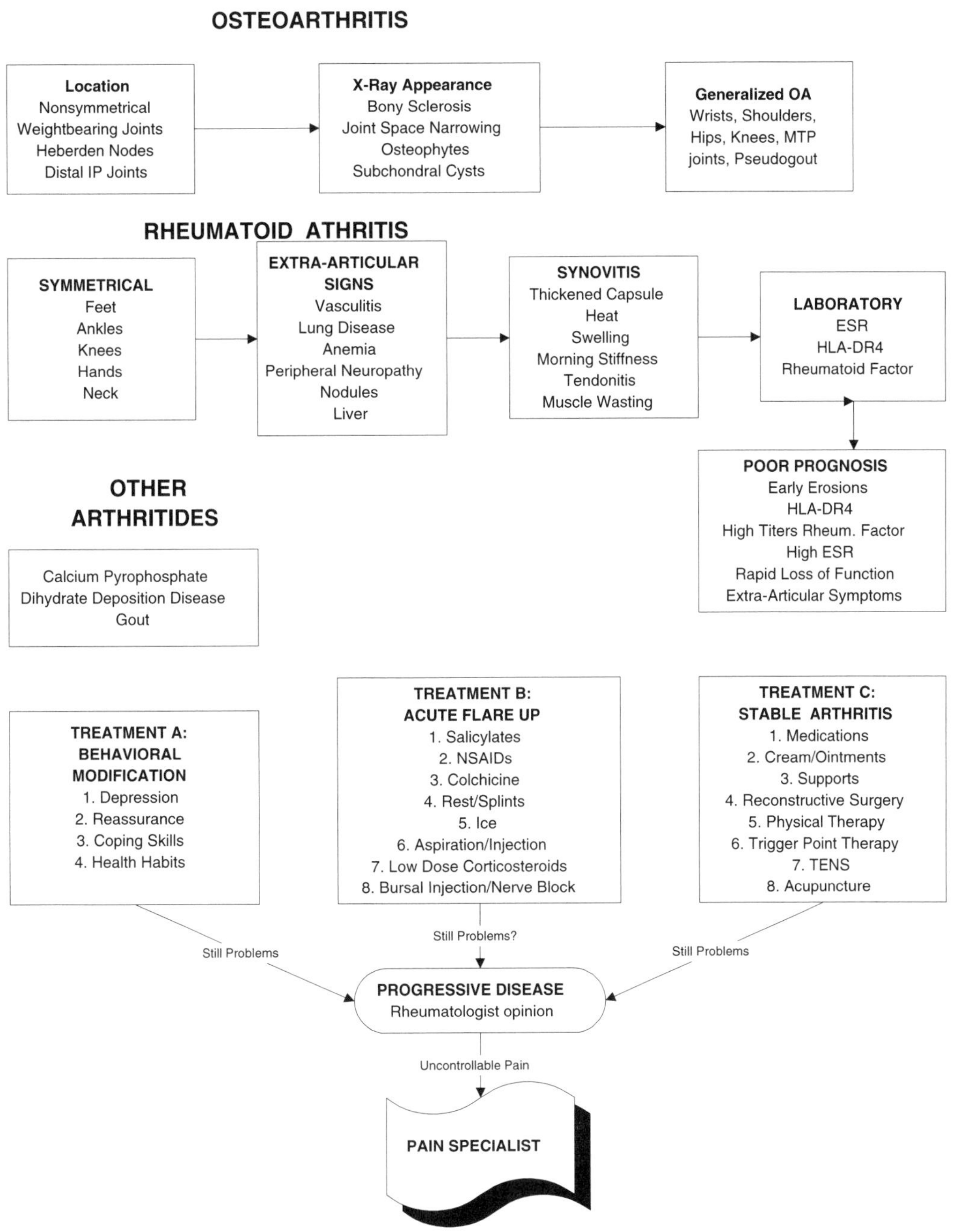

OSTEOARTHRITIS

Location	X-Ray Appearance	Generalized OA
Nonsymmetrical	Bony Sclerosis	Wrists, Shoulders,
Weightbearing Joints	Joint Space Narrowing	Hips, Knees, MTP
Heberden Nodes	Osteophytes	joints, Pseudogout
Distal IP Joints	Subchondral Cysts	

RHEUMATOID ATHRITIS

SYMMETRICAL	EXTRA-ARTICULAR SIGNS	SYNOVITIS	LABORATORY
Feet	Vasculitis	Thickened Capsule	ESR
Ankles	Lung Disease	Heat	HLA-DR4
Knees	Anemia	Swelling	Rheumatoid Factor
Hands	Peripheral Neuropathy	Morning Stiffness	
Neck	Nodules	Tendonitis	
	Liver	Muscle Wasting	

POOR PROGNOSIS
Early Erosions
HLA-DR4
High Titers Rheum. Factor
High ESR
Rapid Loss of Function
Extra-Articular Symptoms

OTHER ARTHRITIDES

Calcium Pyrophosphate
Dihydrate Deposition Disease
Gout

TREATMENT A:
BEHAVIORAL
MODIFICATION
1. Depression
2. Reassurance
3. Coping Skills
4. Health Habits

TREATMENT B:
ACUTE FLARE UP
1. Salicylates
2. NSAIDs
3. Colchicine
4. Rest/Splints
5. Ice
6. Aspiration/Injection
7. Low Dose Corticosteroids
8. Bursal Injection/Nerve Block

TREATMENT C:
STABLE ARTHRITIS
1. Medications
2. Cream/Ointments
3. Supports
4. Reconstructive Surgery
5. Physical Therapy
6. Trigger Point Therapy
7. TENS
8. Acupuncture

Still Problems → Still Problems? → Still Problems

PROGRESSIVE DISEASE
Rheumatologist opinion

Uncontrollable Pain

PAIN SPECIALIST

Fig. 10-1. Pain management for the arthritides. IP, interphalangeal; OA, osteoarthritis; MTP, metatarsophalangeal; ESR, erythrocyte sedimentation rate; NSAIDs, nonsteroidal anti-inflammatory drugs; TENS, transcutaneous electrical nerve stimulation.

Anemia. The anemia of RA is usually normocytic and normochronic; sometimes it is hypochronic and, less commonly, microcytic. The degree of anemia usually correlates with the erythrocyte sedimentation rate (ESR). Use of nonsteroidal anti-inflammatory drugs (NSAIDs) may create a continual loss of blood from the gastrointestinal tract, causing an added iron deficiency anemia.

Peripheral neuropathy. Peripheral neuropathy may be caused by nerve entrapment, usually at the wrist (carpal tunnel syndrome) or ankle (tarsal tunnel syndrome) in more severe cases of RA. With vasculitis there may be a sudden loss of sensory and motor power in a nerve distribution.

Sensory loss in a glove and stocking or specific peripheral distribution may also occur. Cervical myelopathy with generalized motor weakness may occur from atlanto-occipital subluxation.

Nodules. Nodules are usually found in areas subjected to recurrent mechanical stress, such as the olecranon, tips of fingers, and sacrum. They are usually not tender unless they ulcerate and become infected. Occasionally they occur in other tissues, such as sclera, lung, pleura, and myocardium. They are diagnostic of RA as well as indicating a poorer prognosis.

Liver. Hepatic enlargement, usually asymptomatic, occurs in 11% of RA patients. Drug causes should be ruled out.

Septic arthritis. Usually *Staphylococcus aureus* can be potentially fatal. It may present as an acute onset with fever, swelling, and severe pain, or much more insidiously. Awareness and early treatment is vital.

SYNOVITIS

Inflammation of the synovial capsule causes heat and swelling. "Gelling" or stiffness of the joint occurs with inactivity, hence the early morning joint stiffness. Tendinitis and muscle wasting may occur rapidly around the inflamed joint.

Laboratory Findings

Erythrocyte sedimentation rate. The ESR and C-reactive protein gives an indication of the severity of the disease and can be used to monitor therapy.

HLA-DR4. The *HLA-DR4* genotype appears to influence the severity of the disease.

Rheumatoid factor. The lgM rheumatoid factor is positive in 75% of individuals with RA. High titers are associated with a poorer prognosis.

OTHER ARTHRITIDES

Calcium Pyrophosphate Dihydrate Deposition Disease

Calcium pyrophosphate dihydrate deposition disease (CPPD) occurs clinically in about 1 in 1,000 adults, usually the elderly. It usually affects one joint—knees, wrists, and metacarpophalangeal joints are the most common sites. Examples of CPPD are as follows:

1. Pseudogout: acute redness, heat, swelling, and severe pain in one or a few joints; attacks last from 2 days to several weeks, with no pain between attacks
2. Pseudorheumatoid arthritis: deep aching and swelling in multiple joints with attacks lasting weeks to months
3. Pseudo-osteoarthritis
4. Pseudoarthritis with acute attacks: osteoarthritislike symptoms with superimposed acute painful joints

CPPD may be associated with hyperparathyroidism, hemochromatosis, or metabolic causes.

Diagnostic Criteria

1. Demonstration of CPPD crystals in tissues or synovial fluid by x-ray diffraction
2. D crystals demonstrated by compensated polarized light microscopy
3. Typical calcifications seen on radiograph

If 1 or 2 and 3 are present, the diagnosis of CPPD is definite; if 2 or 3 is present, the diagnosis is probable.

Gout

Gout causes paroxysmal attacks of severe pain from monarticular joint irritation due to monosodium urate crystals. The most common sites are the first metatarsophalangeal joint (50%), midtarsal joints, ankles, knees, wrists, fingers, or elbows. The affected joint is red, swollen, and hot.

Diagnostic Criteria

1. Demonstration of intracellular sodium urate monohydrate crystals in synovial fluid leukocytes
2. Demonstration of sodium urate monohydrate crystals in an aspirate or biopsy of a tophus
3. Rapid resolution of monarticular arthritis, in the presence of hyperuricemia, following colchicine administration

If any of the above are present, the diagnosis of gout is definite.

TREATMENT OF THE ARTHRITIDES

Behavioral Modification

TREATMENT A

Depression. Early recognition and aggressive treatment of depression is important. Suicidal ideation should be inquired about and, if present, the patient referred to a psychiatrist. Depression will worsen any pain syndrome and can produce further pain anywhere in the body. If the arthritis worsens or other emotional stressors affect the individual adversely, depression may occur. The treating physician should be aware of mood swings, which may signal the onset of depression, at any time during the course of the patient's therapy.

Reassurance. Although 40% of rheumatoid arthritis patients have continued disease activity, only 10% of individuals become severely incapacitated. Approximately 25% of patients recover completely, and a further 25% have slight residual joint damage that usually does not interfere with their ability to work. Osteoarthritis usually runs a slower course than RA, and the functional disability caused will depend on the damage to the weightbearing hip or knee joints. If surgery becomes necessary, it usually involves replacement of these joints or removal of osteophytes impinging on spinal nerves.

Coping skills. Poor coping skills may be manifested by excessive pain behavior. Muscle relaxation exercises, stress management techniques, and methods of coping with environmental and social stressors can be taught. A psychologist trained in pain management is usually the most appropriate referral. Biofeedback can assist the patient in gaining the ability to relax muscles and increase circulation to the affected area.

Health habits. *Smoking.* Nicotine worsens inflammatory arthritis. Smoking cessation must be strongly encouraged.

Weight reduction. Any extra load placed on inflamed or damaged weightbearing joints will have an adverse effect on the individual's pain. These patients should attain their optimal weight by healthy eating habits, which initially may include a low-calorie diet.

Diet. There are many anecdotal stories and popular books relating the efficacy of specific diets. Most stress the avoidance of preservatives and caffeine as well as various foodstuffs. While the scientific evidence for such diets is lacking, for the most part they encourage healthy eating habits. If an individual has an allergy to a foodstuff, it may manifest itself in joint swelling and pain. Avoidance of that food type would obviously be of benefit.

Exercise. Exercise is important in maintaining joint nutrition and healthy muscles. General exercise is also important in giving the individual a coping skill for stress management. The release of various neurotransmitters within the central nervous system by exercise may also diminish pain perception. In acute flare-ups, painful exercises should be stopped.

Acute Flare-Up

TREATMENT B

The acute flare-up is more common in RA. In OA, inflammatory changes secondary to cartilage degeneration or an increase in intraosseous pressure is usually the cause, and it is seldom necessary to progress beyond NSAIDs for pain relief.

Salicylates. Salicylates inhibit prostaglandin synthesis in high doses of 4 to 5 g per day. This gives a blood level of 20–30 mg/ml. Enteric slow-release salicylates cause less gastrointestinal irritation. Tinnitus and hearing loss indicate that toxic levels are being reached. However, if there is preexisting hearing loss, these toxic signs will not be exhibited. Side effects include heartburn, nausea, and epigastric distress. Occasionally, a worsening of asthma or sinus problems is seen. Nonacetylated salicylates do not interfere with platelet function, unlike aspirin, which inhibits platelet aggregation for the life span of the platelet (±10 days).

Nonsteroidal anti-inflammatory drugs. NSAIDs inhibit prostaglandin synthesis. They have an effect both peripherally and centrally. There are many different types, but there is no evidence that one is more effective than another. These drugs should be given for 2 to 3 weeks before their effectiveness can be evaluated. They have a maximum effect, and increasing the dose above this plateau usually increases side effects and cost, but not efficacy. Side effects include gastritis, peptic ulcer, hematemesis, bloating, diarrhea, anemia due to chronic blood loss, and interstitial nephritis.

Colchicine. Specific for the treatment of gouty arthritis, 1–2 mg colchicine in 20 ml saline can be given intravenously over a 5-minute period. An additional 1 mg IV can be given 6-hourly, with a maximum total treatment dose of 4 mg. It should be given in reduced dosage to patients with renal compromise, as it is mainly excreted unchanged in the urine. Colchicine is extremely irritating to the tissues, and care must be taken to avoid extravasation during injection. Pain relief usually occurs within 12 hours, with redness and joint swelling subsiding over the next 5 to 7 days.

Patients with recurrent attacks of gouty arthritis can often abort an acute attack by taking 0.6 mg colchicine by mouth for 4 to 6 doses at the first sign of joint pain.

Rest/splinting. In the acute inflammatory stage, activities will need to be restricted. Splints may help where tendinitis is prominent. The only exercises tolerated at this stage may be passive range of movement performed by trained therapists or gentle isometrics. Gentle stretching and more active range of movement can be done as the acute phase remits.

Ice. Cryotherapy can be given as ice massage (a polystyrene cup filled with water and frozen), frozen polyglycol gel bags, or ice and water baths into which the feet can be placed. Treatment should be limited to a minimum of 20 minutes hourly.

Aspiration/intra-articular injection. Removal of fluid from an acutely swollen joint can decrease pain. Corticosteroid injections can decrease joint swelling and pain. No more than three injections of corticosteroids at intervals of 6 months or longer should be given because of the danger of accelerating further cartilage destruction. Strict asepsis must be used in any procedure where the joint is entered owing to the risk of septic arthritis.

Low-dose corticosteroids. For a severe flare-up, a short course of corticosteroids may be very effective. Once the patient has been started on corticosteroids, however, it is often very difficult to take him or her off. The decision to start long-term corticosteroids may be best undertaken by a rheumatologist.

Bursal injection/nerve block. If a bursa is inflamed and causing pain, aspiration and injection of a local anesthetic with a corticosteroid can be tried. Common sites of bursitis are the trochanteric bursa at the hip, the anserine bursa at the knee, and the calcaneal bursa at the ankle. If the painful area is in the distribution of an easily blocked peripheral nerve (e.g., posterior tibial nerve for large toe pain), a local anesthetic block may decrease the pain significantly for several days.

Stable Arthritis

TREATMENT C

Medications. *Simple analgesics.* Simple analgesics can be taken on an as-necessary basis, or around the clock, if the pain is causing severe dysfunction. Simple analgesics include acetaminophen up to a maximum dose of 4 g per day, tramadol up to 400 mg per day, or a combination of weak opioid/acetaminophen preparation up to a maximum acetaminophen dosage of 4 g per day.

Nonsteroidal anti-inflammatory drugs. If inflammation or synovitis is not present, NSAIDs are probably best avoided. This is due to their side effects, especially the risk of gastric bleeding, and their potential to cause further damage to articular cartilage.

Tricyclic antidepressants. If sleep is disturbed due to pain, a TCA such as amitriptyline or nortriptyline, given at night, should be trialed. The starting dose is 10–25 mg, depending on the age of the patient. It should be increased every three nights until a good night's sleep is achieved, 100–125 mg dose is reached, or side effects prevent further trial. If no improvement in pain or sleep is seen, a blood level should be measured. If the level is subtherapeutic for depression, the TCA should be increased to give therapeutic antidepressant levels for 4 weeks. If no improvement in the patient's pain or mood is evident, the TCA should be stopped. Weight gain, which may remain even when the TCA is stopped, is a major problem with these medications. If significant weight gain is noticed, the TCA should be discontinued.

Creams/ointments. *Capsaicin.* Capsaicin 0.075% and 0.025% are creams derived from red peppers. Rubbed on the skin over the painful area every 6 hours for 3 to 6 weeks, they will deplete the neurokinin transmitter substance P and desensitize the subcutaneous nociceptors. If there is no benefit after 3 to 6 weeks, the treatment should be stopped. Capsaicin often causes burning initially in the treatment, which may be severe enough to prevent continued use. It is proving to be very effective in the treatment of OA pain.

Anti-inflammatory creams. When anti-inflammatory creams are rubbed on the skin overlying the joint, the active ingredient from the creams can be found in the joint fluid. Skin reactions are common, and it becomes impractical if several joints are affected.

Herbal/homeopathic creams. There are many over-the-counter antiarthritic preparations available, as well as those prescribed by licensed herbalists or homeopaths. Double-blinded, placebo-controlled studies as to their efficacy are lacking. However, if the patient claims that these creams help his or her condition, if they do not contain toxic substances and if they are not financially crippling to the individual, tacit encouragement of the substance should not be withheld.

Supports. Supports and braces are important if functional deformities and joint instabilities develop after arthritic damage. These include orthotic devices and custom-made footwear.

Reconstructive surgery. Reconstructive surgery includes nerve transpositions where entrapment has occurred and artificial large joint replacement (e.g., hip and knee). Small joint replacements have had some success, depending on how well the ongoing active arthritic process can be suppressed.

Physical therapy. *Exercises.* Exercise to strengthen a muscle should be individualized and given together with range of motion exercises for the joint. Exercise should be daily and frequent to maintain function, but should not be of sufficient intensity to trigger a "flare-up." Resistive isotonic exercises using Theraband or surgical tubing are useful and inexpensive. A BAPS board (a wobble board on which the patient stands and tries to maintain balance) is useful for weightbearing and proprioceptive exercises. Water exercises are also useful, and organizations like the YMCA often have inexpensive group water exercises for arthritis sufferers. At home a total gym-type machine, properly set up and used, can provide safe resistance exercises. All exercises should ideally be given and followed up by a trained therapist. Other instruction should also be given at these sessions, including the use of energy-sparing devices for home use and supportive equipment.

Heat. Warmth, by relaxing the tissues, can assist in maintaining movement of the joints. The heat should not be higher than can be tolerated by facial skin, otherwise skin damage may occur. To prevent excessive drying of the skin, a lanolin-type moisturizing cream can be rubbed on before the heat treatment.

Trigger point therapy. Massage, cold spray and stretch techniques, ice massage and stretch, dry needling, and local anesthetic injections may have a role where localized trigger points in the muscles proximal to the joint refer pain to the arthritic area. Any trigger point treatment must be accompanied by a home stretching and range of movement exercise program.

TENS. Transcutaneous electrical nerve stimulation (TENS) can be of benefit. The patient should be instructed on placement and frequencies to be trialed. The TENS electrode can be placed over the peripheral nerve serving the painful area, on trigger or acupuncture points proximal to the painful joints, or around the painful joints themselves. A burst mode on the newer machines supposedly prevents tissue accommodation to the frequencies used. If a 1-week trial does not help, it is unlikely TENS will be of benefit (see Fig. 33-1).

Acupuncture. If acupuncture is to be successful, 50% of patients will respond within three treatments and probably 90% within six treatments. If no improvement occurs after six treatments, given initially biweekly and then weekly, therapy should be discontinued. Acupuncture may be performed with needles only or with electrical stimulation. If the patient responds well to acupuncture, the duration of pain relief varies. Periodic booster treatments are usually required.

Progressive Disease

If the first-line anti-inflammatory drugs and therapies do not control the active disease, the patient should be referred to a rheumatologist. For rheumatoid arthritis the rheumatologist may commence treatment with the following agents.

Gold salts. Approximately 60% of patients who use gold salts improve significantly without toxicity; 20% respond but have toxic effects; 20% do not respond.

Penicillamine. Penicillamine has a similar efficacy to gold. Most patients respond within 6 months. Multiple toxicities, including autoimmune deficiency, due to the drug have been reported.

Antimalarial agents. Hydroxychloroquine is the most commonly used antimalarial drug. Eye toxicity is the most serious side effect. Treatment requires monitoring by an ophthalmologist every 6 months.

Sulfasalazine. The efficacy of sulfasalazine is similar to gold, but fewer patients respond.

Immunosuppressive agents. Azathioprine, methotrexate, and cyclophosphamide may be used in patients in whom conventional therapies have failed. Toxic effects include bone marrow suppression, liver damage, and blood dyscrasias.

High-dose corticosteroids. Although high-dose corticosteroids are usually successful initially, it is difficult to withdraw them. Maintenance therapy with steroids carries the risk of psychoses, osteoporosis, diabetes, and lowered immunity.

PAIN SPECIALIST

Although the pain specialist is not usually involved in the treatment of pain in the arthritic patient, he or she has a role if pain continues to be incapacitating, despite conventional therapy. Diagnosis and treatment by the pain specialist may include the following procedures.

Lumbar sympathetic blockade or phentolamine infusion. A lumbar sympathetic blockade or a phentolamine (an alpha-1 receptor blocker) infusion will assess the involvement of the sympathetic system in the pain syndrome. If sympathetic blockade reduces the pain significantly, prazocin (an oral alpha-1 receptor blocker) or clonidine (an alpha-2 agonist) may be trialed.

Nerve blockade. A nerve blockade may identify nerves that have been damaged or entrapped by the arthritic process. Subsequent treatment will depend on the duration of the pain relief. Neurolysis, for example, by radiofrequency ablation of sensory nerves to the facet (zygapophyseal) joints of the spine, can be effective in creating long-term relief of back pain. Before any destructive lesioning of nerves, the patient should have had 75% pain relief by accurate local anesthetic blockade of the nerve on at least two occasions.

Differential spinal or epidural block. If a spinal or epidural sensory and motor block to T10 does not relieve the patient's pain in the lower limbs, the pain is considered to be centralized. This pain may have a strong emotive content, and a multidisciplinary approach involving physicians and psychologists or psychiatrists is recommended.

Multidisciplinary pain management program. A multidisciplinary pain management program incorporates many features already discussed in the conventional treatment. It brings a pain team to focus on the individual and his or her problems. The pain team usually includes a pain physician, psychologist or psychiatrist, physical therapist, and occupational therapist. Other members may include a social worker and vocational rehabilitation counselor. The objectives are to rationalize medication, teach coping skills, educate, and give vocational guidance where appropriate. The long-term objective is to allow the individuals to control their pain and not let the pain control them.

CASE STUDY

Mrs. Y, a 50-year-old business executive, had been complaining of pain and swelling in her fingers for the last 5 years. The pain and stiffness were worse in the morning and were helped by anti-inflammatory drugs. The latest flare-up had been more severe than previously and had limited her ability to perform her job. She was anxious about the arthritis spreading to other joints and of her ability to keep her job if she was not 100% fit. She was sleeping poorly over the last few months. She had recently divorced and required her income, as she had two dependents and poor financial support from her ex-husband. She smoked two packs of cigarettes a day and drank alcohol on social occasions only.

On examination, she was an overweight woman with swollen and hot metacarpophalangeal joints of both hands. There were no subcutaneous nodules or tendinitis evident. Breath sounds were normal and full neurologic examination revealed normal sensation in the extremities.

Impression   Arthritis, probably rheumatoid.

Plan

1. Increase the nonsteroidal anti-inflammatory to the maximum daily dose and use frequent ice baths for the swelling and pain.
2. Send blood for ESR, HLA-DR4 and complete blood count.
3. Advise her to rest her joints during the flare-up by avoiding typing or using the fingers excessively.
4. Reassure her that it is very unlikely she will become severely handicapped.
5. Consider putting her on nortriptyline at night, working up to antidepressant levels.
6. Discuss her overweight problem and suggest a sensible diet plan. Discuss referral to a dietitian or a weight loss program.
7. Strongly advise her to stop smoking, as this could be exacerbating her problem.
8. See her again in 1 week.

She returns, complaining of no improvement. If anything, the pain is getting worse, and she is becoming more dysfunctional. Her sleep was greatly disturbed and she had had to take sick leave from work because of the discomfort. She has decreased her smoking to one pack a day and is taking 75 mg nortriptyline at night with no significant side effects. She is having gastric discomfort from the NSAID.

On examination the fingers do appear more swollen. Her blood work showed a high ESR and the HLA-DR4 was positive. There was a mild microcytic anemia.

Plan

1. In view of the blood tests and her worsening clinical status, which indicate an "aggressive" type of rheumatoid arthritis, she was referred to a rheumatologist as a matter of urgency.
2. Nortriptyline was increased to 100 mg at night.
3. Total smoking cessation was again stressed.
4. Capsaicin cream 0.025% was prescribed to rub on the joints four times a day.
5. The NSAID was changed to another type.

See her again in 3 weeks after ensuring she had an appointment with the rheumatologist the next day.

The rheumatologist put her on high-dose corticosteroids initially with a tapering dose schedule. She was also placed on gold salts. The remainder of the treatment remained unchanged. On her follow-up appointment she appeared much more comfortable, her joint swelling was less, and she was sleeping better. She had stopped smoking. She found the capsaicin cream caused too much "burning," so she had stopped using it. She was back at work, although not functioning at "full speed." She still appeared depressed regarding her general situation, not only her illness.

Plan

1. Advise her to continue seeing the rheumatologist.

She was eventually weaned to low-dose steroids, and the gold salts were stopped after 6 months.

A blood test for ESR and nortriptyline levels were taken. The ESR had decreased by over 50%, a good prognostic sign. The nortriptyline levels were below the therapeutic range for depression. Nortriptyline dosage was increased to 175 mg.

She eventually did well on low-dose corticosteroids, and the occasional few days of NSAID for a flare-up. The nortriptyline was maintained for 6 months.

She began to socialize more and changed her job to one with less typing. She continued to be followed at regular intervals.

SUGGESTED READINGS

Grennan DM, Jayson MIV: Rheumatoid arthritis. pp. 397–407. In Wall PD, Melzack R (eds): Textbook of Pain. 3rd Ed. Churchill Livingstone, New York, 1994

McCarthy C, Cushnaghan J, Dieppe P: Osteoarthritis and rheumatoid arthritis. pp. 387–396. In Wall PD, Melzack R (eds): Textbook of Pain. 3rd Ed. Churchill Livingstone, New York, 1994

Cancer Pain

Pain is the most common symptom of cancer. The incidence of pain in all stages of cancer and in advanced cancer is 30% to 40% and 65% to 80%, respectively. Cancer pain can be acute, chronic, or intermittent, and frequently the patient suffers from more than one area of pain. Unfortunately, cancer pain is widely undertreated. Of the cancer patients who suffer from pain, approximately 80% to 90% can be adequately managed with oral analgesics, using the algorithm shown in Figure 11-1. The majority of the remaining 10% to 20% can be managed with more invasive techniques performed by pain specialists.

There are many causes of cancer pain: 70% of cancer pain results from bone metastases, nerve compression, visceral distention, soft tissue infiltration, and mucous membrane ulceration; 15% of cancer pain results from anticancer therapy, such as surgery, chemotherapy, and radiation; and the remaining 15% of the pain is unrelated to the cancer.

It is important to determine the cause of the pain, as this will influence treatment. Cancer may cause both neuropathic pain and nociceptive pain. If the tumor invades neural structures, the resulting neural damage creates neuropathic pain. In general, neuropathic pain is relatively opioid-resistant and will require treatment with the co-analgesics (i.e., antidepressants, antiarrhythmics, anticonvulsants). By contrast, nociceptive pain is opioid- and NSAID-sensitive. An example of nociceptive pain is the pain of bone metastasis or visceral cancer.

Chronic benign pain should be dealt with only during clinic hours, but it may be necessary to deal with cancer pain as an emergency. Cancer pain should be dealt with more aggressively than chronic nonmalignant pain, but the goals of treatment should agree with the goals of the patient and the patient's family regarding the acceptable amount of side effects for the degree of pain relief.

Figure 11-1 presents an algorithm for the management of cancer pain.

TREATMENT PLANS FOR CANCER PAIN

TREATMENT A

Tricyclic antidepressants. The antidepressants may be very helpful in the treatment of cancer pain resulting from nervous system injury. Although the TCAs are the drugs of choice, treatment should not be limited to these, as the newer antidepressants may prove to be beneficial. The choice of antidepressant will depend on the patient's sleep pattern and tolerance. If the patient has disturbed sleep, a more sedating antidepressant, such as amitriptyline, should be chosen. If no sleep disturbance is present, a less sedating antide-

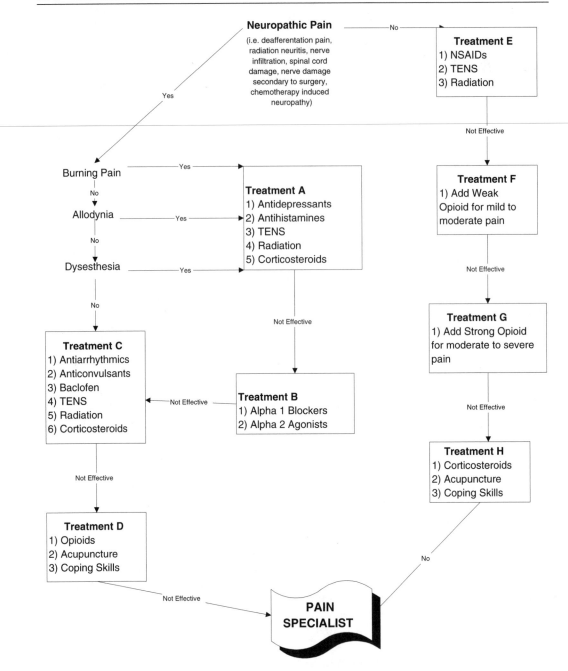

Fig. 11-1. Pain management in cancer. NSAIDs, nonsteroidal anti-inflammatory drugs; TENS, transcutaneous electrical nerve stimulation.

pressant, such as nortriptyline, may be beneficial. Doses up to 150 mg per 24 hours have been reported effective. A combination of amitriptyline and fluphenazine may be tried if a TCA alone is ineffective. A 2- to 4-week trial of therapy should be attempted before the decision is made that it will be ineffective.

Antihistamines. The addition of hydroxyzine at bedtime may improve the patient's symptoms and also improve sleep.

TENS. Transcutaneous electrical nerve stimulation (TENS) may improve the patient's pain. If no benefit is seen after a week of using different frequencies on a set regimen, it is doubtful that it will be of long-term benefit (see Fig. 33-1).

Radiation. If the pain is the result of tumor compression of neural structures, a course of radiation therapy to decrease the tumor size may reduce the pain.

Corticosteroids. A course of corticosteroids may provide temporary relief by decreasing the swelling within and around the tumor.

TREATMENT B

Alpha-1 blockers. Cancer pain may result from sympathetic instability and may be sustained by the sympathetic nervous system. Because of this, alpha-1 blockers may be beneficial. The drugs of choice are prazosin, phenoxybenzamine, or terazosin titrated to effect. Significant improvement should be noticed within 1 to 2 weeks if effective.

Alpha-2 agonists. Clonidine may improve cancer pain by preventing the release of norepinephrine. Clonidine may be administered via the oral route or transdermal patch. Significant improvement should be noticed within 1 to 2 weeks if effective.

TREATMENT C

Antiarrhythmics. Mexiletine may improve the spontaneous lancinating pain sometimes seen in these pain syndromes. It can be titrated up to a maximum of 10 mg/kg per day. Tocanide is another antiarrhythmic that may be effective. Significant improvement should be noticed within 1 to 2 weeks if effective.

Anticonvulsants. Carbamazepine is currently the anticonvulsant of choice. However, gabapentin may be a reasonable first-line drug because of the low side effect profile of this drug. Others that may be effective are phenytoin, valproic acid, and clonazepam for neuropathic pain. Significant improvement should be noticed within 1 to 2 weeks if effective.

Baclofen. Baclofen is an antispasmodic agent that may be of benefit in neuropathic pain. This drug can be titrated to effect. Significant improvement should be noticed within 1 to 2 weeks if effective.

TENS. A transcutaneous electrical nerve stimulator may improve the patient's pain. If no benefit is seen after a week of using different frequencies on a set regimen, it is doubtful that it will be of long-term benefit (see Fig. 33-1).

Radiation. If the pain is the result of tumor compression of neural structures, a course of radiation therapy to decrease the tumor size may reduce the pain.

Corticosteroids. A course of corticosteroids may provide temporary relief by decreasing the swelling within and around the tumor.

TREATMENT D

Opioids. If treatment regimens A–C fail, a trial of opioids should be undertaken. Neuropathic pain syndromes are often less responsive to opioid therapy. If a reasonable dose of opioids is not effective in pain treatment, referral to a pain specialist should be considered.

Acupuncture. By central neuromodulation and decreasing local muscle spasm, acupuncture should logically help in central pain. Unfortunately, there are no controlled studies showing it to be effective.

Coping skills. Inquiry should be made into mood and suicidal ideation. Patients with overt depression or active suicidal thoughts should be referred to a psychiatrist for therapy to run in conjunction with other therapies. Simple coping skills should be taught and family support encouraged in all instances where these are found to be lacking.

TREATMENT E

Nonsteroidal anti-inflammatory drugs. NSAIDs can be very helpful in nociceptive cancer pain. They are especially useful in pain secondary to bony metastasis and should be used in the early treatment.

TENS. Transcutaneous electrical nerve stimulation may improve the patient's pain. If no benefit is seen after a week of using different frequencies on a set regimen, it is doubtful that it will be of long-term benefit (see Fig. 33-1).

Radiation. If the pain is the result of tumor compression of neural structures, a course of radiation therapy to decrease the tumor size may reduce the pain.

TREATMENT F

Weak opioids. If treatment E is unsuccessful, the addition of a weak opioid such as codeine or hydrocodone is indicated. These opioids usually contain acetaminophen and should be limited to 4 g acetaminophen per day. If there is inadequate pain relief with this dose, a strong opioid is indicated.

TREATMENT G

Strong opioids. The strong opioids such as morphine, methadone, or hydromorphone are indicated for moderate to severe cancer pain. A dosing regimen should be developed that will maintain stable blood levels and avoid breakthrough pain. See Chapter 3 on opioid analgesics.

TREATMENT H

Corticosteroids. A course of corticosteroids may provide temporary relief by decreasing the swelling within and around the tumor.

Acupuncture. By central neuromodulation and decreasing local muscle spasm, acupuncture should logically help in central pain. Unfortunately, there are no controlled studies showing it to be effective.

Coping skills. Inquiry should be made into mood and suicidal ideation. Patients with overt depression or active suicidal thoughts should be referred to a psychiatrist for therapy to run in conjunction with other therapies. Simple coping skills should be taught and family support encouraged in all instances where these are found to be lacking.

PAIN SPECIALIST

If pain persists despite the above regimens, referral to a pain specialist is indicated. The pain specialist should evaluate the patient both physically and psychologically. Therapies may include the following procedures.

Medication optimization or withdrawal. Frequently, the pain specialist will optimize medications by adjusting doses or trying different combinations. In cases where the excessive or improper use of medications interferes with the patient's ability to function, the pain specialist may withdraw the medications.

Diagnostic blocks to evaluate the pain mechanism. If the pain is localized to a specific area of the body, a local anesthetic block to the nerve that supplies this area will give information on the pain pathway taken. An example is abdominal pain that results from pancreatic cancer. A block of the celiac plexus will often result in dramatic pain relief. If the pain is significantly decreased with this procedure, neurolytic ablations may be tried. Depending on the life expectancy of the patient, stimulatory techniques may also be tried.

Intravenous drug infusions. Pain specialists frequently use intravenous drug infusions to evaluate the response of the pain to various classes of drugs. These include lidocaine, phentolamine, or opioid infusions. These infusions give the pain specialist information on the physiologic aspects of the pain and help guide therapy.

Differential spinal or epidural block. If the patient suffers from pain in the trunk or lower extremity, a spinal or epidural injection of local anesthetic can provide information on the pain pathways. If a sensory and motor block occurs in the painful area but the patient continues to report pain, the pain is considered centralized.

Epidural steroid injections. If the pain results from a nerve root compression secondary to metastasis, epidural steroid injections may provide temporary relief.

Intraspinal drug therapy. Infusion of opioids, baclofen, or local anesthetics into the intrathecal or epidural space may provide excellent pain relief in selected cases. Internalized systems allow for long-term drug therapy.

Spinal cord stimulation. Depending on the patient's life expectancy, spinal cord stimulation may be an option for extremity pain. Spinal cord stimulation can also be performed for trunk pain, although it is more difficult to achieve good stimulation than with extremity pain.

Psychological counseling. Cancer pain can create suffering for both the patient and family. Psychological counseling may be of benefit in teaching coping skills for patient and family. A pain psychologist can also prepare the patient and family for the possible need for home or hospice health care.

CASE STUDY

Mrs. X is a 57-year-old woman who was diagnosed with breast cancer 6 months previously. She underwent a modified radical mastectomy and had chemotherapy postoperatively. She now presents with low back pain. She describes the pain as a dull ache in her mid-lower back. The pain was constant and worse with sitting and activity. The average visual analog scale (VAS) is 60/100 (0 = no pain to 100 = worst pain imaginable). On examination there is diffuse tenderness of the lower back with some muscle tightness of the paraspinous muscles. Neurologic examination of her lower extremities was unremarkable. A bone scan revealed metastatic disease of her lumbar spine.

Impression Metastatic cancer to lumbar spine.

Plan

1. NSAIDs.
2. TENS.
3. See patient in 1 week.

Patient returned stating her VAS has decreased from 60/100 to 40/100; however, she requested additional pain relief.

Plan

1. Add tramadol 50 mg increasing to 100 mg q 6 h.
2. See patient in 1 week.

Patient returned stating her pain score was 20–30/100 most of the time but tolerable. However, she had intermittent exacerbation when she tried to increase her activity.

Plan

1. Add an opioid for mild to moderate pain (i.e., codeine or hydrocodone).

Patient did well with the above regimen for approximately 2 months. The NSAIDs were discontinued because of severe gastric upset and guaiac-positive stools. On discontinuing the NSAIDs, the pain increased.

Plan

1. Start a time-contingency opioid for moderate to severe pain. A reasonable regimen would be MS Contin every 8 to 12 hours with immediate-release morphine for breakthrough pain.

Patient returned stating that, although she was obtaining adequate pain relief, she was having a lot of nausea/vomiting with the increase in morphine.

Plan

1. Add an antinauseant drug.

In spite of multiple antinauseant trials, the patient continued to have nausea and vomiting.

Plan

1. Give a trial of corticosteroid therapy and decrease the dose of the opioids.
2. Since the patient had guaiac-positive stools with NSAIDs, coadminister an H2 blocker.

The above measures should be instituted on a primary care level. If they fail to produce relief, a consultation with a pain specialist should be considered. Early referral is recommended when the usual treatment modalities as outlined above are proving inadequate.

SUGGESTED READINGS

American Pain Society: Principles of Analgesic Use in the Treatment of Acute Pain and Cancer Pain. 3rd Ed. APS, Skokie, IL, 1992

Rowlingson JC, Hamill RJ, Patt RB: Comprehensive assessment of the patient with cancer pain. pp. 23–40. In Patt RB (ed): Cancer Pain. JB Lippincott, Philadelphia, 1993

Storey, P: Primer of Pallative Care. Academy of Hospice Physicians, Florida, 1994

12 | Central Pain

Pathologic lesions to the central nervous system may result in pain. This usually occurs after traumatic or vascular lesions and results in a very painful condition that may be very difficult to manage. The pain syndromes usually occur with lesions at or near the main pain pathways. An example is a stroke involving the ventral posterolateral thalamus, which is an area where ascending pain pathways connect with thalamic nuclei (see Ch. 2). Another example is a spinal cord injury with resulting pain in the distal lower extremities. The distal limbs are the most common sites of intense pain, although the pain may occur anywhere in the body. The type of pain that results from central nervous system lesions is very similar to that which results from a peripheral nervous system lesion. The patients often complain of burning pain, spontaneous lancinating pain, hyperalgesia, and allodynia.

Lesions to the peripheral nervous system can lead to a central pain syndrome. An example is phantom limb pain after an extremity amputation. In these cases, the central nervous system exhibits plasticity in which changes occur within the dorsal horn and supraspinal regions of the brain. The dorsal horn cells continue to send pain messages to the brain in the absence of ongoing tissue damage. These changes may persist beyond the normal healing period and result in chronic pain.

The mechanism behind central pain is poorly understood. Many studies suggest that there is a loss of central inhibition that results from these lesions, but it is likely that many factors play an important role in the pathogenesis of central pain. These pain syndromes can be extremely difficult to manage.

Occasionally, spinal cord-injured patients will present with mechanical pain from the injured vertebral column. This pain is usually radicular and can be treated as back pain with radiculopathy. Mechanical causes of the pain should be ruled out before diagnosing central pain. These patients may also present with abdominal pain. Before declaring this pain as central, intra-abdominal pathology should be ruled out.

An algorithm for management of central pain is presented in Figure 12-1.

TREATMENT PLANS

TREATMENT A

Tricyclic antidepressants. Antidepressants may be very helpful in the treatment of central pain syndromes. Although the TCAs are the drugs of choice, treatment should not be limited to these, as the newer antidepressants may prove to be beneficial. The choice of

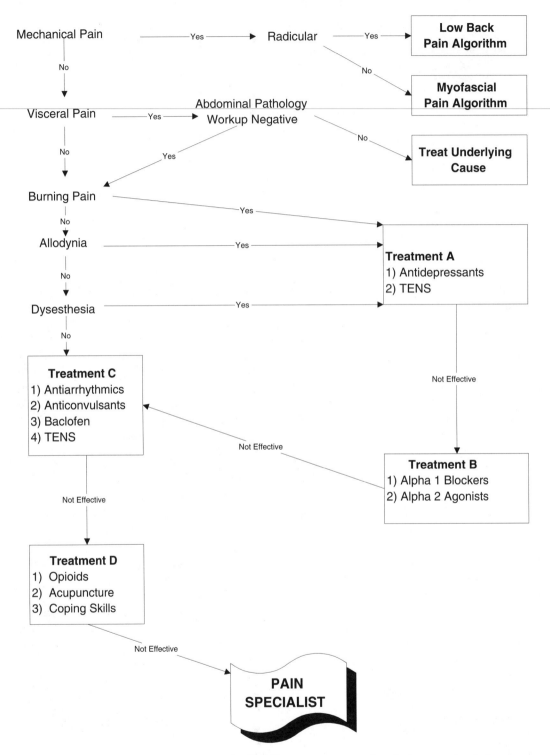

Fig. 12-1. Management of central pain. TENS, transcutaneous electrical nerve stimulation.

antidepressant will depend on the patient's sleep pattern and tolerance. If the patient has disturbed sleep, a more sedating antidepressant, such as amitriptyline, should be chosen. If no sleep disturbance is present, a less sedating antidepressant, such as nortriptyline, may be beneficial. Doses up to 150 mg per 24 hours have been reported effective. A combination of amitriptyline and fluphenazine may be tried if a TCA alone is ineffective. A 2- to 4-week trial of therapy should be attempted before the decision is made that it will be ineffective.

TENS. A transcutaneous electrical nerve stimulator (TENS) may improve central pain, but the pads should not be placed over areas of sensory deficit (i.e., paraplegia). In these cases, the TENS unit can be placed just above the level of the spinal cord injury. If no benefit is seen after a week of using different frequencies on a set regimen, it is doubtful that it will be of long-term benefit (see Fig. 33-1).

TREATMENT B

Alpha-1 blockers. Central pain may result from sympathetic instability and may be sustained by the sympathetic nervous system. Because of this, the alpha-1 blockers may be beneficial. The drugs of choice are prazosin, phenoxybenzamine, hydantoin, or terazosin titrated to effect. Significant improvement should be noticed within 1 to 2 weeks if effective.

Alpha-2 agonists. Clonidine may improve central pain by preventing the release of norepinephrine. Clonidine may be administered via the oral route or transdermal patch. Significant improvement should be noticed within 1 to 2 weeks if effective.

TREATMENT C

Antiarrhythmics. Mexiletine may improve the spontaneous lancinating pain sometimes seen in these pain syndromes. This drug can be titrated up to a maximum of 10 mg/kg per day. Tocanide is another antiarrhythmic that may be effective. Significant improvement should be noticed within 1 to 2 weeks if effective.

Anticonvulsants. Carbamazepine is currently the anticonvulsant of choice; however, gabapentin may be a worthwhile first-line drug, since it has a low side effect and toxicity profile. Others that may be effective include phenytoin, valproic acid, and clonazepam. Significant improvement should be noticed within 1 to 2 weeks if effective.

Baclofen. Baclofen is an antispasmodic drug that may be of benefit in neuropathic pain. It can be titrated to effect. Significant improvement should be noticed within 1 to 2 weeks if effective.

TENS. TENS may improve the patient's pain. If no benefit is seen after a week of using different frequencies on a set regimen, it is doubtful that it will be of long-term benefit (see Fig. 33-1).

TREATMENT D

Opioids. If treatment regimens A–C fail, a trial of low-dose opioids may be of benefit. Unfortunately, neuropathic pain syndromes such as central pain are less responsive to opioid therapy. If a reasonable dose of opioids is not effective in pain treatment, a referral to a pain specialist should be considered.

Acupuncture. Central neuromodulation and decreasing local muscle spasm by acupuncture should logically help in central pain. Unfortunately, there are no controlled studies showing it to be effective.

Coping skills. Inquiry should be made into mood and suicidal ideation. Patients with overt depression or active suicidal thoughts should be referred to a psychiatrist for therapy to run in conjunction with other therapies. Simple coping skills should be taught and family support encouraged in all instances where these are found to be lacking.

PAIN SPECIALIST

If pain persists despite the above regimens, referral to a pain specialist is indicated. The pain specialist should evaluate the patient both physically and psychologically. Therapies may include the following procedures.

Medication optimization or withdrawal. Frequently, the pain specialist will optimize medications by adjusting doses or trying different combinations. In cases where the excessive or improper use of medications interferes with the patient's ability to function, the pain specialist may withdraw the medications.

Diagnostic blocks to evaluate the pain mechanism. If the pain is localized to a specific area of the body, a local anesthetic block to the nerve that supplies this area will give information on the pain pathway taken. In partial spinal cord injuries, peripheral diagnostic blocks can help differentiate between peripheral and central causes of the pain. If the pain is significantly decreased with this procedure, neurolytic techniques may be tried.

Intravenous drug infusions. Pain specialists frequently use intravenous drug infusions to evaluate the response of the pain to various classes of drugs. These include lidocaine, phentolamine, or opioids. These infusions may give the pain specialist information on the physiologic aspects of the pain and help guide therapy.

Differential spinal or epidural block. If the patient suffers from pain in the trunk or lower extremity, a spinal or epidural injection of local anesthetic can provide information on the pain pathways. If this technique does not provide pain relief, then the pain may be originating from supraspinal areas.

Intraspinal drug therapy. Infusion of opioids, baclofen, or local anesthetics into the intrathecal or epidural space may provide excellent pain relief in selected cases. Internalized systems allow for long-term drug therapy.

Spinal cord stimulation. Spinal cord stimulation may be an option for central pain. Adequate coverage of paresthesia with a single electrode may prove difficult, and twin electrodes may have to be trialed. The trial period should be of adequate duration to assess efficacy, for example, 5 to 10 days.

Psychological counseling. Psychological counseling may be of benefit in teaching coping skills for patient and family.

CASE STUDY

Mr. X, 35 years old, was involved in a motor vehicle accident 1 year previously, which resulted in a T10 paraplegia. He presented with complaints of burning pain in his left foot. He described the pain as a continuous burning pain with an occasional sharp jab in the left great toe. The average visual analog pain score (VAS) is 80/100. The VAS was from 0 (no pain) to 100 (worst pain imaginable). The pain interferes with his sleep. Medication includes extra strength acetaminophen without any pain relief. On examination he was mentally alert and in no obvious distress. Sensory examination showed complete loss of sensory and motor function below the T10 level. The patient suffered from mild spasticity in both lower extremities.

Impression

1. Central pain syndrome.

Plan

1. Stop the acetaminophen, as this drug has little efficacy in this syndrome.
2. Start a tricyclic antidepressant.
3. Trial of TENS.
4. See him in 10 days.

Patient returned stating his sleep has improved, but he still suffered from intense burning pain. The TENS had not helped.

Plan

1. Stop TENS.
2. Continue the tricyclic antidepressant.
3. Choose one of the following: prazosin, phenoxybenzamine, terazosin, clonidine.
4. See him in 10 days.

Patient returned stating his burning pain was much improved on prazosin 1 mg tid, but he still suffered from intermittent sharp stabbing pains.

Plan

1. Continue the TCA and prazosin.
2. Start one of the following: gabapentin, mexiletine, tocanide, carbamazepine, phenytoin, valproic acid, or clonazepam.

The above measures should be instituted on a primary care level. If they fail to produce relief, a consultation with a pain specialist should be considered. If you have access to acupuncture or a psychologist within your system, these may be tried before referral to a pain specialist. Early referral is recommended when the usual treatment modalities as outlined above are proving inadequate.

SUGGESTED READINGS

Likavec MJ: Pain secondary to paraplegia or quadriplegia. pp. 224–227. In Raj PP (ed): Practical Management of Pain. Mosby Year Book, Philadelphia, 1986

Tasker R: Pain resulting from central nervous system pathology (central pain). pp. 64–283. In Bonica JJ (ed): The Management of Pain. Lea & Febiger, Philadelphia, 1990

13 | Diabetic Neuropathy

Diabetic neuropathy (DN) is a metabolic disorder that results from damage to peripheral nerve fibers secondary to hyperglycemia. In spite of its fairly high incidence, it is a poorly understood pain syndrome, and not all patients with diabetic neuropathy suffer from pain. The neuropathy is thought to result from ischemic neuronal damage. Some diabetic neuropathy patients have signs of large myelinated fiber disease, while others show small unmyelinated fiber disease. These are probably variants of the same disease. Many will have sensory abnormalities without pain. DN can be divided into acute and chronic phases.

Chronic DN patients will typically show a gradual onset of bilateral dysesthesias and pain in the distal legs and feet. This neuropathy may occur anywhere from months to years after the onset of the diabetes. The incidence and prevalence of painful diabetic neuropathy is proportional to the duration of the disease; 35% of the diabetics who have their disease for 10 years will have a painful neuropathy. Initially these patients will demonstrate sensory changes in the distal extremities, which may progress to frank numbness. This numbness occurs because of demyelination of distal nerves, which may be complemented by a loss of small axons and peripheral sympathetic control. It is not uncommon for patients to have a sensory loss in the distal extremities and yet suffer from severe pain.

Acute DN is characterized by a sudden onset of severe pain, with constant burning in the feet, dysesthesias, allodynia, and lancinating leg pains. The pain may also follow the distribution of individual cranial or peripheral nerves. Despite these symptoms, neurologic examination may be unremarkable. This type of neuropathy usually remits when the blood sugars are controlled.

A treatment algorithm for management of diabetic neuropathy is given in Figure 13-1.

TREATMENT PLANS

TREATMENT A

Antidepressants. Antidepressants have been demonstrated to be effective for DN in clinical trials with the tricyclic antidepressants (TCA) being the agents of choice. Treatment should not be limited to TCAs, as the newer antidepressants may also prove to be beneficial. The choice of the antidepressant will depend on the patient's sleep pattern and tolerance. If the patient has disturbed sleep, a more sedating antidepressant, such as amitriptyline, should be chosen. If no sleep disturbance is present, a less sedating antidepressant, such as nortriptyline, may be beneficial. Doses up to 150 mg per 24 hours have been reported effective. A combination of amitriptyline and fluphenazine may be tried if a TCA alone is ineffective. A 2- to 4-week trial of therapy should be attempted before the decision is made that it is ineffective.

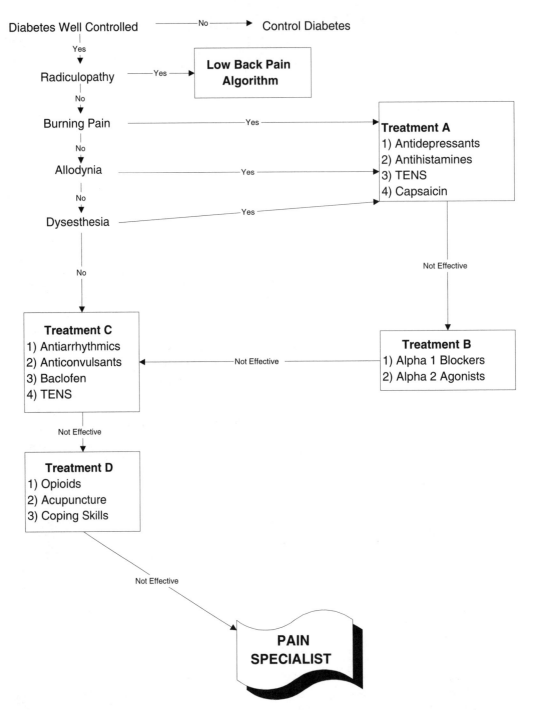

Fig. 13-1. Management of pain from diabetic neuropathy. TENS, transcutaneous electrical nerve stimulation.

Antihistamines. The addition of hydroxyzine at bedtime may improve the patient's symptoms and also improve sleep.

TENS. A transcutaneous electrical nerve stimulator (TENS) may improve the pain of DN, but the pads should not be placed over an area of severe sensory deficit. If the patient suffers from a severe sensory deficit, more proximal placement such as behind the knee may prove helpful. If no benefit is seen after a week of using different frequencies on a set regimen, it is doubtful that it will be of long-term benefit (see Fig. 33-1).

Capsaicin. Capsaicin cream may be helpful in DN. It is suggested that initially 0.025% capsaicin is tried. If this is unsuccessful, then a 0.075% cream can be tried. Initially, this cream may burn after application; however, this will disappear with continued use. As significant depletion of the substance P from the peripheral nerve terminals takes up to 3 weeks, treatment must be continued for this minimum period of time before efficacy can be gauged. The patient must use this cream 3 to 4 times per day to be effective.

TREATMENT B

Alpha-1 blockers. DN may result from sympathetic instability and may be sustained by the sympathetic nervous system. Because of this, the alpha-1 blockers may be beneficial. The drugs of choice are prazosin, phenoxybenzamine, or terazosin titrated to effect. Significant improvement should be noticed within 1 to 2 weeks if effective.

Alpha-2 agonists. Clonidine may improve the pain of DN by preventing the release of norepinephrine. It also acts centrally to inhibit central pain pathways. Clonidine may be administered orally or transdermally. Significant improvement should be noticed within 1 to 2 weeks if effective.

TREATMENT C

Antiarrhythmic drugs. Mexiletine has proved effective for DN in clinical trials. This drug can be titrated up to a maximum of 10 mg/kg per day. Tocanide is another antiarrhythmic agent that may be effective. Significant improvement should be noticed within 1 to 2 weeks if effective.

Anticonvulsants. Carbamazepine is currently the anticonvulsant of choice. However, the newer anticonvulsant, gabapentin, may prove more effective; it lacks many of the side effects of the older drugs. Others that may be effective include phenytoin, valproic acid, and clonazepam. Significant improvement should be noticed within 1 to 2 weeks if effective.

Baclofen. Baclofen is an antispasmodic drug that may be of benefit in neuropathic pain. This drug can be titrated to effect. Significant improvement should be noticed within 1 to 2 weeks if effective.

TENS. TENS may improve the pain of DN, but the pads should not be placed over an area of severe sensory deficit. If the patient suffers from a severe sensory deficit, more proximal placement, such as behind the knee, may prove helpful. If no benefit is seen after a week of using different frequencies on a set regimen, it is doubtful that it will be of long-term benefit (see Fig. 33-1).

TREATMENT D

Opioids. If treatment regimens A–C fail, a trial of low-dose opioids may be of benefit. Unfortunately, neuropathic pain syndromes such as DN are less responsive to opioid therapy. If a reasonable dose of opioids is not effective in pain treatment, then a referral to a pain specialist should be considered.

Acupuncture. Central neuromodulation and decreasing local muscle spasm by acupuncture should logically help in DN. Unfortunately, there are no controlled studies showing it to be effective.

Coping skills. Inquiry should be made into mood and suicidal ideation. Patients with overt depression or active suicidal thoughts should be referred to a psychiatrist for therapy to run in conjunction with other therapies. Simple coping skills should be taught and family support encouraged in all instances where these are found to be lacking.

PAIN SPECIALIST

If pain persists despite the above regimens, referral to a pain specialist is indicated. The pain specialist should evaluate the patient both physically and psychologically. Therapies may include the following procedures.

Medication optimization or withdrawal. Frequently, the pain specialist will optimize medications by adjusting doses or trying different combinations. In cases where the excessive or improper use of medications interferes with the patient's ability to function, the pain specialist may withdraw the medications.

Diagnostic nerve blocks to evaluate the pain mechanism. If the pain is localized to a specific area of the body, a local anesthetic block of the nerve that supplies this area will give information on the pain pathway taken. If the pain is significantly decreased with this procedure, neurolytic or neurostimulation techniques may be tried.

Intravenous drug infusions. Pain specialists frequently use intravenous drug infusions to determine what type of drug the pain may respond to. These infusions include lidocaine, phentolamine, or opioids. They give the pain specialist information on the physiologic aspects of the pain and help guide therapy.

Differential spinal or epidural block. If the patient suffers from pain in the trunk or lower extremity, a spinal or epidural injection of local anesthetic can provide information on the pain pathways. If a sensory and motor block results in the painful area without relieving the patient's pain, the pain is considered centralized.

Spinal cord stimulation. Patients who suffer from pain in the extremities may benefit from spinal cord stimulation. Because of the symmetry of diabetic neuropathy, spinal cord stimulation with twin electrodes may be necessary.

Intraspinal drug therapy. Infusion of opioids, baclofen, or local anesthetics into the intrathecal or epidural space may provide excellent pain relief in selected cases. Internalized systems can provide long-term drug therapy.

A multidisciplinary pain management program. A multidisciplinary approach involves a group of specialists trained in pain management. Each member of the team addresses specific problems the patient faces. The team usually includes a pain physician, psychologist or psychiatrist, and physical therapist. Other members may include a social worker and vocational rehabilitation counselor. The objectives are to rationalize medication, teach coping skills, educate, and give vocational guidance where appropriate. The long-term objective is to allow the individuals to control their pain and not let the pain control them.

CASE STUDY

Mr. X, 55 years old, has a 10-year history of insulin-dependent diabetes that has been well controlled. Approximately 5 years ago, the patient began noticing sensory loss in his toes, which progressed to involve both of his feet in a stocking distribution. He now complains of pain in the area of sensory loss. He describes the pain as a constant burning with some mild dysesthesia. The average visual analog pain score (VAS) is 80/100. The VAS is from 0 (no pain) to 100 (worst pain imaginable). The pain interferes with his sleep. Medication includes ibuprofen 400 mg q 6 h without any pain relief. On examination he was mentally alert and in no obvious distress. The patient stated light touch of his feet created an unpleasant sensation. Sensory examination showed decreased sensation to temperature, touch, and pinprick in both feet below mid-calf. His random blood sugar was 140 mg/ml.

Impression Painful diabetic neuropathy.

Plan

1. Stop the ibuprofen, as the NSAIDs have little efficacy.
2. Start a tricyclic antidepressant. If the TCA is not too sedating, and the patient continues to complain of pain, instruct the patient to add hydroxyzine at bedtime.
3. See him in 10 days.

Patient returned stating he had noticed some decrease in his pain but requested some more pain relief.

Plan

1. Continue the above medications.
2. Trial of capsaicin cream 0.025% rubbed on the area qid for 3 weeks. Also consider adding a TENS unit.
3. TENS trial.
4. See patient in 1 week for results of TENS and again in 3 weeks.

Patient returned stating that 3 weeks of capsaicin cream therapy had not proven effective. He was continuing to use the TENS unit with about 20% relief of pain. He continued to use the TCA and hydroxyzine at nighttime.

Plan

1. Discontinue the capsaicin.
2. Continue the TENS.
3. Start clonidine.
4. See patient in 10 days.

Patient returned stating the burning pain was much decreased but the dysesthesias were persisting.

Plan

1. Add either gabapentin, carbamazepine, phenytoin, valproic acid, or clonazepam.

The above measures should be instituted on a primary care level. If they fail to produce relief, consultation with a pain specialist should be considered. Early referral is recommended when the usual treatment modalities as outlined above are proving inadequate.

SUGGESTED READINGS

Loeser JD: Peripheral nerve disorders (peripheral neuropathies). pp. 211–219. In Bonica JJ (ed): The Management of Pain. Lea & Febiger, Philadelphia, 1990

Wynn-Parry CB, Withrington R: The management of painful peripheral nerve disorders. pp. 395–401. In Melzack R, Wall PD (eds): Textbook of Pain. Churchill Livingstone, New York, 1984

CHAPTER 14 | Geriatric Pain

Of the 4,000 medical articles published each year on pain, less than 1% address geriatric pain. Of 11 medical textbooks on geriatrics reviewed, only two chapters discussed pain. Of eight geriatric nursing textbooks reviewed, a total of 5,000 pages, only 18 pages (0.36%) were related to pain and its treatment.

Yet, population reviews report a pain prevalence of 73% to 80% in the elderly population. If this high pain prevalence is correct, pain centers should have a large clientele of the elderly, with a proportionate amount of research and articles dealing with their pain problems. This is not the case. Suggested reasons for the high prevalence and low referral rates are the following:

1. Specialist therapy is expensive, and the elderly often have poor insurance coverage.
2. Both the primary physician and the patient may believe that pain is a natural process of aging, thereby creating a negative referral bias.
3. Some pain centers have a cap on the upper age of a patient, because their main focus of pain management is a return to work outcome.
4. There may be a change in pain perception with age. The elderly may believe that pain is normal for their age, and they do not wish to bother the doctor. Perhaps the poor memory experienced by some older people can affect their pain perception. However, studies on memory and concentration show no difference between the young and the elderly populations on the effect that pain has on these two variables.
5. Pain could yield some secondary gains. The elderly individual might justify his or her loss of mobility because of pain to legitimize dependence. In the nursing home setting, pain might legitimize obtaining love, contact, or attention.
6. The elderly tend to have more bereavement, may have a lowered sense of self-worth, and often have poor general health; in theory, this should make them more susceptible to pain.
7. There is evidence that depression may mimic or worsen chronic pain. The elderly have a high incidence of missed depression. Could depression be the reason for the high incidence of reported pain?

Whatever the reason, a large number of geriatric patients may be suffering excessive pain unnecessarily.

The practitioner who deals with the elderly patient in pain should do the following:

1. Pace the presentation, task relevance, and difficulty level to the patient's skill.
2. Increase the time expected for a response.
3. Increase the time given to the patient to study the visual material.
4. Slow the pace of speech when talking to the individual.
5. Ensure that social supports are available, especially if the patient is living alone.
6. Nurture the patient's hope in medical care and treatment.
7. Arrange home visits and involvement of significant others and support groups.

Algorithms for the approach to geriatric patients and for the treatment of their pain are given in Figures 14-1 and 14-2.

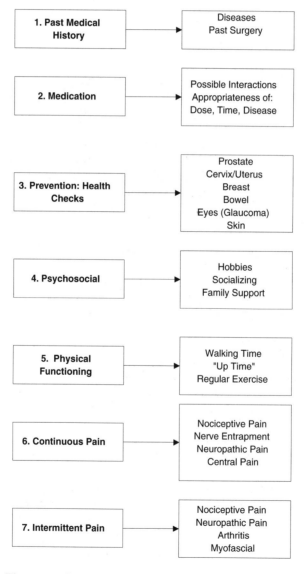

Fig. 14-1. General principles of geriatric pain management.

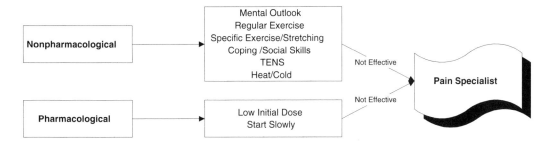

Fig. 14-2. General principles of pain treatment. TENS, transcutaneous electrical nerve stimulation.

GENERAL PRINCIPLES OF GERIATRIC PAIN

Past Medical History

With the increasing number of diseases that often accompany aging, pain may be an unwelcome companion. Previous operations can contribute to or be responsible for the pain syndrome due to ongoing degeneration, scar neuroma formation, or altered biomechanics.

Medications

The elderly have differences in absorption, breakdown, and excretion of medications, which makes them more sensitive to drugs. They may be taking several medications for different chronic disease processes. These drugs can interact with each other or with the analgesic regimen.

Older people often have difficulty remembering what to take and when; only 45% of them take medications as prescribed. A careful history from both the patient and a close relative or companion, and a review of the number of tablets left, may reveal gross discrepancies between optimum dosages and what is actually being taken. Ideally, the medication bottles should be carefully labeled or color-coded with clear instructions written in large letters as to when they should be taken. A regular review of medications and their potential side effects should be undertaken and, where possible, treatment regimens simplified or stopped.

Prevention: Health Checks

Annual routine health checks should include, but not be limited to, rectal examination, Pap smear (every 5 years when over 60 years of age), breast examination (mammography is recommended in women over 50), with teaching of self-breast examination, proctoscopy in patients with a high risk or with blood in the feces, and glaucoma check. At each visit blood pressure measurement and a check on any suspicious skin lesions should be carried out.

Psychosocial Functioning

Many studies have pointed out that a healthy lifestyle for the elderly means remaining mentally and physically active. Obtaining a baseline of social functioning and hobbies (before the pain) the patient is interested in maintaining is important information. Social services, occupational therapists, and local clubs and groups are ancillary aids in assisting the individual to retain, or regain, an acceptable quality of life. Family members, if present, should be enrolled into the treatment plan so they can assist and perhaps gently cajole the patient into taking action in becoming more socially interactive, if appropriate.

Physical Functioning

How much exercise and "up time" the patient engages in shows the extent to which he or she can be considered housebound. Daily regular exercise is to be encouraged, ideally outside the house. Some will find it easier and more pleasant to exercise in a group. Many communities have exercise programs specifically for the elderly.

Continuous Pain

Nociceptive Pain

Nociceptive pain is usually NSAIDs- and opioid-sensitive and is eased by position (mechanical), warmth, or cold. If the pain is associated with a fever, weight loss, or systemic symptoms such as nausea or vomiting, the possibility of infection or neoplasm should be thoroughly investigated. The treatment depends on the cause.

Neuropathic Pain

Neuropathic pains are usually not NSAIDs-sensitive and may be resistant or relatively resistant to opioids. The pain is often described as a continuous burning or aching pain not influenced by body position. It may also be shooting or lancinating, lasting a few seconds. This type of pain is usually partially sensitive to anticonvulsants, tricyclic antidepressants, or sodium channel blockers [Mexitil (mexiletine), Tegretol (carbamazepine), Dilantin (phenytoin), Depakote (sodium valproate)].

Central Pain

When pain has been present for several months, it is unlikely to be "cured." This is possibly due to hyperexcitation (wind-up) of the dorsal horn nociceptors.

Intermittent Pain

Nociceptive Pain

Nociceptive pain is usually mechanical and is exacerbated by certain movements or overuse. Often caused by joint degeneration, it can be treated initially by rest and NSAIDs if severe. Gentle range of movement and stretching exercises should be introduced as soon as practical to prevent further joint damage. Early referral to a physical therapist for joint mobilization, stretching, and a home exercise program is important. Joint mobilization is very important. Physical therapy that concentrates on heat and massage is of little value.

Neuropathic Pain

Neuropathic pain is usually radicular, causing shooting pains in a nerve distribution. It may or may not be related to posture or movement. It usually indicates nerve or nerve root irritation. Treatment options include medications such as anticonvulsants, sodium channel blockers, and tricyclic antidepressants, as well as surgery if entrapment or impingement of a nerve root is the pain provoker. Electromyography (EMG), magnetic resonance imaging (MRI), or computed tomography (CT) scan and diagnostic blocks can be helpful in diagnosing these conditions.

Arthritic Pain

Arthritic conditions are common in the elderly but are not necessarily painful. Acute inflammatory flare-ups occur, however, usually necessitate relative rest of the joint and a short course of NSAIDs. Flare-ups may be precipitated by acute overuse.

Myofascial Pain

Myofascial pain is common and is usually secondary to other causes but may perpetuate restrictive joint movement as well as create painful trigger points. Acupuncture, dry needling, cold, self-pressure, specific stretching, and range of joint movement techniques are all useful in maintaining healthy joints.

GENERAL TREATMENT PRINCIPLES

Nonpharmacologic Therapy

Mental outlook. Baselines should be reevaluated in the elderly patient, before and while a new therapy is trialed. One useful memory test is FOGS: F = family story; O = orientation for date and place; G = general information, for example, name of the president, recent events; S = spelling of a word forward and backward.

Regular exercise. A regular exercise program should be encouraged even in those confined to the home, chair, or bed. Exercise programs are available for specific arthritic and myofascial pains, or a specific program may be developed by the physical therapist or occupational therapist.

Coping skills. The elderly can develop new coping strategies, although socialization problems, isolation, and set behavior patterns may make it harder to implement them.

TENS. Transcutaneous electrical nerve stimulation (TENS) can be very effective and allows the patient to retain an external focus of control.

Heat/cold. Thermal modalities carry little risk, although the skin of the elderly is thinner and more fragile. Creams should be used on the skin before heat or cold application. Any heat used should not be greater than can be comfortably tolerated by the face.

Pharmacologic Therapy

The elderly have differences compared to the healthy adult population with respect to absorption, breakdown, and excretion of medications. This makes them more sensitive to most medications. All pain medicines should be started at a low dose and increased slowly to efficacy.

Summary

It is important that physical, psychological, and social aspects of the geriatric patient should be taken into consideration when dealing with an elderly patient in pain. A diagnosis of the cause of the pain should take secondary importance to the effective treatment of it, and the comfort and functioning of the patient.

Headaches

Headache is the most common pain syndrome. The Nuprin Pain Report of 1985 reported that 73% of those surveyed suffered from headaches: 20% had headaches for 6 to 10 days a year, 22% for 11 to 30 days, 11% for 31 to 100 days, and 7% had headaches for more than 100 days of a year. The incidence of headache in women is approximately 10% greater than in men.

Headaches may be caused by organic lesions such as displacement or inflammation of cranial vascular structures, contraction of the head and neck muscles, cervical zygapophyseal joint dysfunction, or direct pressure on the cranial and upper cervical nerves. Pain afferents of the face, head, and neck converge on the nucleus caudalis in the brain stem. Stimulation of this nucleus and of the trigeminal complex increases extracranial blood flow. This causes extravasation of plasma in the dura and release of peptides that stimulate the nociceptors. These effects may explain the vascular type of pain in both tension and migraine headaches.

Using the International Headache Society criteria for migraine, Rausmussan in 1992 reported the lifetime prevalence of common migraine was 8% (female:male ratio 7:1) Women were more likely to have classical (with aura) migraine.

Over 95% of headaches seen by a family physician have no structural lesion. The pain and dysfunction is strongly influenced by environmental stressors and past experiences. These must be addressed in any treatment plan. Using a headache diary (Fig. 15-1) for two or three headache cycles can assist both patient and therapist in identifying environmental stressors and medication efficacy.

A headache pain treatment algorithm is presented in Figure 15-2.

HEADACHES OF RECENT ONSET OR INCREASING SEVERITY WITHOUT TRAUMA

Raised Intracranial Pressure

1. Headaches of abrupt onset may signify raised intracranial pressure due to spontaneous intracranial hemorrhage, hydrocephalus, or tumor. They may be accompanied by a change in personality, worst in the morning, aggravated by sitting or standing, and relieved by lying down.
2. Acute meningeal irritation due to subarachnoid hemorrhage, encephalitis, or meningitis causes fever, stiff neck, and a positive Kernig sign, and is usually accompanied by severe head pain with vomiting and photophobia.

HEADACHE DIARY

Fill in each day at the hour you are having a headache, its intensity, what you ate, drank and smoked, as well as medications taken. Note your activity just before the headache started.

Headache Score: 0 = no headache; 1 = mild; not interfering with daily activities; 2 = moderate; some interference with daily activities; 3 = severe; significant interference (have to lie down, return home).

Date_____   DAY_____   NAME_____

Hour	Headache Score	Activity at time of headache	Food/drink taken	Pain medications taken	COMMENTS
0-1					
1-2					
2-3					
3-4					
4-5					
5-6					
6-7					
7-8					
8-9					
9-10					
10-11					
11-12 noon					
12-1					
1-2					
2-3					
3-4					
4-5					
5-6					
6-7					
7-8					
8-9					
9-10					
10-11					
11-12 midnight					

SUMMARY: No. Of headache hours _____   Headache Score (on average) _____
            Total No. Of cigarettes smoked._____

Fig. 15-1. Headache diary.

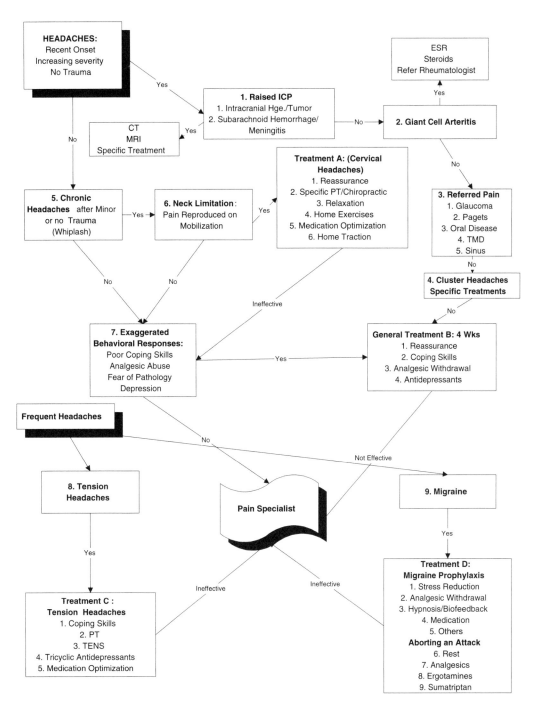

Fig. 15-2. Management of headache. ICP, intracranial pressure; CT, cat scan; MRI, magnetic resonance image; Hge, hemorrhage; ESR, erythrocyte sedimentation rate; TMD, temporomanidibular dysfunction; TENS, transcutaneous electrical nerve stimulation.

3. Hospital admission for computed tomography (CT) scanning and magnetic resonance imaging (MRI) to exclude mass lesions or hydrocephalus is mandatory. A lumbar puncture, if not contraindicated after the CT/MRI, is also mandatory. Subarachnoid hemorrhage can be missed by CT on admission in 20% of patients.

Giant Cell Arteritis

Giant cell arteritis, or temporal arteritis, is a preventable cause of blindness and stroke and must be excluded. For diagnosis, three the following criteria need to be satisfied:

1. Age 50 or older at onset.
2. New onset localized headache.
3. Temporal artery tenderness or decreased pulsation.
4. ESR more than 50 mm/hr.
5. Biopsy shows necrotizing arteritis.

Scalp tenderness and claudication of the jaw or tongue with swallowing or eating are also often present.

Temporal arteritis may be associated with polymyalgia rheumatica. This should be considered if the patient presents with associated aches and pains in the shoulder and pelvic muscles with fever, sweats, and masseter claudication. Blood should be drawn for an ESR (erythrocyte sedimentation rate) and steroids started immediately. Steroids do not affect the temporal artery biopsy changes for at least 48 hours. Initially 60 mg of prednisone per day is given. The dosage is decreased as the ESR and symptoms decrease. Maintenance prednisone may be necessary for life.

Referred Pain

Glaucoma

Glaucoma often presents as a localized pain in the eye and forehead in middle-aged and elderly patients. In acute attacks it is associated with vomiting and visual impairment. The cornea may be cloudy with discoloration of the iris and a dilated pupil. An urgent referral to an ophthalmologist is required. Diagnosis is by tonometry and treatment is with miotics, topical beta blockers, acetazolamide, or iridectomy.

Paget Disease

Paget disease of the skull may present with diffuse headaches, somnolence, and deafness due to enlargement of the skull. Hydrocephalus may also occur with accompanying nausea and vomiting. Radiographs of the skull, long bones, and ribs show patchy sporadic thickening and irregular changes. The alkaline phosphatase level is raised. Treatment includes calcitonin or bisphosphonates.

Oral Disease

Tooth abscesses, dental decay, glossodynia, a cracked tooth, gingival disease, or inflammation of the jaw may all cause headaches. These must be carefully looked for and referred to a dentist if found.

Temporomandibular Joint Dysfunction

Pain from the temporomandibular joint (TMJ) can refer pain to the side of the face and to the temporal area and behind the eye, usually on the ipsilateral side. It is often worse on awakening. Asking the patient to open the mouth wide and palpating the TMJ usually identifies the problem. Restriction of jaw opening, with or without deviation of the jaw and tenderness over the masseter muscles, is found. Treatment often has to be multidisciplinary. Stretching of the masseters and increasing the jaw opening is encouraged by home exercises. A dental arthrosis for sleeping helps if bruxation (grinding one's teeth) is a problem or malalignment of the joint, usually after trauma to the jaw, has occurred. Many patients exhibit features of primary fibromyalgia and require antidepressants, relaxation, and coping skills. Most patients will continue to have symptoms indefinitely.

Chronic Sinus Disease

Sinusitis is not a cause of persistent facial headache pain. However, acute sinusitis, usually in the presence of coryza and purulent nasal discharge, can present as an acute dull aching or throbbing pain over the infected sinus. Tenderness is usually present on the upper molar and premolar teeth and over the cheek. The pain is postural, worse on bending, or with the head in certain positions. Sinus headaches seldom last for more than a week or two. They are treated by decongestants and antibiotics. If allergies are causing ethmoidal congestion, prophylaxis may include regular nasal chromoglycate.

Cluster Headaches (Migrainous Neuralgia, Horton Syndrome)

Cluster headaches occur predominantly in men (10:1) between the ages of 20 and 40. For a definitive diagnosis at least five attacks of pain fulfilling the following three criteria should have occurred.

1. The pain should be severe, unilateral, orbital, supraorbital, or temporal. It is often described as a knifelike or burning sensation in the eye. It should last 15 to 180 minutes if left untreated.
2. The ipsilateral headaches are associated with at least one of the following: conjunctival injection, lacrimation, nasal congestion, rhinorrhea, forehead or facial sweating, miosis, ptosis, eyelid edema. The pain is only on one side; however, the side may change even within a cluster period.
3. The frequency of attacks varies from every other day up to eight per day.

Cluster headaches usually occur at night within an hour or two after sleep. In contrast to migraines, most patients get out of bed and pace the floor, often crying and banging their heads due to the severe pain. Nausea and vomiting rarely occur during an attack. The acute episodic cluster attack lasts 1 to 4 months with a range of less than 1 week to 12 months. There is usually one cluster period per 6 to 18 months. Some patients will experience headaches with no periods of remission or with remission periods of less than 15 days. These types of clusters are usually refractory to conventional forms of prophylactic therapy. There is usually no family history. The patients tend to smoke and drink rather heavily. Sensitivity to alcohol occurs during the cluster period. There is a high incidence of peptic ulcers.

Specific Treatment of Cluster Headaches

Prevention. Ergotamine 1 to 2 mg by suppository or sublingually should be given 1 hour before the expected daytime attack. If night attacks occur, this dose should be taken before sleep. Ergotamine (a 5-hydroxytryptamine antagonist) is not well absorbed orally, often producing subtherapeutic levels. Suppositories (1–2 mg), inhalation (0.36 mg), or sublingual (1–2 mg) are the most effective forms of administration. Good control occurs in 75% of patients. The drug should be stopped each Sunday to see if the headache recurs. If this regimen is unsuccessful, before the onset of a headache, a trial of sumatriptan 6 mg subcutaneously or 25 to 50 mg orally, methylsergide 1 to 2 mg tid, or verapamil 40 to 80 mg tid should be given.

Treatment. The treatment of cluster headaches includes *oxygen*, 5 to 10 L/min for 10 minutes, at the onset of the headache. This is often effective. A *local anesthetic* sprayed to the rear of the nasopalatine fossa, or *viscous lidocaine* placed on a wick and inserted to the back of the nasopalatine fossa (both block the sphenopalatine ganglion), may abort an attack. *Sumatriptan* orally or by injection may also abort an attack. Surgery is rarely indicated, but *sphenopalatine ganglion ablation* and *trigeminal gasserian ablation* have been successful in some resistant cases.

Lithium carbonate has been used successfully in some chronic cluster headache patients. Serum lithium levels should be maintained between 0.7 and 1.2 mEq/L. Care must be taken in prescribing other medications that may interfere with lithium metabolism or excretion.

Capsaicin cream applied once a day to the ipsilateral nostril approximately 1.5 to 2 cm from the external orifice has been reported as breaking the cycle in over 50% of patients. The capsaicin causes burning and rhinorrhea initially. These effects diminish with the second and subsequent applications and usually disappear after 5 to 8 applications.

Calcium antagonists, verapamil and nifedipine, have also been used for chronic cluster headaches.

Chronic Headaches After Minor or No Trauma (Whiplash)

Headaches after a knock on the head are common and usually due to local bruising and abrasions. These headaches settle in 3 to 10 days, but recovery may be influenced by compensation and litigation issues. Most patients with severe head injury or after major craniotomies seldom have headaches lasting more than 7 days. However, patients with minor head injuries (<20 minutes loss of consciousness, Glasgow coma scale on admission >13/18, and a hospital stay of less than 48 hours) with no organic signs, often have minor cognitive deficits with a high incidence of headaches. These headaches seldom persist for more than 6 months. Head trauma may cause a temporary increase in preexisting migraine attacks.

Treatment is with reassurance soon after injury and encouragement to an early return to work. Anxieties, phobias, resentments, and depression are common and often require counseling. Analgesics are ineffective for these headaches and further investigations after the initial injury are usually unwarranted.

Neck Movement Limitation, Pain Reproduced on Mobilization ("Cervical" Headache)

Neck pain accompanied by headaches is common following a whiplash injury. Moving or mobilizing a damaged, or dysfunctional, zygapophyseal (Z) joint may reproduce the headache. The patient presents with neck stiffness and reduced range of movement, with pain anywhere from the occipital to the frontal and temporal areas. The pain is usually unilateral and may be felt behind the eyes. If the lower cervical Z joints are involved, pain is felt over one shoulder, between the shoulder blades, and occasionally down the arm in a nonradicular pattern. Neck stiffness with headache, not settling after 2 to 3 weeks of home exercises, should be referred to a physical therapist or chiropractor for specific Z-joint mobilizations. Occasionally, associated symptoms may include nausea, vomiting, photophobia (not marked), dizziness, and difficulties on swallowing.

TREATMENT A

Reassurance. Reassuring the patient that there does not appear to be any serious pathology such as a tumor or "brain infection" is important. A good history, physical examination, and logical treatment plan can do much to allay anxiety and help the patient's pain.

Specific physical therapy/chiropractics. Mobilizations of the cervical Z joints should gently stretch tight joint capsules and thus encourage a greater range of neck movement. Improvement should be seen within 3 weeks, or the therapy should be changed or stopped.

Relaxation. The ability to relax is important in preventing tightening of muscles around painful cervical joints. There are many self-help books or courses on the market from which the individual can learn effective relaxation techniques.

Home or work exercises. Specific exercises for the neck should include rotation of the head to both sides and side flexion to both sides. These four movements should be repeated with the head in extension, neutral, and flexion. The exercises should be performed 3 to 4 times a day.

Medication. Most medications are ineffective for these headaches and should be withdrawn. A careful history will reveal those patients who are taking frequent prescription or over-the-counter analgesics.

Home traction. Traction can be trialed for a week at home. If effective, it can be used 2 to 4 times a day initially and then on an as-needed basis.

Exaggerated Behavioral Responses to Headaches

The following questions may be helpful in the assessment of headache severity and the behavioral response.

What do you do when you get a headache?
Do you have to leave work?
Do you escape to a bedroom, or dark room, turn off the radio, instruct children to be quiet,
    and your spouse not to smoke?
Do you put a cold cloth over your eyes?
Can you eat with your headache?

A headache diary (see Fig. 15-1) continued for a week or two during two or three headache periods may give a clue to precipitating factors as well as behavioral responses.

TREATMENT B

Reassurance. The physician should be honest but reassuring when it is unknown why a symptom has developed or changed. He or she should see the patient repeatedly until the headache is controlled. Over 95% of patients who present with headaches have no structural lesions.

Coping skills. Symptoms and behaviors are strongly influenced by social environment, past experiences, and family problems. The individual's coping skills, use or abuse of medication, and anxieties should be addressed and appropriate treatment undertaken.

Analgesic withdrawal. Ergotamine should never be used on a daily basis. If it is used without at least 4 days between treatments, rebound headaches can occur. Caffeine-containing medications and drinks should also be limited along with any regular intake of over-the-counter analgesics. Drug-induced headaches are associated with sleep abnormalities. Regular use of analgesics may reduce the effect of prophylactic headache medication. When analgesics are withdrawn, for at least 5 to 7 days, the patient should be warned of the possibility of severe rebound headaches, nausea, cramps, diarrhea, sleeplessness, and emotional distress.

Antidepressants. The depressed patient with headaches often has many other physical complaints, severe insomnia, early awakening, appetite changes, and a decrease of sexual activity. The headache is usually biphasic, being worse in the morning and the evening, which may coincide with the periods of greatest family stress. Tricyclics with sedative effects such as amitriptyline, or nortriptyline in large night doses should be tried in those patients with sleep disorders.

Monoamine oxidase inhibitors such as phenelzine or isocarboxazid can be trialed in those refractory to conventional treatment. The patient must be warned to avoid tyramine-containing foods such as cheese, and to check before taking any new prescription or over-the-counter medication to avoid serious drug interactions. Referral to a psychiatrist or psychologist should be sought if improvement is not rapid.

FREQUENT HEADACHES

Tension Headaches

Tension headaches are the most common type of headache. They often have obvious precipitating events such as overwork, lack of sleep, or emotional crises. Chronic tension headaches occur at least 15 days a month. The headache may start in the forehead or neck and is usually, but not always, bilateral. It is often described as a heavy feeling, or tightness like a clamp or band around the head. It is usually a steady nonpulsatile ache fluctuating during the day. Another common description is a creeping sensation, or burning, felt under the scalp. Visual disturbances, photophobia, and vomiting are rare, and most people continue to work despite their headache.

Inquiry should be made into and reassurance given about fears of brain tumors, clots, or hypertension. If the headache is long-standing, there is unlikely to be a complete cure, and the patient should be informed of this. If possible, stressors should be identified and a plan to decrease them worked out. Stressors could include work, sleep disturbances, sexual problems, and psychological factors, such as anxiety, depression, hysteria, compulsivity, and family problems.

TREATMENT C

Treatment of tension headaches includes the following procedures.

Coping skills. Learning coping skills, referral for hypnosis, biofeedback, or relaxation training may be necessary.

Physical therapy. Physical therapy for home exercises and mobilization of the neck is often useful.

TENS. Transcutaneous electrical nerve stimulation (TENS) should be trialed with the electrodes over the nuchal muscle insertions and the trapezius.

Tricyclic antidepressants. TCAs, if effective, should be continued for a minimum of 6 months and then weaned slowly. Other antidepressants can be trialed if the TCAs are ineffective or cause intolerable side effects.

Medication optimization. Sumatriptan can be tried for severe headaches resistant to other treatment; however, it should not be given more than twice per week. Buspirone, a $5HT_1A$ serotonin receptor partial agonist with minimal sedation effects, can be trialed.

Prolonged use of buspirone does not cause habituation. Owing to the chronic nature of the headaches, habituating analgesics or sedatives (especially benzodiazepines) should be avoided. Detoxification from analgesics and anxiolytics is important to end the vicious cycle of dependence and withdrawal headaches.

Migraine

Classical migraine with aura occurs in less than 20% of migraine patients. The aura, which usually lasts 20 to 25 minutes is generally visual and includes flashing zigzag lines and lights starting at the peripheral of the eye, moving centrally. Paresthesias of the hand and mouth occur sometimes with dysphasia or aphasia. There may be a pain-free interval before the migraine commences, or the aura may overlap the pain. Occasionally the aura occurs without the headache or the headache occurs without the aura. The pain is typically unilateral but may be bilateral. It may alternate sides during and between attacks. An untreated migraine headache may last from 4 to 72 hours. The headache is usually throbbing, made worse by stooping or physical activity. Exacerbations often occur during times of emotional distress.

Common migraines (migraines without aura) present with similar paroxysmal attacks but without the aura. The headache is similar to a tension headache, and is usually described as throbbing, nonspecific, dull, and aching. Untreated it may last 1 to 2 days or longer. It is usually not associated with photophobia or nausea, but may awaken the patient from sleep. Both classical and common migraines occur at various times in the same patient. In 5% of patients, migraine may present with hemiplegia or ophthalmoplegia.

Migraine may coincide with estrogen withdrawal, which occurs after each menses or after delivery. The mechanism is probably mediated by neurotransmitter changes rather than direct effect of the estrogens.

TREATMENT D

Prophylaxis

If attacks occur more than twice a month, prophylaxis should be considered. This includes the following procedures.

Stress reduction. It is important to assess the patient's precipitating stresses. When possible, advise the patient to keep a diary. Stressors include fatigue, overwork, bright lights, discos, sleep excess or shortage, missing meals, occasionally a food sensitivity (usually chocolates, citrus fruits, or ripe cheese), alcohol or red wines, menstruation, exercise, nitrite or nitrate (found in most cured meats), monosodium glutamate, and cigarette smoke.

Analgesic withdrawal. Any analgesic taken daily should be withdrawn. Ergotamines in particular can cause withdrawal rebound headaches if they have been taken regularly. Ergotamines have no place in migraine prophylaxis. If the patient is on numerous medications, including opioids, hospitalization for short-term sedation may be required to ensure successful withdrawal.

Relaxation. Hypnosis, biofeedback, and/or relaxation training has been used successfully to decrease the incidence of headaches.

Medication. Amitriptyline or nortriptyline 75 to 150 mg q hs introduced gradually has been reported to be effective in up to 60% of patients. The beta blockers propranolol 120 mg per day, atenolol 50 mg per day, or metropolol 100 mg per day (atenolol and metropolol are more beta-1 selective with less effect on bronchi or diabetes) are often effective if the patient is very anxious, hypertensive, or has tachycardia associated with the headaches.

Cyproheptadine, 4 mg tid, is a calcium channel blocker and inhibits serotonin and histamine activity. Pizotifen 0.1 mg bid or 1.5 mg q hs is modestly effective and free from major side effects other than sedation and weight gain. Methylsergide, 1 to 2 mg, is often effective but should only be used under careful supervision and for periods not exceeding 3 to 4 months; pleural, pericardial, and retroperitoneal fibrosis are rare but serious side effects that curtail its prolonged use. Other calcium channel blockers, for example, flunarizine and verapamil, may also be used in prophylaxis.

Gynecologic techniques. Although there are general trends toward improving headache with increasing estrogen or absence of estrogen withdrawal, for example, pregnancy or menopause, the results of hysterectomy or oophorectomy have been disappointing. In some studies, headaches have worsened, and these operations are not recommended as a treatment.

Aborting an Attack

The following techniques can be used to abort a migraine attack.

Rest.   Rest in a dark, quiet room.

Analgesics.   Simple analgesics at the onset of the attack and 4 hours later, if necessary, should include acetaminophen 1 g, or aspirin 600 mg, or a nonsteroidal in the first instance. Their absorption is improved by giving metoclopromide 10 mg or dromperidone 10 to 20 mg concurrently. Caffeine and tranquilizers combined with an analgesic add to the expense but not the efficacy of the analgesic. If vomiting is severe, suppositories of dromperidone, prochlorperazine, or chlorpromazine should be used.

Ergotamines.   Ergotamines should be given by suppository (1–2 mg), sublingually (1–2 mg), or by inhalation (0.36 mg). No more than two doses should be given at intervals of 2 to 6 hours.

Sumatriptan.   Sumatriptan is a selective $5HT_1$ receptor agonist, causing vasoconstriction. It does not penetrate the blood-brain barrier and therefore has no CNS side effects. If 6 mg is given subcutaneously, approximately 77% of individuals with migraines will have relief within 60 minutes and 83% within 2 hours. For 70%, the oral preparation (25–50 mg) will provide relief in 2 hours. Headaches recur within 48 hours in more than 40% of patients and may require a further injection. Sumatriptan may precipitate angina in the patient with ischemic heart disease.

PAIN SPECIALIST

If the patient continues to suffer significant headaches that affect his or her quality of life, referral to a multidisciplinary pain center is appropriate. Here the following may be suggested.

1. Further investigations or specialist referrals based on an extensive history and physical examination.
2. Diagnostic greater or lesser occipital nerve or cervical zygapophyseal joint blocks to assess the "cervicogenic" component of the headache. If effective in reducing the headache more than 75%, more focused PT or chiropractics may be ordered. If PT/chiropractics is unsuccessful and a second Z-joint block with local anesthetic again removes the headache, radiofrequency ablation of the sensory branches to the Z joints may be recommended.
3. Diagnostic sphenopalatine ganglion blocks or trigeminal gasserian blocks for intractable cluster headaches. If successful, neurolysis may be recommended.

4. Diagnostic stellate ganglion block if the sympathetic nervous system is thought to be involved.

5. A multidisciplinary pain management program. A multidisciplinary team consisting of at least a psychologist or psychiatrist, physician, physical therapist, and occupational therapist approaches the various headache therapies as a team and integrates them for the individual. Thus, medication optimization, psychotherapy (individual, group, and family), biofeedback, relaxation and coping skills, focused physical therapy, and work station or work site analysis can all be done.

CASE STUDY

Mrs. Y is a 38-year-old, single mother with three children. She presents with a history of severe daily headaches from the age of 16. The headaches have become increasingly worse over the last month. She describes the headaches as occasionally unilateral but usually as a viselike band around her head. She states that she has mild photophobia and nausea, but she manages to eat and go to work despite the headaches because, economically, she "has to." She has neck stiffness associated with the headache. The neck stiffness has worsened since she had a whiplash injury when her stationary car was rear-ended 4 weeks ago. At that time she suffered no loss of consciousness or other injuries. She is seeking legal advice regarding this incident. She has noticed no precipitating factors that cause her headache. When she gets upset, she notices that the headache can become more severe. During the interview she breaks down in tears but denies suicidal ideation. She states her sleep is disturbed by anxiety with frequent early morning awakening.

She takes an acetaminophen plus codeine combination, approximately 10 tablets per day, and ergot medication, 2 to 4 tablets, approximately 3 times a week. She takes the ergot tablet for her "migraine" headaches, which she describes as a throbbing unilateral headache, different from the daily constant headache. Other medications include Valium 10 mg q hs and ibuprofen 200 mg, at least 6 per day if the headache is severe. She has previously tried numerous other over-the-counter medications and NSAIDs with minimum success. She states her Verbal Analogue Pain score (VAS) is at best 25/100, at worst 100/100, and on average 50 to 60/100. She has had no investigations for her headache or her neck pain.

She is a clerical worker who admits to severe financial difficulties partly due to nonpayment of maintenance by her husband for the upkeep of her three children. There is a strong family history of migraines. There is no other medical or family history of relevance.

The neurologic examination was normal, with normal power, sensation, and reflexes in the upper limbs. Fundoscopy was normal. She was able to open her mouth wide to reveal poor dental hygiene. There was no nasal discharge. Her neck rotation was limited to the right and left to 60 degrees due to pain. Her neck flexion was limited. Her chin reached three fingers from the chest. Neck extension was also markedly limited due to pain. Her neck was tender to palpation. Pressure on the upper cervical Z joints reproduced her headache. Pressure on the back of the head over the greater occipital nerve also produced pain traveling to the vertex. She had numerous tender and trigger points in the muscles of trapezius, neck, and sternocleidomastoid.

Impression

1. Chronic tension headache with probably some vascular component.
2. Possible analgesic abuse causing worsening of headaches.
3. Possible Z-joint strain following the whiplash causing the recent worsening of the headaches.
4. Poor coping skills to various stressors.

Plan

1. Reassure the patient that there is no evidence of brain tumor or cervical disc herniation evident.
2. Carefully explain to the patient various potential precipitating reasons for her headache. These include social and financial problems, analgesic abuse, neck stiffness possibly due to Z-joint dysfunction.
3. Be honest in stating that medications and medical treatments are unlikely to cure her headaches, but there are many nonpharmacologic ways of improving her ability to cope.
4. Address the social and economic problems with referral to the appropriate social worker.
5. Work out a tapering schedule for decreasing her analgesics, approximately 20–50% per day. All analgesics should be given on a round-the-clock basis. No analgesic should be given on a prn basis. Stop the ergotamine. Be available for reassurance to any frantic calls regarding initial exacerbation of headaches. Reassurance, and not extra analgesia, is needed. A beta blocker can be useful at this stage, both as prophylaxis and to decrease feelings of anxiety.

    The patient may have to have a short-term admission to a hospital for withdrawal of the analgesics, with short-term sedation if a taper at home does not succeed. Have the patient repeat the instructions to ensure she understands the therapy and the reasons for the withdrawal of the analgesics. She should be aware that her headaches may increase temporarily during the withdrawal phase, but it is very important that she come off these medications entirely.
6. Commence nortriptyline at night up to antidepressant dosage levels. The sedation effect should help normalize her sleep pattern, and the tricyclic should be useful for her headache pain.
7. Continue the benzodiazepine at the present time. This drug should later be withdrawn, but only after she has successfully been weaned off the other analgesics. Weaning from any benzodiazepine may be very protracted.
8. Order physical therapy, or chiropractics, consisting of neck mobilizations and a home neck exercise program.
9. See her again in 3 days.

The patient was seen in 3 days. She was in tears, stating that the taper had made her headache far worse. She was now taking acetaminophen/codeine combination, two tablets q 8 h. She was sleeping slightly better with the nortriptyline, 25 mg q hs. She was requesting something stronger for headaches to tide her over. She had heard that Stadol (buprenorphenol) was "good."

Plan Reexamine and reassure that no neurologic symptoms are developing. Increase her nortriptyline up to 100 mg q hs and up to antidepressant range (as assessed by blood levels) if side effects are tolerated. Avoid the use of any new opioids. Continue her analgesic withdrawal. Positive reinforcement of gains made and sticking to the taper are very important.

The patient should be seen frequently until the analgesics are weaned off and the headaches under better control. In this patient, a referral for some kind of relaxation therapy such as biofeedback would be useful. Referral to a psychiatrist for formal evaluation of her depression should be pursued if the patient is obviously not coping. If there is deterioration of psychosocial functioning, referral to a psychologist, preferably with training in the treatment of chronic pain, should be made.

Results Long-term, this patient did well on propranolol 120 mg/day, with nortriptyline 150 mg at night. She took the occasional (1–2 tablets per week) acetaminophen 500 mg for "severe" headaches. The Z-joint mobilizations by the physical therapist made her neck feel "looser" and markedly lessened her headaches. She was seen by a psychologist for biofeedback and coping skills training.

Referral to a multidisciplinary pain center would be indicated if the analgesic weaning was unsuccessful; adequate physical therapy with mobilization of her Z joints continued to reproduce her headaches without relieving them; she continued to cope poorly with her various stressors; her continued employment was in jeopardy; or her family dynamics were becoming dysfunctional despite appropriate primary treatment.

Physical interventions by the Pain Specialist may include cervical Z-joint blocks, which, if successful, may be followed by radiofrequency ablation of the sensory nerves to the joints. Occipital nerve blocks on occasion may be useful in aborting a prolonged severe headache.

SUGGESTED READINGS

Bogaards MC, ter Kuile MM: Treatment of recurrent tension headache: A meta-analytic review. Clin J Pain 10:174–190, 1994

Pearce JMS: The clinical management of headache. Pain Rev 1:89–101, 1994

Herpes Zoster and Postherpetic Neuralgia

Postherpetic neuralgia is a sequela of acute herpes zoster. Although acute herpes zoster is very painful, the normal course of the disease is resolution of both lesions and pain. However, some individuals will have pain that persists well beyond the acute herpes zoster phase. These patients suffer from a persistent and agonizing pain (postherpetic neuralgia).

Postherpetic neuralgia is defined as pain persisting more than 1 month. It is rare under the age of 40 and is common in the elderly (15–70%). Probably because of lowered immune responses in the elderly population, the resulting severe acute herpes zoster infections lead to more inflammation in the affected neural tissue, which in turn increases the likelihood of postherpetic neuralgia. This stresses the importance of early treatment of acute herpes zoster in the elderly.

The clinical manifestations of postherpetic neuralgia are typical of neuropathic pain. The patient often complains of allodynia, dysesthesia, hyperesthesia, and hyperpathia to the extent that it is difficult for the patient to wear clothing over the affected area. They also complain of intermittent shooting pain that may last from seconds to minutes. Depending on the severity of the initial zoster infection, some patients may have a loss of skin sensation in the affected areas. Systemic symptoms of acute herpes zoster include fever, nuchal rigidity, headache, nausea, and adenopathy. Sacral nerve involvement may cause urinary retention. Facial nerve motor deficits may occur.

There are many theories on the pathogenesis of postherpetic neuralgia. It is thought the pain arises from both peripheral and central (spinal cord) mechanisms. The gate control theory of pain (see Ch. 2 on anatomy) may explain some of the features of the pain of postherpetic neuralgia, as there is a loss of large myelinated fibers and a relative preservation of small unmyelinated fibers from the affected area. The large myelinated fibers are thought to inhibit the small unmyelinated pain fibers. Loss of these large fibers means a lack of inhibition to dampen the pain sensation. Direct damage by the virus to neurons in the dorsal horn may also lead to spontaneous activity, which is perceived as pain.

An algorithm for the treatment of postherpetic neuralgia is given in Figure 16-1.

TREATMENT PLANS

Acute Herpes Zoster

Pain, paresthesia, and dysesthesia in a dermatomal distribution usually precedes the vesicular eruption of herpes zoster (HZ) by a few days. The prodromal pain may be

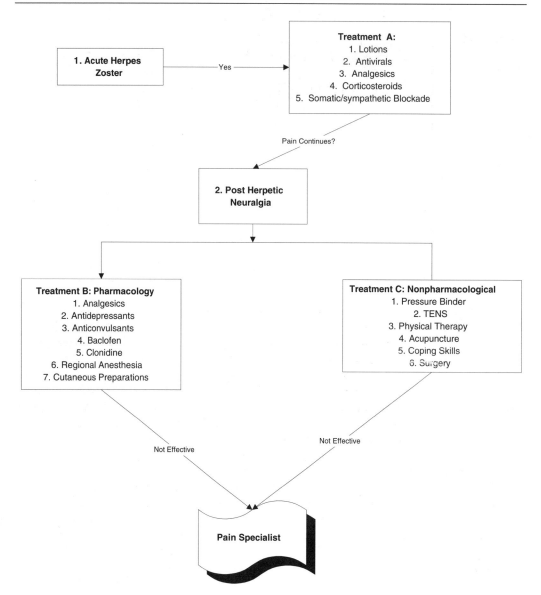

Fig. 16-1. Management of postherpetic neuralgia. TENS, transcutaneous electrical nerve stimulation.

severe and mimic other pathology. The vesicles usually crust within 1 week and heal within 1 month. Secondary infection of the vesicles may occur and needs to be treated. During the vesicular stage susceptible contacts may develop chickenpox if in contact with the exudate. Dermatomal pain without a rash has been described. Older patients are more likely to have severe pain than younger patients. Generalized zoster is seen almost exclusively in immunocompromised persons. The thoracic dermatomes are most commonly affected (more than 50% of patients). Extensive diagnostic evaluation for an occult malignancy is unwarranted in patients with segmental herpes. Recurrent attacks of herpes are uncommon (1–5%) and often indicate a malignancy or immunosuppressive disorder.

TREATMENT A

Lotions. Lotions, compresses of Burrow's solution, or calamine lotion decrease the intense itching discomfort.

Antiviral agents. Famcyclovir 500 mg tid for 7 days slightly decreases the duration of rash and intensity of pain. However, more importantly, it significantly decreases the incidence of postherpetic neuralgia. To be effective, Famcyclovir must be commenced within the first 72 hours of the vesicular eruption. Interferon may attenuate HZ in immunocompromised patients.

Analgesics. If acetaminophen or nonsteroidals are inadequate or are contraindicated, more potent analgesics, such as tramadol, acetaminophen/opioid combinations, or opioids, are indicated.

Steroids. Systemic steroids have some effect on pain and may decrease the incidence of postherpetic neuralgia. There is no evidence of increased risk of causing disseminated herpes zoster with their use. Intradermal steroid/local anesthetic injections into the rash have been used with uncontrolled studies reporting success.

Sympathetic or somatic blockade. Local, epidural, and sympathetic blocks, if administered within the first 2 weeks of the disease, have been reported to decrease pain and the incidence of postherpetic neuralgia. The blocks are repeated, often at daily intervals, for 5 to 7 days. Unfortunately, most studies have been uncontrolled. Stellate ganglion blocks are advocated for herpes zoster affecting the ophthalmic branch of the trigeminal nerve to decrease both the incidence of pain and corneal ulceration. Intrapleural injections of local anesthetic via an indwelling catheter can reduce both the severity and duration of pain of thoracic herpes zoster.

Postherpetic Neuralgia

Pain persisting 4 to 6 weeks after the vesicular eruption has healed is called postherpetic neuralgia (PHN). Although it usually remits spontaneously, some patients have pain for life. Risk factors for PHN include age, ophthalmic herpes, diabetes mellitus, cancer, severity of the acute herpes, and immunocompromise.

Pharmacologic Therapy

TREATMENT B

Antiviral agents have no role to play in PHN. They must be used in the first 72 hours of the acute lesion to have any effect. There is no clear evidence of benefit of corticosteroids in PHN given either systemically, intradermally, or into the epidural space.

Analgesics. Weak opioids, opioid/acetaminophen combinations, or tramadol trialed to maximum should be used. If the weak analgesic is ineffective or has excessive side effects, strong opioids should be trialed. Unfortunately, even opioids are often ineffective, and it should be made clear to the patient that these are given on a trial basis only. When trialing opioids, set goals must be agreed upon to include function as well as decreased pain. The patient should be aware that the opioids will be discontinued if they are ineffective, that is, if the goals are not reached, or if there are excessive side effects.

Antidepressants. Tricyclic antidepressants are the first-line choice, either amitriptyline or nortriptyline, usually at a dose of 75 mg q hs. Desipramine, 25 mg increasing to a maximum of 200 mg in the morning, has also been successfully used. Fluphenazine, up to 8 mg per day in divided doses q 6 h, has been reported to be successful in some patients when combined with a tricyclic antidepressant.

Anticonvulsants. Although commonly used, there are no controlled studies showing their efficacy. Carbamazepine and diphenylhydantoin are the most frequently used. Gabapentin may be the more logical first choice because of its low side effect profile.

Baclofen. Baclofen has been reported to help some patients.

Clonidine patches. Clonidine patches have been reported to help some patients. The patch is placed over the most allodynic area. With renewal of the patch (weekly) a new site is chosen; there should be a marked reduction in allodynia over the previous site of application. If, after 3 to 4 weeks of treatment, there is no improvement, or there are side effects, usually hypotension, this therapy should be stopped.

Regional anesthesia. Although pain may be temporarily decreased, there is little evidence of long-term improvements in PHN following peripheral nerve blocks. The persistent dull ache felt with some of the scars produced by the herpes eruption may occasionally be relieved by infiltration of the scar with local anesthetic and steroids. Sympathetic blocks and epidural steroids are less and less effective as the duration of PHN increases. The best results are produced when the pain is less than 2 to 3 months old.

Cutaneous preparations. Capsaicin 0.075% cream rubbed on the area qid may help. If burning on application is excessive, the lower dose of 0.025% capsaicin cream should be used. It is thought to work by enhancing the release of substance P from type C fibers and preventing its reaccumulation. It may also have a weak neurolytic effect. This causes a total decrease in substance P both peripherally and centrally, thus affecting peripheral and central mediated pain mechanisms. As significant depletion takes 3 to 6 weeks, treatment must be continued for this minimum period of time before efficacy can be gauged.

A salve can be made by making a paste of soluble aspirin (3 or 4 of the 650-mg tablets) in a small amount of water and adding it to 5 to 10 ml of alcohol (or ether). After dabbing this paste on the affected area, it is allowed to dry. Pain relief should occur within 20 to 30 minutes. Lack of relief indicates other treatments should be used. If pain relief occurs, the salve should be dabbed on three times a day. Nonsteroidal creams have also been used to good effect in some patients. Local anesthetic creams, such as 5% lidocaine-prilocaine cream (EMLA) and 5% or 10% of lidocaine gels, have been used effectively in short trials. They are well tolerated and appear to be effective in selected individuals.

Nonpharmacologic Therapy

TREATMENT C

Pressure binder. If the patient states that firm pressure (not light touch) over the affected area decreases the pain and the affected area is accessible to having a binder placed on it (mid- or lower thoracic area), a neoprene-type binder can give significant pain relief. The action may be stimulating the low threshold A beta receptors to "close the gate."

TENS. There is no way of anticipating which patients may benefit from transcutaneous electrical nerve stimulation (TENS). As it is relatively inexpensive and free from side effects, apart from local skin irritation, it is worth a week's trial. The TENS electrodes must not be placed on the touch-sensitive (allodynic) area or the patient's pain may be worsened. If no benefit is seen after a week of using different frequencies, it is doubtful if it will be of long-term help (see Fig. 33-1).

Physical therapy. The pain of acute herpes followed by PHN often causes myofascial pain with subsequent restriction of joint movements. Both the myofascial restriction and joint dysfunction add to the pain of PHN and may become a major cause of it. Physical therapy, concentrating on mobilization of the affected joints and treatment of myofascial pain, should be ordered and a home exercise program given (see Ch. 18 on myofascial pain).

Acupuncture. Acupuncture, by central neuromodulation and decreasing local muscle spasm, may help in PHN. Unfortunately, there are no controlled studies showing it to be effective.

Coping skills. Inquiry should be made into mood and suicidal ideation. Patients with overt depression or active suicidal thoughts should be referred to a psychiatrist for therapy. This is supplemental to other therapies. Simple coping skills should be taught and family support encouraged in all instances.

Surgery. There is no proven consistent surgical cure for PHN despite many different neurosurgical approaches, including cordotomy, rhizotomy, sympathectomies, gasserian ganglion ablation, stereotactic thalamotomy or mesencephalotomy, resection or undermining of the skin of the involved area, or cryotherapy. Dorsal root entry zone (DREZ) lesioning may help some patients in the short term, but long-term results are not promising, and there is at least a 10% risk of neurologic complication. Deep brain (thalamic) stimulation also appears helpful in a small series of patients, but it has about a 15% complication rate.

Long-Term Medications

If treatment is successful, tapering and possible cessation of medications should be tried after a further month of effective pain relief. PHN has a natural tendency to remit spontaneously in most cases. In a small proportion of resistant cases, long-term continuation of medication is necessary.

PAIN SPECIALIST

If pain persists despite the above regimens, a referral to a pain specialist is indicated. A pain specialist may try the following treatments:

1. Review previous treatments and trial possible modifications.
2. Administer phentolamine or lidocaine infusions to establish whether the pain is sympathetic-mediated or lidocaine-sensitive neuropathic pain. Appropriate oral medications could then be trialed.
3. Intercostal nerve or paravertebral root block will block the pain if peripheral mechanisms are causing the patient's pain. Unfortunately, the pain of PHN is often centralized. This means the central neurons are excited and triggering pain impulses to the brain. These neurons lie within the spinal cord. This "centralization" of pain means neurolytic procedures on peripheral nerves are rarely indicated and even less frequently successful.
4. If none of the above therapies is successful, numerous more invasive methods have been tried, unfortunately with poor long-term results, for example, epidural steroids, spinal cord stimulators, indwelling intrathecal morphine or intrathecal/epidural morphine/bupivacaine catheters and pumps, dorsal root entry zone (DREZ) neurosurgical lesioning, and intrathecal neurolysis.

Despite all therapies, there remains 5% to 10% of patients in whom no therapy is effective. These patients require additional psychological support and coping mechanisms to help them deal with their intractable pain. Pain due to PHN remains a leading cause of suicide in the elderly.

CASE STUDY

Mrs. X, a 70-year-old woman with postherpetic neuralgia of the 8th and 9th right thoracic dermatomes, presents with intractable pain. She had had acute herpes in that area 6 months previously. Medications for the pain included an opioid/acetaminophen 4 per day, amitriptyline 25 mg at night, and ibuprofen 400 mg q 6 h. She stated the pain was burning, constant, and her Verbal Analog Score (VAS) was 80/100 on average. The VAS was from 0 (no pain) to 100 (worst pain imaginable). The pain interfered greatly with her sleep. On further questioning, she stated that coughing, twisting, and deep breathing made the pain worse. She received some comfort by holding her side. She did not appear to be depressed and denied any suicidal ideation. Examination showed a mentally alert, obviously distressed lady with scars of old herpetic lesions over the 8th and 9th ribs on the right. Touching the skin lightly caused pain, but holding a hand firmly on the area was perceived as comfortable. Thoracic rotations (sitting with arms folded while the examiner rotated the upper chest) was limited by pain. The thoracic spine was tender over T8–T9.

Impression Postherpetic neuralgia with a secondary musculoskeletal (myofascial) component.

Plan

1. Stop the anti-inflammatory drugs (ibuprofen) as these have little efficacy.
2. Use the fact that pressure over the area decreased her pain by suggesting she wear a neoprene-type binder most of the time.
3. Increase the amitriptyline by 25 mg every three nights until a satisfactory sleep pattern is achieved, intolerable side effects occur, or 100 mg is reached. If, after 3 weeks at 100 mg, there is still no sleep improvement, the blood level should be checked. If the blood level is below therapeutic antidepressant range, the amitriptyline should be increased to antidepressant levels for a further 3 to 4 weeks. After this period, if there is no improvement in mood, function, or sleep, it should be discontinued.
4. A salve made with aspirin (3 to 4 soluble tablets) in alcohol was dabbed onto the painful area. After 20 to 30 minutes she stated her skin felt less sensitive. The salve was given to her with instructions to apply it three times a day.
5. If the aspirin salve did not work, capsaicin cream 0.025% rubbed on the area qid for 3 to 6 weeks may decrease the pain by depleting substance P. If this is successful, continue the cream for a further 2 to 3 months. Tell the patient to avoid rubbing her eyes after application because of the intense eye irritation capsaicin causes.
6. See the patient in 1 week.

The patient returned stating she was sleeping well on 50 mg amitriptyline, but was constipated, felt very tired during the day, and had a very dry mouth, which she found uncomfortable. Her pain was generally improved at rest to 40–50/100 but still increased when she was active.

Plan

1. Change the amitriptyline to nortriptyline 25 mg at night. This has less anticholinergic and sedating effects. The dose is reduced initially to see if the pain relief was related to wearing the neoprene binder.
2. Give a laxative and instruction on increasing fluid and roughage intake.
3. Physical therapy to relieve the muscle spasm by mobilizing the spine can decrease the pain dramatically. Dry needling or trigger point injections may also be of value. Effects should be apparent within 3 weeks if physical therapy is going to work. If no improvement is seen after 3 weeks, stop the physical therapy.

If the above measures failed to work, stronger analgesics, starting with round-the-clock tramadol or opioid/acetaminophen combinations, and going on to oral or transdermal (skin patch) opioids, should be trialed. The patient must be made aware that these are being trialed only (see Fig. 6-3). If no improvement in pain or function is seen or side effects occur, the medications should be tapered and stopped. A prescription for laxatives should always be given concurrently and constipation should be inquired about at each follow-up.

If the pain was lancinating in nature, a trial of different anticonvulsants can be used. Gabapentin 100 mg tid, increasing gradually to a maximum of 600 mg tid, may be the logical first choice because of its low side effect profile. Carbamazepine (Tegretol), phenytoin (Dilantin), and clonazepam (Klonopin) can be trialed, starting at low doses, and increased every 3 to 5 days until efficacy or side effects occur. If one anticonvulsant does not work, another may prove to be effective. Unfortunately, they are often ineffective and poorly tolerated in PHN.

The above measures should be instituted at a primary physician level. If they fail to produce relief, a consultation with a pain specialist should be asked for. As a general rule, results of therapy are much poorer for any chronic pain condition, including PHN, which lasts longer than 6 months before adequate therapy is instituted. Early referral is therefore recommended when the usual treatment modalities as outlined above are proving inadequate.

SUGGESTED READING

Loeser JD: Postherpetic neuralgia. pp. 257–263. In Bonica JJ (ed): The Management of Pain. Lea & Febiger, Philadelphia, 1990

Low
Back Pain

Back pain is the second most common reason for physician visits in the United States. "Medical back problems" and "back and neck procedures age under 70" are the third and thirtieth most common reasons, respectively, for U.S. hospital admissions. The annual incidence of low back pain (LBP) is estimated to be 5% of the adult population, with a lifetime incidence or risk of 60% to 85%.

Most back pain problems are nonspecific, self-limited, and resolve in a few weeks. Significant LBP lasting longer than 7 to 12 weeks needs to be evaluated carefully from both physical and psychological aspects. The disability from back pain is often unrelated to the medical explanation. It is the individual as a whole who needs to be treated and, except for the very small percentage with definable pathology, such as a herniated disc causing neurologic sequelae, surgery is rarely indicated. The individual needs to be actively encouraged to return to a functional role in society. If he or she expresses an intense dislike of his job, that person is more likely to spend a longer period off work than the individual who enjoys his employment. Worry about what might happen to their LBP symptoms were work to be resumed also influences return to work often more than symptom presence or severity.

Thus, the patient with LBP who continues to be disabled with his or her pain needs to be evaluated in the knowledge of the individual's environment and work. An active approach with minimal medication and with responsibility placed on the patient to function despite discomfort has been shown to be much more effective than a more passive bed rest and medication as requested approach.

A treatment algorithm for low back pain is given in Figure 17-1.

PRINCIPLES OF EVALUATION OF
LOW BACK PAIN

Continuous Low Back Pain Unrelieved by Position

Continuous low back pain may indicate a herniated disc. The herniated nucleus pulposus causes a foreign protein reaction due to phospholipase A_2 activation. The resultant inflammation around the nerve root, in the epidural space, or even within the disc, creates the continuous pain felt by the individual.

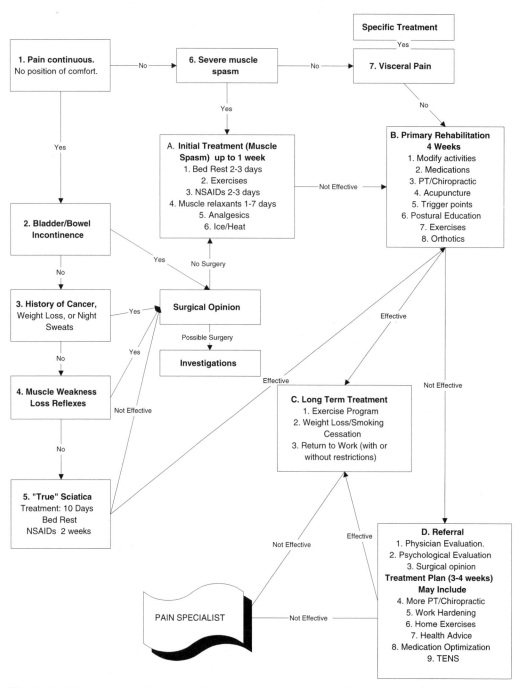

Fig. 17-1. Management of back pain. NSAIDs, non steroidal anti-inflammatory drugs; PT, physical therapy; TENS, transcutaneous electrical nerve stimulation.

Bladder or Bowel Incontinence

Onset of these symptoms must be treated as an emergency with early investigations and surgical opinion. Delayed treatment of a space-occupying lesion, such as a large herniated disk, causing these symptoms may render the individual permanently incontinent.

Previous History of Cancer, Unexplained Weight Loss, or Night Sweats

The possibility of a bone tumor or infection is suspected when a patient presents with a previous history of cancer, unexplained weight loss, or night sweats in association with continuous pain. Relevant investigations (e.g., complete blood count, blood markers for malignancy, radiographs, possible bone scan) should be ordered and the appropriate referral made.

Muscle Weakness or Absent Reflexes

Muscle weakness or absent reflexes should occur in the appropriate nerve supply for the affected nerve root. If the whole of the leg is stated to be weak and no localized muscle weakness is found, this may be a nonanatomic presentation (Waddell's nonorganic sign).

"True" Sciatica

Radicular pain down the sciatic nerve distribution (back of thigh, lateral side of leg and foot) exacerbated by straight leg raising (both sitting and standing), with more leg pain than back pain, may indicate a disk herniation at the L5-S1 or L4-L5 level. Examination of the patient for an L5-S1 or L4-L5 herniated disk should reveal severe back and leg pain at less than 45 degrees straight leg raise (positive Lasègue sign). Pain may be referred down the affected side with straight leg raise of the nonpainful leg (crossover Lasègue sign). Referred pain on pressure over the popliteal fossa with the knee bent at 90 degrees indicates an irritated sciatic nerve at the root level (positive bowstring sign). Complete rest in bed for 10 days is indicated to allow the disk to stabilize and "seal off" from the nerve root by collagen deposition. Severe radicular pain continuing after this period of bed rest and anti-inflammatory drugs indicates the need for investigation and possible surgical opinion.

Severe Muscle Spasm

Careful palpation of the paravertebral muscles of the lower back allows the area of greatest pain to be identified. Together with the history, palpation may differentiate between a soft tissue or a zygapophyseal (facet) joint strain where muscle tenderness is the main presentation and a disk herniation with neurologic signs and symptoms.

Visceral Causes of Low Back Pain

A careful history should be taken and examination made to rule out visceral causes of low back pain. These include urinary tract infection, pelvic inflammatory disease, dysmenorrhea, or a leaking abdominal aneurysm. Specific treatment should be undertaken if these pathologies are found.

TREATMENT PLANS

Initial Treatment [One Week or Less]

TREATMENT A

Muscle spasm is the principal symptom.

Bed rest. The initial bed rest should be as total as possible to allow any inflammation to subside without further exacerbation. There is no evidence that rest more than 72 hours is effective. Longer periods of rest cause muscle weakness and may encourage a sick role. It is important to encourage early mobilization of the individual despite his or her discomfort.

Exercise. Gentle flexion repetitions (knees to chest), or extension exercises (lying prone, doing modified push-ups), should be undertaken after the initial bed rest. As well as possibly preventing the rapid deconditioning that occurs with bed rest, exercises can encourage the patient to play a positive role in the self-management of pain. Exercises should be gentle and should not increase the pain for more than 10 to 15 minutes after completion. They should be done at regular intervals, ideally 4 to 5 times per day.

Nonsteroidal anti-inflammatory drugs. NSAIDs can be used for the initial 2 to 3 days to cover the acute inflammatory stage. Thereafter, long-term use should be avoided because of fostering the concept of reliance on medication as well as potential side effects. There is no evidence that any one nonsteroidal drug is more effective than another.

Muscle relaxants. In severe muscle spasm a trial of muscle relaxants, limited to a maximum of 7 days, can be prescribed. There is little evidence of their long-term effectiveness, and because of their misuse and addiction potential, longer periods should be avoided. Their sedative side effects may be an advantage in the initial few days when rest is encouraged.

Analgesics. As with other medications, analgesics such as the opioid/acetaminophen combinations simply provide a respite from suffering while healing is progressing. The patient should understand that these medications do not cure their back pain as an antibiotic might cure an infection. A date for their termination should be discussed with the patient and given with the initial prescription.

Ice/heat. Ice in a plastic bag, with cream rubbed on the skin to prevent ice burn, can be very effective in decreasing the initial muscle spasm and lessening pain. After about 20 minutes ice loses its efficiency. The treatment can be repeated, on an as-needed basis, hourly or 2-hourly.

Heat should also be applied only to skin that has had cream rubbed on it to prevent skin damage. The heat should not be more than can be tolerated by placing it next to a sensitive skin area such as the face.

There is no objective way of knowing whether ice or heat will be more effective after the initial 48 hours when ice only is recommended. Both ice and heat should be trialed over the first week.

Primary Rehabilitation [Four Weeks]

Modify activities. Early return to work, with some restrictions, where heavy manual labor is involved, should be encouraged. Objects should be lifted close to the body with twisting, bending, and reaching minimized. Frequent changes in posture, from sitting to standing, should be emphasized, as these mobilize tight muscle and joints. The ability to take rest periods or working a shorter hour week should be investigated. A work site evaluation by an occupational therapist can be extremely valuable, especially if recurrent back injuries are occurring. Guidelines for sitting and unassisted lifting for people with LBP have been suggested. (AHCPR, Dec 1994.)

SYMPTOMS	SEVERE	MODERATE	MILD	NONE
Sitting time	20 min	20 min	20 min	50 min
Unassisted lifting				
Man	20 lb	20 lb	60 lb	80 lb
Woman	20 lb	20 lb	35 lb	40 lb

Medications. If medications such as NSAIDs or analgesics such as the opioid/acetaminophen combinations are prescribed, they should be on a fixed time, round-the-clock basis, with a limit on the number and duration of therapy.

Physical therapy/chiropractics. Mobilization of the joints and myofascial treatments should be combined with home exercise programs to encourage strength and flexibility of the affected part. After the initial 48 to 72 hours of back pain, when muscle spasm is intense, passive treatments such as ultrasound, or interferential, must be supplemented or replaced with more physical joint and soft tissue mobilizations and stretching. Improvement should be rapid. If no improvement is apparent after 3 weeks, the type of therapy should be reviewed and either changed or stopped.

Acupuncture. The use of acupuncture needles, either at classical acupuncture meridian points or in myofascial tender and trigger points, has a large and often enthusiastic following. Any method of decreasing muscle spasm should be supplemented with a home exercise program of stretching and range of movement exercises. Within four sessions approximately 50% of those who will benefit will have done so. Within six treatment sessions 90% will probably have responded, if the pain is susceptible to acupuncture. Treatments are usually done twice a week for 2 weeks and weekly thereafter.

Trigger point injections. Trigger point injections may be effective if localized pressure over the tender point reproduces the patient's pain (a trigger point). Stretches and range of movement exercises must be given after successful deactivation of any trigger point. The patient should be taught ischemic compression and cold methods of deactivating trigger points, together with specific stretches. Ideally, these should be taught by the therapist who treats the trigger points.

Postural education. Continued poor postural habits while sitting may be a factor in the onset and continuation of low back pain. A soft support placed on the chair to support the small of the back can help. Chairs should allow the individual to get up to the work surface without leaning forward. Working surface heights should be corrected for the individual by either lowering the chair or raising the work surface. The latter can be achieved inexpensively by using wooden blocks. Special kneeling or "posture" chairs, which encourage maintenance of a normal lumbar lordosis may be effective in diminishing postural discomfort. A brief ergonomic review of the work or home environment with specific emphasis on correct sitting with regular intervals of standing and mobility exercise should be undertaken. It would be appropriate to refer to an occupational therapist for more specific advice. The physical therapist should include general postural advice as part of their therapy.

Exercises. Exercise should include general conditioning aerobic exercise such as walking, cycling, or swimming. This can be done at home or at a commercial gym and does not need trained therapists to supervise. The duration of exercise should be increased with time until the patient is doing 20 minutes 3 to 4 times a week. The 20 minutes daily can be completed in two sessions, that is, 10 minutes in the morning, 10 minutes in the evening. Following simple advice such as using the stairs or walking around the block when arriving at work, at lunch time, and in the evening will probably give an adequate workout if followed conscientiously. Physical therapists and chiropractors should give the patient a home program as part of their treatment plan. Specific exercises for the back often include back extension exercises performed lying prone, 3 to 4 times a day, progressing to back extensions standing. There is no evidence to suggest that back-specific exercise machines are any more effective than ordinary exercises.

Orthotics. A leg length discrepancy or significant biomechanical imbalances (pronation or supination) may require orthotics to improve gait and weightbearing. A temporary corrective heel raise (up to 1 cm) can be easily made out of newspaper and placed in the shoe of the patient's short limb. If patients place one in every shoe they wear, back pain should improve within a few days, if unequal leg lengths are affecting the LBP.

Long-Term Treatment

TREATMENT C

Long-term exercise program. Ideally, a regular lower back stretching program should be done one to two times per day. This should last no more than 5 minutes in most instances or patient compliance will be poor. Abdominal and back-strengthening exercises should be done three times per week. Aerobic exercise for a minimum of 3 to 4 times a week, 15 to 20 minutes, should be encouraged. Although walk and jog programs may give more strength to the back, swimming is often the most comfortable because of the buoyancy support of the water. Walking up and down stairs and not using elevators should be encouraged. Whatever exercise program is undertaken, it should be seen as fun. Other general health benefits, as well as those for the low back, should be emphasized to the patient. Joining a regular exercise group is one way to maintain interest, but self-motivation is still a crucial factor.

Weight loss/smoking cessation. A formal weight loss program together with regular exercise should be undertaken for any overweight individual with low back pain. Weighing the patient at each visit and positive acknowledgment of any weight loss should be an important motivation for the patient. An initial low-calorie diet followed by a calorie-restricted regular eating plan may help the patient lose the weight quickly initially and then maintain it. A dietary referral or recommendation for a weight loss program should be considered.

Smoking cessation is very important. Smokers have a higher incidence of LBP; stopping smoking may improve oxygenation to the tissues or reduce coughing. The weight gain that is often associated with stopping smoking should be carefully monitored. A formal exercise program often assists smoking cessation by replacing an unhealthy habit with a healthy one.

Return to work. The more a practitioner knows of the type of job the patient does, the more specific the advice can be regarding job modification. Dislike of one's job has been found to be a major predictor of low back pain. This emphasizes the close link between the environment and chronic pain perpetuation. Reported claims for low back pain among those who lift heavy objects are more prevalent when the objects are held away from the body while lifting and when associated with bending and twisting. Office workers whose jobs rarely involve lifting heavy loads have been reported as having a higher incidence of sciatic pain if they work in a bent or twisted posture. Vibration, particularly from motor vehicle driving, is associated with a high incidence of back pain. Encouragement of a review of job positions and a positive mental outlook are important for successful long-term reintegration of the individual with chronic back pain into the workforce. Where the employer takes pro-active measures in preventing and treating LBP and institutes transitional work programs to get the worker back to full-time employment, days lost due to injury are dramatically reduced.

Referral [Three to Four Weeks]

TREATMENT D

If the primary treatments have not effectively returned the individual to work by 6 weeks, and it is unlikely he will be back at work within the next 2 weeks, a referral to a multidisciplinary for reevaluation for a specific diagnosis should be considered. This reevaluation should provide a logical rationale for further focused treatment.

Physician evaluation. The full history and physical examination should include the following:

1. Special reference to environmental factors, nature of injury, and psychosocial stressors.
2. Examination should include Waddell's nonorganic signs, pain behavior mannerisms, and other signs of an exaggerated response to injury.
3. A review of all investigations performed. Substandard or equivocal investigations should be repeated where clinically relevant.
4. A review of the previous treatments tried and investigations done should indicate their effectiveness.

Psychological evaluation. Psychological evaluation should include standardized acceptable psychomimetric testing and an individual interview. As well as depressive symptoms and overt psychopathology, specific environmental and psychosocial stressors, which may be hindering a return to work, should be evaluated. A history of previous employment and educational levels attained should be obtained. The patient's medication intake should be enquired about. This should be compared to the medication intake history as obtained by the physician.

Surgical opinion. The surgeon's opinion should be given only after he or she has done the following:

1. Reviewed the history, physical examination, and the investigations.
2. Examined the patient.
3. Ideally reviewed the evaluation of a psychologist.
4. Is satisfied the relevant investigations are of adequate standard, if surgery is contemplated.

If surgery is not performed, any treatments undertaken in this phase should last 3 to 4 weeks or less before being reviewed. These therapies should be stopped or modified if significant functional improvement is not shown, or if a return to work is not imminent within the next 3 to 4 weeks. These therapies may include, but are not limited to, the following:

More physical therapy/chiropractics. Based on a focused physical examination and possibly other investigations, a tentative diagnosis can be made. This may allow specific physical therapy or chiropractics to be prescribed. This treatment should emphasize manual mobilization of joints, which have become tight due to disuse, as well as an individualized home exercise program. If significant improvements do not occur within 3 to 4 weeks, therapy should be stopped.

Work hardening. A work hardening program should concentrate on the skills, strengths, and abilities the patient requires for his or her specific job. Specific restrictions are usually given before the return to work. How diligently restrictions are followed and how meaningful they are has yet to be fully evaluated. This is partly due to the wide range of occupations and varying job requirements that are available.

Home exercises. Specific injury rehabilitation stretching and strengthening exercises, which should have already been taught, should be continued on a daily basis. If the individual is returning to the workforce at this stage, the type and the time that is spent stretching should be modified to fit in with the individual's schedule. Simple aerobic conditioning, such as walking the stairs instead of using the elevator and walking more at lunch time or before and after work, must be encouraged. Unlike other treatments, it should be emphasized that home exercises should become part of a lifelong program.

Health advice. If the individual is greatly overweight, or if he or she smokes, both of which increase the likelihood of back pain, he or she must be encouraged to take appropriate steps to diet and stop smoking. These steps may include joining smoking cessation or weight reduction classes. Taking responsibility for one's general health can have a major effect on the individual's disability.

Medication optimization. At this stage in the individual's rehabilitation, all medications being used for back pain should be carefully reviewed. This includes both prescription and over-the-counter medications. There is little use for the muscle relaxants and benzodiazepines and they should be withdrawn if possible. The need for opioids and NSAIDs on a regular basis should be assessed individually. The risk:benefit ratio of any medication should be reviewed periodically. Other medications specific for certain chronic pain syndromes such as sympathetic maintained pain or neuropathic pain may be trialed at this stage. Any trials of new medication should be time-contingent and allow the effective dose to be reached, or the lack of effect or significant side effects to be evident within 3 to 4 weeks.

TENS. Modern transcutaneous electrical nerve stimulation (TENS) units are small portable devices powered by a 9-volt battery. Most units have two channels, each controlling a pair of electrodes placed on the painful body area. The output frequency pulse width and intensity can be varied. Other features may include automatic modulation and burst modes. TENS is thought to work by neuromodulation at the spinal cord level. The stimulated release of substances such as endorphins produce analgesia.

TENS is safe and nonaddictive. The immediate effectiveness of TENS in pain control is reported to be 60% to 80%.

Unfortunately, its efficacy decreases with time to 25% to 30%.

PAIN SPECIALIST

The pain specialist or team should review the history, and the degree of deactivation and psychosocial distress. After careful examination, treatment plans may include the following procedures.

Medication optimization or withdrawal.

Lumbar epidural steroids. Lumbar epidural steroids can be used for radicular pain referral in an attempt to settle down any ongoing inflammation presumably caused by a herniated nucleus pulposus.

Lumbar zygapophyseal (facet) joint injections. Lumbar zygapophyseal joint injections will estimate the significance of the Z joint in the pain process. If pain is significantly relieved by two local anesthetic injections given at different times, and if specific physical therapy to mobilize the joint does not help, radiofrequency ablation of the sensory nerves to the Z joint may help the individual considerably. Anecdotally, steroid injections into the facet joints occasionally have been found to help. However, in controlled studies no difference has been shown between the effect of local anesthetic plus steroids and local anesthetics alone. There is little evidence of the therapeutic effect of repeated zygapophyseal joint injections.

Sacroiliac joint injection. Unilateral low back pain, worse on sitting, with decreased sacroiliac (SI) joint mobility and pain on SI joint provocation maneuvers, may indicate an SI joint irritation. A painful SI joint is often associated with piriformis and lumbar paravertebral muscle spasms on the painful side. Confirmation by a significant decrease in pain with a fluoroscopically guided SI joint injection, and possibly piriformis injection or dry needling, will enable a treatment plan to be devised. Treatment should consist of physical therapy mobilizations of the SI joint, lumbar Z (zygapophyseal) joints, and piriformis stretching. A home exercise program should also be given.

Diagnostic nerve root blocks. A small amount of local anesthetic, placed accurately onto the nerve root under fluoroscopy, which removes the individual's pain, indicates that the pain source may be the nerve root. Further views of the exit foramina of the root for surgically amenable obstruction may be indicated.

A multidisciplinary approach. A multidisciplinary assessment by a pain-trained psychologist or psychiatrist and physician, with or without a physical therapist, will facilitate an individual treatment plan that emphasizes education, coping skills, and specific exercises, plus vocational guidance. Coping skills may be enhanced by biofeedback and hypnosis. The objective is to give the individual control over his or her pain and not have the pain control the individual.

CASE STUDY

Mr. A., a 37-year-old, obese, semiskilled laborer, slipped on some oil at work and landed on his back. He was able to get up and go to the rest room to clean the oil off his trousers, but shortly thereafter complained of increasing pain with radiation down the back of his right leg as far as his knee. He left work early and that evening was unable to sleep because of muscle spasm. This was despite taking several acetaminophen tablets. The next day he did not go to work because of the pain and again had a somewhat disturbed, but slightly easier, night. He presented the next day with the following history and examination. He stated that the principal area of pain was in his right lower back. On a verbal analog score (VAS) he counted it as 90/100, which would decrease to 70/100 with acetaminophen. He stated that the pain was helped by heat (a hot bath) and complete rest, which would decrease the pain to 20/100. He denied any incontinence or leg weakness. There was no previous history of note except for a possible history of gastric ulcer related to excessive alcohol intake. He was a smoker (20 to 40 cigarettes a day) on antihypertensive medication.

On examination all back movements standing were painful with some possible bruising and spasm over his right lower back. His sitting straight leg raise on the right was 70 degrees, and his lying straight leg raise was 60 degrees with pain referred to the low back. He had normal power, sensation, and reflexes in both limbs. Palpation of his abdomen revealed no masses. Palpation of the back revealed a very tender area over the right lower back and the L4-L5-S1 area.

Impression Probable soft tissue injury, possible zygapophyseal (facet) joint strain.

Plan

1. Complete bed rest 24 hours.
2. Nonsteroidal drugs for 48 hours (no longer because of history of ulcer).
3. Muscle relaxant for 2 days.
4. Analgesic for 5 days.
5. See patient again in 3 days.

Patient returned and appeared to be much improved but still stated that the pain was as severe as before. He stated that he was unable to work and requested more pain tablets. Straight leg raise sitting on the right was again 70 degrees, but lying was reduced to 30 degrees with pain in his low back. There were no other new findings.

Plan

1. Encourage movement around the home and start light home exercises, including back flexions and extensions.
2. Tramadol 50 mg every 6 hours was prescribed.

3. No further muscle relaxants or NSAIDs were prescribed.
4. To see him again in 3 days.

The patient returned still complaining of pain. He stated that he had minimal pain on lying down but severe pain on walking or exercising. He could sit and watch TV relatively comfortably on a recliner. The examination showed, as previously, no neurologic abnormalities but tenderness over the paravertebral area on the right.

Plan

1. Obtain a radiograph to exclude transverse process fracture (this was done and the result was negative). Physical therapy was prescribed.
2. Possible trigger point injection.
3. Encourage exercises.
4. Discuss with him a weight loss and smoking cessation program.
5. No more medications given at this stage.
6. To see patient again in 1 week.

The patient returned still complaining bitterly of pain. The physical therapist stated that she was unable to treat him with mobilizations because of patient resistance. The patient was discussing litigation against his company. Further questioning revealed that the patient disliked his work, describing it as mundane and boring.

The above patient, while initially having a significant soft tissue injury with bruising and spasm, was beginning to exhibit pain behavior. Objective evidence of a significant disc herniation was lacking in that there was no neurologic fallout; on sitting, the straight leg was 70 degrees, but on lying the patient stated there was pain at 30 degrees (Waddell's nonorganic sign). Pain was minimal on reclining but extremely high on movement. There was little objective muscle spasm to feel. The relative lack of muscle spasm was confirmed by the physical therapist. The patient himself was requesting stronger medication and more time off work.

Plan The patient needs to be firmly informed that further investigations, MRI/CT, are unnecessary. He should be informed that a return to work is his best option. A discussion of the patient's job prospects, if possible with a job supervisor, may reveal potential work change.

If the patient continues to insist on incapacitation due to his back pain, referral for a multidisciplinary evaluation would be appropriate.

If the patient accepts a return-to-work mandate, a further period of modified activities plus physical therapy and home exercise program should be prescribed. A weight loss and smoking cessation program should also be strongly encouraged.

SUGGESTED READINGS

Fordyce WE: Back Pain in the Workplace. International Association for the Study of Pain (IASP) Press, Seattle, 1995

McKenzie RA: The Lumbar Spine: Mechanical Diagnosis and Therapy. Spinal Publication, New Zealand, 1981

US Department of Health and Human Services, Agency for Health Care Policy and Research (AHCPR), Executive Office Center, Rockville, Maryland, December 1994

18 | Myofascial Pain

Pain in muscles is extremely common. The Nuprin Pain Report of 1985 reported that 53% of respondents experienced muscle pain. Localized areas or bands of muscle tenderness, termed *trigger points*, may be "active," meaning pressure on them refers pain, or "latent," indicating that, although tender, no referral of pain is felt.

The most common cause of myofascial pain is acute muscle overload. The overload may be due to physical exertion, trauma, cold, emotional "stress," or repetitive movements, such as typing. Poor posture and prolonged immobility, as well as nutritional, metabolic, and endocrine factors may play a role.

An important feature of trigger points is that stimulating them with a needle, injecting a local anesthetic into them, or spraying coolant vapor over them can deactivate them, often for a significant period of time.

It is important to examine for trigger points (TPs) and to treat them in all chronic pain syndromes. The TPs may not be the primary cause of the patient's pain, but they can perpetuate it. Medications are usually ineffective in treating TPs.

The treatment algorithm of myofascial pain is presented in Figure 18-1.

PRESSURE REPRODUCES PAIN

The muscle should be positioned so it is slightly on stretch while the examiner uses the finger pads to palpate. A trigger or tender point is felt as a tender, taut band in the muscle. Pressure applied to a trigger point gives pain locally and distally. Pressure should not be too strong (approximately 4 kg of pressure), or held for more than 5–10 seconds or it may confuse the patient's perception of pain. Common trigger point referral zones can be found in the textbooks.

Trigger Points

TREATMENT A

The basic treatment of trigger points and muscle tightness is divided into three distinct parts, all of which have to be followed to achieve good results.

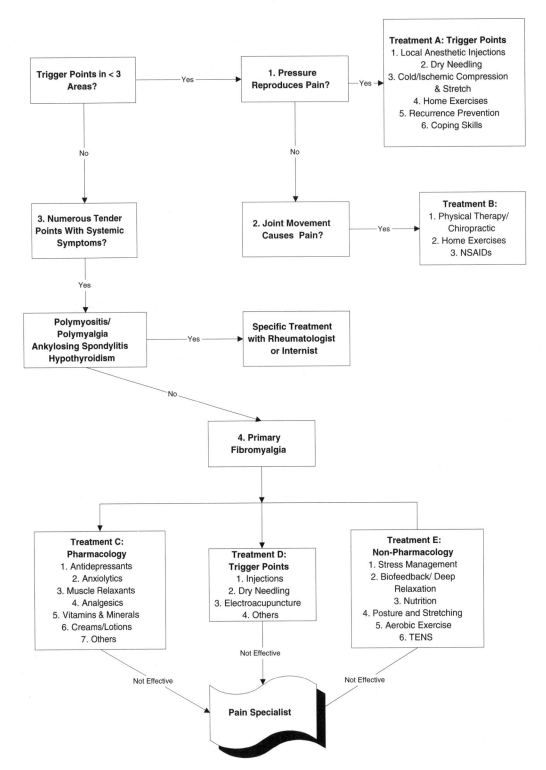

Fig. 18-1. Management of myofascial pain. NSAIDS, nonsteroidal anti-inflammatory drugs; TENS, transcutaneous electrical nerve stimulation.

1. Deactivation of trigger points by local anesthetic injection, dry needling, cold or ischemic compression.
2. Maintenance of the trigger point deactivation by frequent stretching of the muscle and range of movement exercises of the affected joint. After the pain and range of muscle movement has improved, a long-term maintenance exercise program should be prescribed.
3. Prevention of recurrence, if possible, by analyzing the events that triggered and maintained the problem, and giving advice on avoidance.

Local anesthetic injection (bupivacaine 2–3 ml). As the theory of local anesthetic injections into a trigger point is both to stabilize the muscle membrane and to physically damage the muscle fibers in spasm, bupivacaine is a good choice. Bupivacaine is longer acting than lidocaine, and is mildly myotoxic. The injection technique is to hold the trigger point firmly between two fingers of one hand and to introduce a 22- or 25-gauge needle, with the local anesthetic syringe attached, into the muscle band. Reproduction of referred pain should be sought before injection. A muscle twitch is often seen with the correct needle location. There is no evidence that the injection of more than 2–3 ml is any more effective than a larger volume, and it probably causes more pain due to tissue damage and distention when the local anesthetic wears off. Epinephrine should not be added to the injectate. During the injection the patient's pain is often reproduced, but immediately after the injection pain relief should be evident, with an increased range of movement of the joint. The patient should be warned that once the local anesthetic wears off, pain is often increased for 2–3 hours. After this period, pain again decreases. Stretching and range of movement exercises of the joint must be given to the patient to continue at home. These exercises should be frequent while the local anesthetic is still working. Injections should not be repeated more frequently than every 5 to 7 days. In some chronic myofascial states, occasional trigger point injections may have to be done periodically for life.

Dry needling. The insertion of a needle into a trigger or tender point can be as effective as a local anesthetic injection. I use different depths of insertion, depending on the clinical impression with palpation. For tender points (no pain referral on pressure), a shallow insertion of 2–3 mm is used. For trigger points (pain referred to a distal site), insertion of the needle into the trigger point is attempted. Clamping of the muscle around the needle is common and, with agitation of the needle, will relax in seconds. Duration of insertion varies from 30 seconds with shallow insertions, to 5 to 15 minutes for the deeper trigger point insertions. Disposable, sterile, size 32-gauge acupuncture needles are as effective and far less painful than hollow, cutting edge, injection needles. The acupuncture needles are round-bodied and cause only small microhematomas in the muscle, so that the post-muscle soreness is minimal. Significant relief of pain with dry needling should be apparent after the first treatment session. Muscle stretching and joint range of movement exercises must be given immediately after the treatment and continued frequently for a few hours.

Cold, ischemic compression and stretch. Superficially cooling the skin over the affected muscle appears to temporarily decrease muscle spasm. Putting pressure on the tender or trigger point firmly for 2 to 3 minutes also decreases muscle spasm. Cooling can be done by using a fluromethane spray, or rubbing ice over the affected muscle for 2 to 3 minutes. This can be done simply by placing a polystyrene foam cup or "Dixie cup" filled with water into the freezer. When frozen, removal of 1 cm of the cup's rim will make ice available which can be held relatively comfortably because of the container surrounding it. Ischemic compression can be done for 2 to 3 minutes with a finger, lying on a ball, or by using a walking-stick handle. After temporary deactivation by one of these means, stretching and range of movement exercises must be carried out.

Home exercises. Successful deactivation of the trigger point will often be temporary if stretching and joint range of movement exercises are not followed regularly by the patient. Knowledge of the insertion and origin of the affected muscle allows a passive stretch of that muscle to be devised. Stretches should be held to a slow count of 30. The patient should breathe in and out deeply while holding the stretch and at each exhalation should relax and allow the muscle to stretch further. Concentration on breathing slowly also focuses the patient on general relaxation. Stretching should be done as frequently as possible (4 to 5 times a day) during the first 2 weeks of treatment. This allows lengthening of the muscle fibers to occur and gives an active self-help dimension to the individual's therapy. If successful, this gives the patient an exercise program to follow when, as often happens, the muscle spasm recurs. After the initial 2 weeks, a maintenance stretching program of once or twice a day can be instituted. Ideally, frequent stretching should be encouraged 4 or 5 times a day for 3 to 4 weeks to achieve maximum muscle and joint flexibility. However, in clinical practice, 1 to 2 weeks is the longest most patients will perform exercises consistently with any frequency. Any home stretching exercise program should probably not last more than 2 to 3 minutes each time or boredom, lack of time, and patient noncompliance will occur.

Recurrence prevention. Identification of postural problems, work site evaluation—if the problem occurred at work—and general observation of the patient may enable suggestions to be made regarding posture modifications. An occupational therapist may be an appropriate referral at this point.

Coping skills. Emotional stress causes muscles to tighten and may activate trigger points. Learning to deal effectively with stressors is important in preventing recurrence of myofascial pains. Electromyographic (EMG) biofeedback can be very effective in training the individual to appreciate and control the sensation of muscle relaxation. Constant reassurance that the patient's pain is (1) not "all in the head" and (2) not indicating a cancer, or other life-threatening disease, is important.

JOINT MOVEMENT CAUSES PAIN

Mobilization of the joint and gentle repeated movements recreate the patient's pain (concordant pain).

TREATMENT B

Physical therapy/chiropractic. Physical therapy or chiropractics should involve mobilization of the affected joint. These mobilizations should be increased in a graded fashion and, in some areas, such as the thoracic spine, should include manipulation. This, together with a well-controlled home exercise program, can do much to improve the patient's pain and joint movement. Range of movement exercises should be frequent, initially several times a day for 1 to 2 weeks, to encourage maximum rapid improvement. If the patient has had no clinical improvement with physical therapy in 3 weeks, the treatment should be reviewed. If good mobilization and a home exercise program has been carried out diligently, but with no improvement, it is unlikely that further therapy will have benefit, and it can be stopped.

Home exercises. Regular home exercises for stretching and joint range of movement is important.

Nonsteroidal anti-inflammatory drugs. A short course of anti-inflammatories is often necessary during the first week of a physical therapy/chiropractic and home exercise program when tight connective tissue is being stretched and mobilized.

NUMEROUS TENDER POINTS WITH SYSTEMIC SYMPTOMS

The occurrence of numerous trigger points with systemic symptoms is common in patients presenting to outpatient rheumatology clinics.

Polymyositis and Dermatomyositis

Polymyositis and dermatomyositis are inflammatory diseases of skeletal muscles with lymphocytic infiltration causing muscle damage. Dermatomyositis is where the polymyositis affects the skin, giving a characteristic rash of the face, chest, elbows, or knees. The cause is unknown but is thought to be either viral or autoimmune. The disease has an insidious onset and is progressive over the years. It usually starts with weakness rather than pain in the proximal limb muscles, especially the hips, thighs, and shoulder girdles. A deep aching pain in the calves and buttocks can occur in up to 50% of patients, with tenderness on palpation of the thigh muscles. Muscle enzyme creatine phosphokinase levels are raised, and biopsy of the muscles shows infiltrates, inflammatory cells, and widespread destruction of muscle fibers. Referral to a rheumatologist is important. Treatment is with high-dose steroids.

Polymyalgia Rheumatica

Polymyalgia rheumatica usually presents as a diffuse aching pain and stiffness in the neck, hip, and shoulder girdle in a patient over the age of 55. Mastication may cause intermittent claudication, which interferes with chewing in the late phase of meals. The pain is worse with movement, and the patient usually has a markedly raised ESR and chronic anemia. The cause is unknown. Referral to a rheumatologist is important. Concomitant headaches with temporal artery bulging, irregularity, tenderness or decrease in pulsation, with or without a fading of visual acuity, should be treated as an emergency. These symptoms may indicate temporal arteritis, which, if untreated, may result in blindness or a stroke. Treatment is with high-dose corticosteroids and immunosuppressive therapy, for example, azathioprine, which may have to be continued indefinitely.

Ankylosing Spondylitis

Early ankylosing spondylitis may mimic polymyalgia but usually occurs in young males. Chest expansion, when measured from deep inspiration to expiration, is less than 1 inch. Blood tests show the characteristic HLA-B27 subtype.

Hypothyroidism

All patients with generalized muscle pains should have thyroid function tests to exclude thyroid disease.

PRIMARY FIBROMYALGIA

The term primary fibromyalgia and *chronic fatigue syndrome* have been used interchangeably and may be part of a continuum of the same disease. Clinically, fibromyalgia appears to be a musculoskeletal system response to stress. The relationship to viral symptoms and prodroma are not well understood. Generalized body aches and pain should be present on digital palpation in at least 11 of 18 tender point sites (see Table 18-1). This is not related to trauma. Passive movement of the muscles increases the pain. The pain should have been present for 3 or more months. The pain and tenderness are usually at sites of tendon insertion. The symptoms tend to get worse with vigorous physical activity, although morning stiffness may be improved with light exercise. Often the patient is most symptomatic when

Table 18-1. Criteria for Fibromyalgia

Pain, in 11 of 18 tender point sites on digital palpation. Pain, on digital palpation, must be present in at least 11 of the following tender point sites.[a]

Occiput: bilateral, at the suboccipital muscle insertions.

Low cervical: bilateral, at the anterior aspects of the intertransverse spaces at C5–C7.

Trapezius: bilateral, at the midpoint of the upper border.

Supraspinatus: bilateral, at origins above the scapular spine near the medial border.

Second rib: bilateral, at the second costochondral junctions, just lateral to the junctions on upper surfaces.

Lateral epicondyle: bilateral, 2 cm distal to the epicondyles.

Gluteal: bilateral, in upper outer quadrants of buttocks in anterior fold of muscle.

Greater trochanter: bilateral, posterior to the trochanteric prominence.

Knee: bilateral, at the medial fat pad proximal to the joint line.

[a]Digital palpation should be performed with an approximate force of 4 kg. For a tender point to be considered "positive" the subject must state that the palpation was painful. "Tender" is not to be considered "painful." (From the American College of Rheumatology: Criteria for Fibromyalgia. Arthritis Rheum. 33:160–172, 1990)

standing, sitting, or lying still. Warm weather and hot baths tend to improve the pain and cold makes the pain worse. The subject often complains of swelling of the hands and feet with exercise. Females often complain that rings on their fingers become tight. Almost invariably the patients complain of poor sleep. Stage IV sleep is usually most affected. The patient may go to sleep easily but awakens early feeling exhausted. The patients often complain of anxiety attacks and chronic headaches (50%). Symptoms of irritable bowel syndrome are common (30%). Patients also complain of nonradicular and nondermatomal numbness, most often affecting the upper extremities (60%). Rolling of the skin and subcutaneous tissues of the upper scapula area between the examiner's thumb and forefinger elicits tenderness in 60%. After palpation of tender points over the shoulders and neck, reactive hyperemia is seen in over 50% of patients.

An association with previous major depression in patients and families suggests genetic factors may play a role.

A careful examination for other musculoskeletal problems, such as rotator cuff injury, sacroiliac joint, or lumbar facet joint dysfunction should be carried out. Treatment of these separate problems with physical therapy and exercises is important, in conjunction with the treatment of primary fibromyalgia.

Pharmacologic Therapy

TREATMENT C

Antidepressants. Tricyclic antidepressants initially given at night may, by increasing serotonin levels, decrease alpha wave intrusion patterns, and improve the REM (rapid eye movement) and restorative sleep patterns. The tricyclics may need to be trialed up to therapeutic antidepressant dose levels. Improvement in sleep should be seen within 2 weeks of treatment. If no improvement is apparent within 4 to 6 weeks, or side effects are significant, treatment should be stopped. Doxepin hydrochloride often produces a more subjective improvement in sleep.

If excessive drowsiness prevents increasing the doxepin or other tricyclics to antidepressant levels in a clinically depressed patient, continuing the doxepin at 10–25 mg at night and adding Prozac (fluoxetine) 20 mg or paxil 20 mg in the morning can be used. Trazadone 50–100 mg at night has also been reported to improve sleep and decrease tender points.

Anxiolytics. Some patients on antidepressants become extremely agitated with jittery feelings or "restless legs" interfering with their sleep. Alprazolam 0.5–1 mg or perphenazine (2–4 mg) taken in the evening can abolish these effects and improve sleep.

Muscle relaxants. Cyclobenzaprine in small doses of 10–40 mg per day has been reported to be useful. Carisoprodol 350 mg at night can improve sleep and may decrease tender points.

Analgesics. With its central mechanism of action, acetaminophen up to 4 g per day is worth trialing if pain continues to be a significant feature. Nonsteroidal drugs given on an intermittent basis may be useful if there are "flare-ups" associated with exercise. These "flare-ups" are often associated with joint irritation such as lumbar facet or sacroiliac joint strain.

Vitamins and minerals. Vitamin B in large doses and the antioxidants, vitamin E and calciferol, have been claimed to improve muscle pain. Calcium and magnesium tablets, 400–600 mg, taken 45 minutes before sleep, appears to improve the sleep pattern in some patients by decreasing muscle aching.

Creams/lotions. Many creams containing various active substances have been tried. Their moderate success may be partly due to the patient actively rubbing the painful areas and "desensitizing them."

Other agents. Opioids usually are not effective and addiction may become a problem.

Trigger Points

TREATMENT D

Injections. A double-blinded study of trigger point treatment reported that dry needling, saline, or procaine injections were equally effective. Unfortunately, the effects of the injection were usually short-lived.

Dry needling. Placing acupuncture needles into the tender contracted muscle, usually at muscle motor points or musculotendinous junctions, often elicits a cramplike feeling. The muscle often contracts and grasps the fine acupuncture needle. Gradually the muscle contraction relaxes. This can be facilitated by agitation of the needle. Several sites in the same muscle may need to be treated before the whole muscle relaxes. Many of these trigger points correspond to acupuncture points and referral to an acupuncturist may produce benefits.

Electroacupuncture. In one study electroacupuncture was shown to be of some benefit.

Other techniques. Low-intensity laser and auriculotherapy have not been shown to be of use.

Nonpharmacologic Therapy

TREATMENT E

Stress management. Strategies for managing stress should be developed for the patient. Many patients have difficulties verbalizing their deeper emotional conflicts and focus on the obvious ones of family and financial difficulties. Life stressors should be addressed and coping skills discussed. The patient must be reassured that the illness will not render him or her a cripple and treatment can help, but perhaps not cure. Referral to a psychologist, for exploration of and help to resolve deep emotional conflicts, is important in therapy. Hypnotherapy has been used with some success in fibromyalgia. Cognitive and behavioral approaches are used to address the sensory, affective, cognitive, and behavioral aspects of fibromyalgia.

Biofeedback/deep relaxation. The techniques of biofeedback and deep relaxation include focusing on individual muscle groups, tensing each group, and then relaxing. These techniques should be practiced before sleep. A meditation tape with guided imagery can improve relaxation and sleep. EMG biofeedback has also been shown to help train the individual in relaxation techniques.

Nutrition. A high-energy "healthy diet,"—low in fats and processed foods, and high in complex carbohydrates—should be encouraged. Acidic foods such as citrus and tomatoes should be avoided in the late evening as they may disrupt sleep. Alcohol in the evening may induce sleep but can cause awakening in the middle of the night and so should be avoided. Caffeine and nicotine should be avoided after 3 p.m. due to their stimulatory effects. Caffeine is found in chocolate and many soda drinks, as well as coffee and tea. A high fiber, low fat diet with avoidance of dairy products and spicy foods is important if irritable bowel syndrome is present.

Posture and stretching. Correct posture at all times allows efficient muscle functioning and decreases fatigue and strain. Slow stretching exercises after local heat or a hot shower improves muscle flexibility and decreases muscle tension.

Aerobic exercise. A moderate aerobic exercise program is important. Walking, swimming, exercise bike, or gentle aerobics should be done for at least 15 minutes daily. This can decrease anxiety, assist relaxation, and improve sleep. Other benefits of such an exercise program include improved self-esteem and increased energy with a decrease in depression.

TENS. The results of using transcutaneous electrical nerve stimulation (TENS) in primary fibromyalgia is often disappointing. However, localized areas of tenderness can respond favorably to TENS, and with its low side effect profile, it should be trialed. The electrodes can be placed over the major trigger points.

PAIN SPECIALIST

The pain specialist or team should review all therapy and eliminate, as far as practical, primary causes for the myofascial pain, for example, disc pathology, or systemic illness. Withdrawal of most medications, especially opioids, often has a beneficial effect on the individual's motivation and "energy" level. The psychological distress caused by these syndromes should be evaluated and an individualized pain management program devised.

Specific diagnostic or therapeutic local anesthetic nerve or joint injections are usually not indicated in these syndromes. Sympathetic blockade, for example, stellate ganglion blocks, may have a beneficial effect, but it tends to be short-lived.

A multidisciplinary program of education, exercise with coping and relaxation training is recognized as the most effective form of treatment of "resistant" fibromyalgia.

CASE STUDY

Ms. Y., a 35-year-old female, postal delivery worker, with no other significant history, complained of pain in the left shoulder and weakness of her left hand. The problem had arisen following a rear-end collision in a van some 2 years previously. Rest and warmth on the shoulder blade area made the pain easier. She had not tried ice. Carrying her postal bag over her left shoulder, emotional stress and carrying bundles of letters in her left hand all made the pain worse. Her sleep pattern was good and she would awaken refreshed. Her bowels were regular and she did not complain of excessive fatigue. She rated her pain as 50/100 at the worst, 10/100 at the best. She was on regular anti-inflammatory drugs and muscle relaxants on a prn basis. She averaged 2 to 4 muscle relaxant tablets per day.

On examination she had full, pain-free range of movement of her left upper extremity. She had normal power and sensation. It was difficult to confirm her subjective feeling of weakness in her left hand grasp. Her neck movement and thoracic rotation were full and pain-free. She had a marked trigger point of the infraspinatus on the left which referred pain down her left arm to her hand. She stated this was similar to her usual pain. A second trigger point in the left rhomboids at T7–T8 area also triggered a familiar pain into her left arm.

Impression Myofascial trigger points.

Plan

1. Dry needling of the trigger point area.
2. Instruction of frequent stretching of the infraspinatus and rhomboid muscles.
3. To try ice before the stretching.
4. To stop the nonsteroidals and the muscle relaxants.
5. Reassure that there is nothing malignant and nothing sinister. There was also no reason for further investigations, including blood tests, due to lack of systemic symptoms.
6. See her in 1 week.

In 1 week the patient returned. The pain had been easier for 2 to 3 hours following the dry needling but had returned to the previous level. Ice had helped but only while it was on. She was stretching once or twice a day. She had stopped the medications and had noticed little change in her pain.

Plan

1. Repeat the dry needling 2 times per week for 2 weeks.
2. Teach ischemic compression techniques.
3. Encourage the stretching to be done more frequently.

After two dry needling sessions, it was apparent that any improvement was still short-lived (3–4 hours). Local anesthetic (bupivacaine 0.25%, 2–3 ml) was injected into each trigger point. The correct position of the needle in the trigger point was identified by a twitch when the needle touched the muscle and the patient stating that the pain was being reproduced. The trigger points were injected twice more.

TENS, with the electrodes over the rhomboids and infraspinatus, was trialed for 1 week with a moderate, but worthwhile improvement.

After 2 weeks of dry needling and injections, the patient returned stating there had been no further improvement in the pain after the local anesthetic had worn off. This indicated that neither dry needling nor local anesthetic was effective in this particular patient. However, because the patient was functioning well on no medications and was now able to control her pain with ischemic compression, no further treatment was decided upon.

Plan

1. Discharge, to see again if flare-ups occur.
2. Repeated reassurance that there was nothing sinister and there was no sign of arthritis. She had volunteered that she was worried that if it was arthritis, her job might be in jeopardy.

The failure of local therapy of the muscle was possibly due to a central wind-up phenomenon in the spinal cord. The patient, however, was satisfied and was coping well with her pain syndrome. Deep relaxation, biofeedback, and coping skills were considered but were not offered to her because of her minimal disability. If her problem worsened in the future, these would be offered.

SUGGESTED READING

Travell JG, Simons DG: Myofascial pain and dysfunction. The Trigger Point Manual, Vols I and II. Williams & Wilkins, Baltimore, 1992

Neck Pain

Neck pain is an extremely common complaint with or without associated arm and shoulder pain. Plain x-rays are often of little help, except in cases of neck trauma or if a bone lesion is suspected. Severe spondylolysis can be associated with no pain, while a normal cervical radiograph may be associated with severe pain.

Neck pain due to whiplash following a motor vehicle accident (MVA) is estimated to occur in approximately 20% of individuals. Most patients will recover from a whiplash injury in 2 to 3 months.

A careful examination of the neck and neurologic examination should reveal symptoms, if any, which requires further investigation. Most neck pain, however, refers pain in a non-nerve root pattern, and it is the underlying soft tissue cause that needs to be treated. Muscle relaxation techniques and coping skills are important adjuncts in therapy to break the continual pain–tension–pain cycle.

The treatment algorithm for neck pain is presented in Figure 19-1.

NO DIRECT TRAUMA

Whiplash

Rapid deceleration of the head and neck, as often occurs in motor vehicle accidents, can cause damage to the joints and soft tissue of the neck. Sometimes a severe whiplash injury may disrupt a cervical disc. All the above structures have nociceptors and can cause headaches, neck stiffness, and pain referred into the shoulder and down the arm.

Severe Limitation of Neck Movements With Neurologic Involvement

Neck stiffness may be unrelated to significant cervical damage. However, myelopathy indicates the involvement of the cord (increased reflexes, positive Babinski, weakness in the arms or legs) and needs urgent referral to a neurosurgeon. Motor weakness with sensory deficits are usually signs of nerve root impingement and also require a surgical opinion.

Radiculopathy With No Neurologic Deficit

Pain down an arm in a nerve root distribution, with no weakness or objective sensory loss, can be caused by soft tissue damage alone. Initially, conservative therapy should be tried. Referral for a surgical opinion and investigations should be reserved for those failing to improve over the period of primary rehabilitation or if a neurologic deficit occurs.

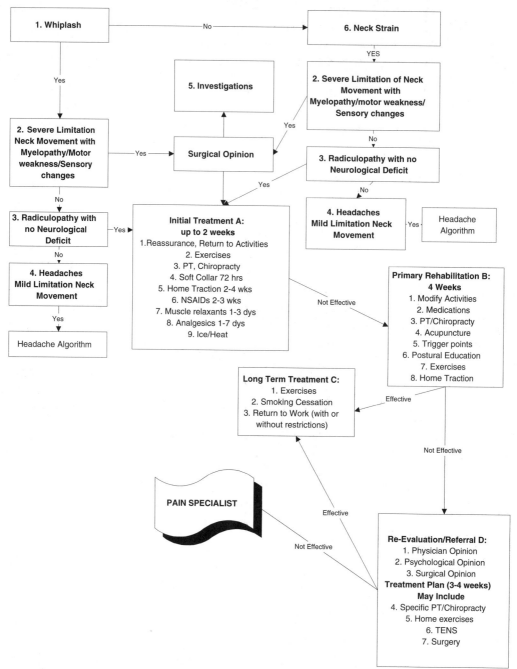

Fig. 19-1. Treatment algorithm for neck pain. PT, physical therapy; NSAIDs, nonsteroidal anti-inflammatory drugs; TENS, transcutaneous electrical nerve stimulation.

Headaches With Mild Limitation of Neck Movement

If the neck movement is full or almost full with no radicular pain down the arm and no neurologic deficit, it is unlikely there is significant pathology in the neck. The zygapophyseal (facet) joints of the neck, however, may be stiff and require mobilization by a physical therapist. A home exercise program is also important (see Fig. 15-2). In neck problems, exercises are usually more beneficial than medication, which tends to be ineffective after a short period of time.

Neck Strain

Certain work positions or previous neck problems (spondylosis, zygapophyseal (Z) joint arthrosis) may predispose the worker to neck pain. Ideally, the worker's head should be in a neutral position while working. At intervals during the work day a full range of active neck movements should be encouraged.

TREATMENT PLANS

INITIAL TREATMENT (TWO WEEKS)

Reassurance and return to activities. Early return to the patient's usual activities should be vigorously encouraged. With mild symptoms no restrictions need be given. With more severe whiplash injuries some work restrictions may be necessary. Restrictions should be reviewed within 3 weeks. The patient should be reassured that the vast majority of these injuries are self-limited.

Exercises. The severe flexion and extension movement of the neck during a whiplash accident causes severe bruising of the muscles and connective tissue. If the neck stiffness due to this bruising is not addressed in the first few days, the zygapophyseal joints can become irritated. This joint pain adds to the patient's overall distress and difficulty of moving the neck.

Physical therapy/chiropractic. An early referral to an experienced physical therapist (PT) or chiropractor for mobilization (not manipulation) of the joints and connective tissue should be made to "free up" stiffened joints and break the "arthrokinetic reflex" which keeps the neck stiff. A single visit can often return a full range of movement (still with some neck discomfort). Regular full range of neck movements every 30 to 60 minutes for the next 3 to 4 days allows the joints to remain mobile and the connective tissue to heal without restriction. Further PT may be required after this stage, but if the patient has been conscientious regarding his or her exercises, recovery is often rapid. The inability of a PT or chiropractor to return full range of movement at the first visit may indicate Z joint or other damage. Multiple, repeated manipulations, without a multidisciplinary evaluation, are not justified.

Soft collar. A soft collar, or Philadelphia, brace may relieve the initial pain of injury. Its use, however, is debatable, and many authorities recommend against it. If used, it should be in conjunction with a full range of neck movement exercises every hour. The use of any neck brace for more than 72 hours may begin to foster a "sickness role" and prolong the disability.

Home traction (2 to 4 weeks). Home traction is effective in unloading the joints and opening the intervertebral foramina. It is especially effective where the patient has radicular pain due to an "inflamed" nerve root. Stretching the mechanoreceptors may also decrease the pain and hasten recovery. Where used, home traction can be done four times a day.

Although traction is useful for possible future flare-ups of neck pain, generally its use should be limited to no more than 4 weeks after the initial injury.

Nonsteroidal anti-inflammatory drugs (2 to 3 weeks). The neck is highly mobile, and relatively minor connective tissue damage or muscle spasm can cause a disproportionate amount of discomfort and disability. NSAIDs, used for both their anti-inflammatory and analgesic effects, make a logical choice of medication. A course of 14 to 21 days may be required. There is no evidence that continuing them for longer after the acute injury has any benefits unless there is active arthritis.

Muscle relaxants (72 hours). Muscle relaxants may be useful in the initial treatment of neck pain. Their use, however, should be limited to the first few days. The patients must be warned of their sedative side effects. There is no evidence that long-term muscle relaxants are of benefit.

Analgesics (1 to 7 days). If NSAIDs are being prescribed, concurrent use of other analgesics is usually not necessary. If NSAIDs are contraindicated because of allergy or ulcer problems, analgesics containing acetaminophen can be used.

Ice/heat. Ice can be used frequently in the first 48 hours of the neck injury. Ice cubes placed in a plastic bag, with cream rubbed on the skin to prevent damage, are probably as effective as commercially available, single-use ice bags. After the initial 48 hours, ice or heat may be used depending on the individual's preference. Ice often decreases pain and spasm but does not help neck stiffness. Heat may decrease spasm and associated pain as well as improve neck mobility.

PRIMARY REHABILITATION (FOUR WEEKS)

Modify activities. Early return to work with minimal restrictions should be strongly encouraged. Frequent active range of neck movement exercises should be emphasized, as these mobilize tight muscles and joints. Taking more rest periods or working a shorter hour week during this initial period should be encouraged, if practical. If initially used, the soft collar should now be abandoned. A work site evaluation by an occupational therapist can be extremely valuable if neck injuries are a common occurrence at the patient's workstation.

Medications. If medications such as NSAIDs or analgesics such as opioid/acetaminophen combinations are prescribed, they should be on a fixed time, round-the-clock basis, with a limit on the number and duration of therapy. Early during this rehabilitation period, these drugs should be stopped.

Physical therapy/chiropractic. Mobilization of the joints and myofascial treatments should be combined with home exercise programs to encourage strength and flexibility of the affected part. Passive treatments such as ultrasound and interferential are ineffective and should be replaced with more physical joint and soft tissue mobilizations and stretching. Improvement should be rapid. If no improvement is apparent after 3 weeks, the type of therapy should be reviewed and either changed or stopped. An important role of the therapist is to encourage frequent range of movement exercises.

Acupuncture. The use of acupuncture needles, either at classical acupuncture meridian points or in myofascial tender and trigger points, has a large and often enthusiastic following. Any method of decreasing muscle spasm should be supplemented with a home exercise program of stretching and range of movement exercises. Within six sessions of acupuncture, a significant improvement should have occurred. If there is no improvement after this period, the acupuncture should be changed or stopped.

Trigger points. Injections of trigger points may be effective if localized pressure reproduces the patient's pain. The trapezius, rhomboid, and sternocleidomastoid muscles are the most common sites of trigger points. Stretches and range of movement exercises must be given after successful deactivation of the trigger point. The patient should be taught ischemic compression and cold deactivation to trial at home together with specific stretches. These should be taught by the therapist who treats the trigger points.

Postural education. Continued poor posture habits, especially with the neck at a fixed angle, may be a factor in the onset and continuation of neck pain. A general ergonomic review of the patient's work or home environment should be undertaken. Specific emphasis should be placed on correct posture and regular intervals of neck mobility exercises. It would be appropriate to refer to an occupational therapist for more specific advice. A physical therapist or chiropractor should include general postural advice as part of their therapy.

Exercises. Exercise should include general conditioning aerobic exercise such as walking, cycling, or swimming. This can be done at home or at a commercial gym. Supervision by trained therapists is not necessary. The duration of the exercise should be increased with time until the patient is doing 20 minutes 3 to 4 times a week. The 20 minutes can be completed in two sessions, that is, 10 minutes morning, 10 minutes evening. Simple advice such as using the stairs or walking around the block when arriving at work, at lunch time, or in the evening, will probably give an adequate workout if followed conscientiously. If the patient has seen a physical therapist or chiropractor, encouragement to exercise and a set home program should have been a part of the treatment plan. Specific exercises for the neck should include active range of movement with rotations of the head to the right and left, and side flexions to the right and left. These movements should be repeated with the head in the flexed and extended positions as well as in neutral. The patient should be encouraged to perform these exercises 3 to 4 times a day. They can be done at any convenient time, waiting in a traffic line, watching commercials, and so on.

Home traction. Home traction can effectively unload the joints and intervertebral foramina of the neck. It can be done up to four times a day. Toward the end of this period, traction should be used less frequently and later only used for "flare-ups."

LONG-TERM TREATMENT

Exercises. Having been taught a program of neck exercises, the patient should be encouraged to repeat them on a maintenance basis at least twice a day. They can be done at any convenient time, but especially if the neck is beginning to get stiff again. Regular aerobic exercise will promote healthy connective tissue, bone, and joints as well as being an effective method of stress management and muscle relaxation.

Smoking cessation. Apart from the obvious health risks of smoking, nicotine irritates synovial joints, coughing can strain the neck, and the associated carbon monoxide poisoning of the red cells diminishes oxygen diffusion to the intervertebral disk.

Return to work (with or without restrictions). An early return to work is important in the treatment of any pain syndrome. Once the initial period of tissue healing has occurred, work should not be detrimental. If the neck has to be held in nonneutral positions, work restrictions or workplace modifications may be necessary. Some of those may be as simple as reorganization of a typist's workplace, to as drastic as a retraining program.

REEVALUATION/REFERRAL

If the primary treatments have not effectively returned the individual to work by 4 to 5 weeks, and it is unlikely that he or she will be at work within the next 2 weeks, a reevaluation and specific diagnosis should be considered. This reevaluation should provide a logical rationale for further focused treatment. The following specialists may be used in the reevaluation process.

Physician opinion. A full history and physical examination should include the following:

1. Special reference to environmental factors, nature of injury, and psychosocial stressors.
2. Examination should include any nonorganic signs, pain behavior mannerisms, and other signs of an exaggerated response to injury.
3. A review of all investigations performed. Substandard or equivocal investigations should be repeated where clinically relevant. An EMG may be requested to evaluate radicular pains.
4. A review of the previous treatments tried and investigations done should indicate the effectiveness or otherwise. Further physical therapy/chiropractic treatments should be based on a fixed time scale with a review before further treatments are authorized.

Psychologist opinion. The psychologist's review should include standardized acceptable psychomimetric testing as well as individual interview. Depressive symptoms, overt psychopathology, and specific environmental and psychosocial stressors, which may be hindering recovery, should be evaluated. A history of previous work employment and educational levels attained, where relevant, should be obtained. The patient's medication intake should be ascertained and compared to the medication intake history as obtained by the physician.

Surgical opinion. An opinion as to whether surgery is indicated should only be given when the surgeon has:

1. Reviewed the H&P and the investigations.
2. Examined the patient.
3. Ideally had a multidisciplinary conference with the involved psychologist and physician.
4. Been satisfied that the relevant investigations are of adequate standard, if surgery is contemplated.

Specific physical therapy/chiropractic. Physical therapy or chiropractic should be focused on the potential causes of the patient's pain. By this stage the Z joints are often tight due to long-standing muscle spasm and need to be mobilized by "hands on" techniques. If mobilization of a joint reproduces the patient's pain, the joint should be stretched and moved to free adherent capsule and connective tissue. Improvement should be evident within 3 weeks. If there is no improvement, therapy should be changed or stopped.

Home exercises. Neck exercises should be continued on a regular basis. Maximum flexibility is probably achieved in six weeks of intensive, frequent stretching; after this period, a maintenance program of twice a day can be followed. "Overpressure" exercises can be introduced cautiously if radicular symptoms or increasing pain does not occur. These exercises are where the patient tries to gently push or pull the head further at end of range of movement, in order to stretch the joint capsules and connective tissue. Recognizing increasing tension in the cervical muscles in times of stress and learning to relax them can prevent Z joint irritation and pain.

TENS. If transcutaneous electrical nerve stimulation (TENS) has not been trialed at this stage, it should be. Electrodes placed on the trapezius muscle or over the painful Z joints for shoulder or neck pain and over the greater or lesser occipital nerves at the base of the occiput for headaches can be very effective. A week's trial will show if it is going to be effective. The stimulation of the TENS must cover the painful area if it is going to be effective. (See Fig. 33-1.)

Surgery. Further investigations and possibly surgery may be advised. It is important that the patient is psychologically stable, and a careful outline of the expected rehabilitation program and outcomes must be presented to them before surgery.

PAIN SPECIALIST

The pain specialist or team should review the history, degree of deactivation, and psychosocial distress. After careful examination, treatment plans may include the following:

1. Medication optimization or withdrawal.
2. Cervical epidural steroids for radicular pain referral. This may be indicated for a relatively acute disc prolapse (less than 6 months) with ongoing inflammation or possibly spinal stenosis with presumed nerve inflammation.

3. Cervical zygapophyseal (facet) joint injections. Where mobilization of the neck reproduces the patient's pain, the Z joints may be the cause. Small volumes of local anesthetic injected under fluoroscopic guidance can confirm the diagnosis and aid in prescribing specific physical therapy. Occasionally, radiofrequency ablation of the sensory nerves to the Z joints may be indicated.

4. Diagnostic nerve root blocks. Accurately placed small volumes of contrast media followed by local anesthetic onto the nerve root may confirm a diagnosis of root entrapment. Concordant pain (pain in the same distribution as the pain complained of) with injection of the irritating contrast dye, followed by cessation of pain on injection of the local anesthetic, is indicative of nerve root compression.

5. Multidisciplinary approach. The pain managment team should consist of a pain physician and a psychologist or psychiatrist, with or without a physical therapist. A pain management program for the patient should include education, coping skills teaching, specific exercises, medication optimization, physical therapy, and vocational guidance. The objective is to give the individual control over his or her pain and regain a quality of life.

CASE STUDY

Ms. Y, age 35, was involved in a motor vehicle accident. She was wearing her seatbelt and was stationary in her car when she was hit in the rear offside. This caused her head to hit the head restrainer. She remained conscious, and only after getting home did she notice her neck was stiff.

She had difficulty sleeping because of occipital headaches and neck and shoulder pain. The next morning she had significant neck movement restrictions with some pain radiating to the right shoulder. Two days later, she arrived at the physician's rooms in a soft cervical collar which she had borrowed from a friend.

Her previous history was significant for occasional migraine headaches for which she took sublingual ergotamine medication. She stated that her neck and right shoulder pain was 90/100 on a verbal analogue pain score and appeared to be increasing. Her headaches were continuous and throbbing over the right occiput, and she had pain referral to the right side of her face.

On examination, rotation, side flexion, and flexion of the neck were all significantly limited, with pain referred principally to the shoulders and into the right upper arm. Her power, sensation, and all reflexes were present and normal. Palpation of her neck revealed marked muscle spasms and tenderness over the zygapophyseal (Z) joints of the midcervical area, right more than left.

Plan

1. The patient was unwilling to have a period of rest because of her work. She was encouraged to discontinue the soft collar.
2. Nonsteroidals were given for 2 weeks to be taken regularly with food.
3. Analgesics were given for 72 hours.
4. She was encouraged to use ice two or three times a day, and to start range of movement neck exercises following the icing. She was given an appointment to be seen again in 3 days' time.

The patient returned, stating that she was unable to sleep because of pain. She also stated that she now had constant headaches and the shoulder referred pain was getting worse, especially in the evening. She described the pain as 85/100. She continued to work full time as a secretary, although her work ability had been limited by her pain. On examination she had some improvement in neck mobility, especially neck rotation. Flexion, however, was still markedly limited with marked muscle tenderness over the midneck and trapezius. Neurologic examination was still normal.

Plan

1. A home traction device was prescribed, and the patient was told to use it 2 to 4 times a day for 15 to 20 minutes at a time.
2. The nonsteroidal was continued but the analgesic was stopped.
3. The patient was instructed on the application of heat, followed by specific stretching exercises of the neck.
4. As the patient was improving in neck mobility with no radicular or myelopathic signs, she was referred to a physical therapist/chiropractor for gentle mobilization of the neck, myofascial release maneuvers, and a home neck exercise program.

The patient was given an appointment to be seen in one week's time.

The patient returned in 10 days still with headaches but with a marked improvement in neck movement. The neck was painful now only at 70–80 degrees of rotation. Side flexion was still limited and caused pain on the right side. She was sleeping better. The neck and shoulder pain averaged 20–30/100, being at worse 80/100 and at best 10/100. She stated that her headache was on average 50/100 and worse 80/100. The headache was associated with more pain in the neck. On examination she still had a normal neurologic examination. Trigger points were noted in the sternocleidomastoid, which referred a headache over the right side of the face and head. She also had trigger points over the greater occipital nerve, at the occiput, and in the trapezius and rhomboids, which referred pain to her neck and shoulder. The pain was aggravated by palpation over the C3-C4, C4-C5 Z joint areas on the right. On further questioning, it appeared that the only physical therapy she was receiving was gentle heat and massage, with no home exercise program.

Plan

1. To give specific instructions for the physical therapist to mobilize the Z joints. If the physical therapist did not, or was not able to, mobilize these joints, another therapist would be recommended.
2. The physical therapist was again requested to give a home exercise program and postural education advice regarding position of computer, chair height, how the phone should be held, and so on.
3. Trigger point injections of the right trapezius, rhomboid, and sternocleidomastoids were performed and stretching excerises given.
4. The patient was taught how to apply ischemic pressure to desensitize the trigger points.

The patient was given an appointment to be seen again in 1 week.

The patient returned after 1 week. Her pain and neck movement had both improved considerably since she had changed physical therapists, rearranged her work space, and started using the neck traction. She was also attending a stress management course given at the local YMCA and had started exercising during her lunch hour. She stated that her neck and shoulder pain was, on occasion, 0/100. This was usually after a period of aerobic exercise. At worst it was 40–50/100, and she noticed this was related to work stress. The headaches were still present but had also improved. She had noticed an increase in the frequency of her migraine headaches since the accident. This worried her, although they were still well controlled by sublingual ergotamines.

On examination, the neurologic examination was normal. Her neck range of movement was almost full, although she was still tender to palpation over the cervical Z joints on the right. Trigger points were present in the trapezius and rhomboids and nuchal muscle insertion.

Plan It was 3 weeks since her injury. She should have stopped her NSAIDs and analgesics and should be decreasing the frequency of use of the neck traction. She should be encouraged to continue to exercise and use the stress management education to recognize and deal with specific stressors as they occur. Physical therapy should be continued. She was reassured that an increase in migraine headaches was common after a neck injury and did not mean anything "sinister." The amount of ergotamine medication should be closely monitored as the risk of rebound migraine headaches due to excessive ergotamines is significant (see Ch. 15).

The trigger points were injected with bupivacaine and her home exercise stretching program was reemphasized.

She was given an appointment for 3 weeks.

She returned in 3 weeks with minimal discomfort and was discharged. Her headache was minimal and she had not taken any ergotamine for 2 weeks. The physical therapist requested a further month of therapy at one session per week. This was prescribed.

SUGGESTED READINGS

Barnsley L, Lord S, Bogduk N: Whiplash injury clinical review. Pain 58:283–307, 1994

Tan JC, Nordin M: Role of physical therapy in the treatment of cervical disc disease. Orthop Clin North Am 23:435–449, 1992

Orofacial Pain

The craniofacial region is one of the most densely innervated areas of the body. It is also an area that is commonly affected by many pain syndromes. It is reported that the temporo-mandibular pain and dysfunction syndrome affects up to 15% of the population. Although the etiology and pathogenesis of temporomandibular dysfunction is still unclear, it is evident that invasive techniques and surgery have overall poor results.

Unfortunately, despite these poor results invasive clinical approaches are common, with considerable financial and in some cases functional cost to the patient. Psychological aspects of any pain syndrome must be carefully reviewed, and this is particularly true in the orofacial region. Many chronic orofacial pains may develop neuronal hyperexcitation within the trigeminal caudalis nucleus of the upper brain stem. Thus central therapy of pain must be pursued. Peripheral treatments such as dental treatments alone are often ineffective. Depression also is one of the most frequently diagnosed disorders in patients with orofacial pain and must be treated aggressively. Referred pain is common in the facial area. Pain from the teeth may refer to remote areas of the head and face and ear. Pain both from neck and masticatory muscles are referred to the oral and facial areas. Cardiac ischemia may refer pain into the jaws. Clinical examination should include examination of the cranial nerves as slow growing tumors may present with a referred pain distribution. Slow-growing cerebellar pontine angle tumors may present with atypical facial pain.

The treatment algorithm for orofacial pain is given in Figure 20-1.

TOOTH PAIN

Pulpal Pain

When a caries lesion invades the tooth pulp an inflammatory process develops. This is associated with acute, intermittent, and spontaneous pain. If microorganisms invade the root apex the tooth becomes sensitive to chewing, touch, and percussion. At that stage the pain becomes continuous and "boring." Pain may increase and throb when the patient lies down. It may wake the patient from sleep. Application of heat and cold to the tooth causes excruciating pain.

Tight Tooth Syndrome

In tight tooth syndrome the enamel is deficient with a crack in the dentine. The patient complains of pain and discomfort associated with cold and hot stimuli in the area.

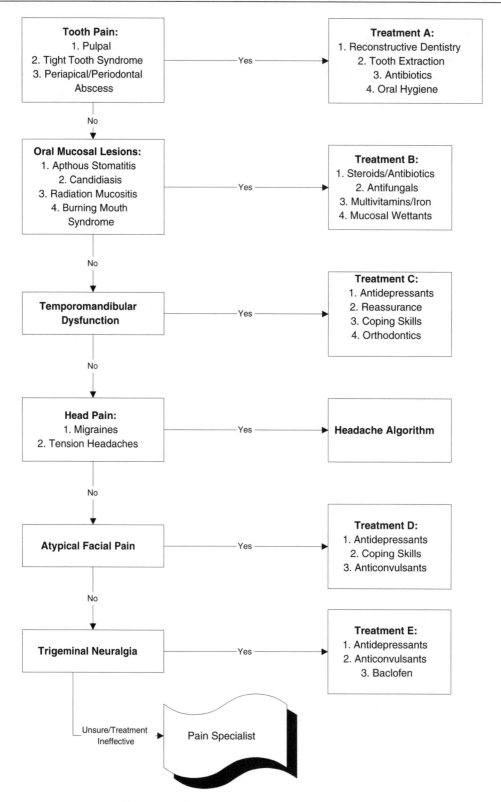

Fig. 20-1. Treatment algorithm for orofacial pain.

Localization is done by trapping the cusp of the suspected tooth, probing around margins of fillings, and applying cold stimuli.

Periapical and Lateral Periodontal Abscess

The tooth is usually loose, and pus may appear around it when a periapical or a lateral periodontal abscess is present. The abscess formation usually results from a blockage of drainage from the periodontal pocket. Cellulitis, fever, and malaise may be present.

TREATMENT A

Reconstructive dentistry. Reconstructive dentistry may include filling of cavities, crowns, or root canal therapy.

Tooth extraction. Extraction should be reserved for teeth that are nonviable or severely damaged.

Antibiotics. Antibiotics and incision drainage should be done for abscesses, especially if systemic signs of infection are present.

Oral hygiene. The patient should be instructed in the correct use of brushing and flossing.

ORAL MUCOSAL LESIONS

Apthous Stomatitis

Apthous ulcers are usually small in diameter (0.3 to 1.0 cm), with healing occurring within 10 days. More severe (major apthous ulcers) deep ulcers may occur that are confluent, are extremely painful, and interfere with speech and eating. Apthous stomatitis is characterized by a prodromal burning sensation 2 to 48 hours before ulceration appears.

Chronic Fungal Infection (Candidiasis)

The patient with candidiasis often has underlying immune suppression either due to disease, such as HIV, or prolonged broad-spectrum antibiotic therapy. Causes of immunosuppression should be sought for in patients presenting with oral candidiasis.

Radiation Mucositis

A severe generalized mucosal pain often occurs following radiation therapy to the head and neck. This is followed by decreased salivary flow as a result of scarring, causing chronic pain and discomfort in the oral mucosa.

Burning Mouth Syndrome

Burning mouth syndrome may occur during menopause or after oophorectomy. Alterations in salivary composition may be a factor. Mechanical irritation due to ill-fitting dentures, or allergy to denture materials, may also play a role. Iron deficiency was observed in 40% of patients with burning mouth syndrome. Low zinc levels have also been reported, as have low serum B1, B2, and B6 levels.

TREATMENT B

Steroids/antibiotics. Topical steroids and oral tetracyclines are used for deep apthous ulcers. Small apthous ulcers require reassurance, with or without topical anesthetic gels, that can be bought over the counter.

Antifungal agents. Nystatin mouth wash for oral candidiasis; amphotericin B may be required for systemic candidiasis.

Multivitamins and iron. For burning mouth syndrome, multivitamin therapy with minerals and iron replacement should be trialed. No caffeinated beverages should be taken for 2 hours after iron therapy, as caffeine chelates the iron and prevents absorption.

Mucosal wettants. Where salivary flow is decreased methylcellulose spray or mouth wash can be used, or sugar-free candy or gum chewed or sucked, to alleviate dryness of the mouth.

TEMPOROMANDIBULAR DYSFUNCTION

Pain of temporomandibular joints following trauma or arthritis (rheumatoid or psoriatic) should be evaluated by an orofacial surgeon and perhaps a rheumatologist. Radiographs may indicate the amount of damage. The jaw pain experienced does not usually correspond to radiographic evidence of damage.

Temporomandibular dysfunction may be localized to the temporomandibular joint area, or may be part of a more generalized pain syndrome such as primary fibromyalgia. Temporomandibular pain typically occurs around the ear and the end of the mandible, but may also be in the jaws, teeth, and diffusely on one side of the face. It may occur bilaterally. The patient's most intense pain is often in the morning or late afternoon. Duration can be from weeks to several years. Pain rarely wakes the patient. Pain may be aggravated during movement, or spontaneous spikes of pain may occur. Examination usually reveals limited mouth opening (less than 40 mm interincisal). Masticatory and neck muscles are usually tender to palpation. Trigger points in the masseter and temporalis muscles are often present.

TREATMENT C

Antidepressants. Antidepressants, in the first instance tricyclics, should be tried. These should be increased to antidepressant levels. If the tricyclic has not improved the pain within a period of 6 weeks a serotonergic-specific reuptake inhibitor (SSRI) should be trialed.

Reassurance. The majority of temporomandibular dysfunctions settle with time. Long-term follow-up indicates a recovery rate of up to 80% independent of whether treatment was active or placebo.

Coping skills. Psychological evaluation and coping skills. The etiology of temporomandibular dysfunction is multifactorial. Psychological stressors play a major role. Stress coping training is important for patients who appear to be coping poorly under stress.

Orthodontics. The role of orthodontics is controversial. Nighttime bruxism appears to be associated with temporomandibular dysfunction. However, there are many studies showing the incidence of displacement of the joint, a grinding habit, unilateral chewing, and lack of posterior tooth support is the same in controls as in those with jaw pain. More studies need to be done regarding the efficacy of orthodontics.

HEAD PAIN

1. Migraines.
2. Tension headaches. For treatment see headache algorithm (Fig. 15-2).

ATYPICAL FACIAL PAIN

Atypical facial pain usually has a chronic, constant intensity plus burning quality that intensifies into a throbbing sensation. The pain is not triggered by remote stimuli, but may be intensified by stimulation of the painful area itself. The pain usually does not wake the patient from sleep. The location is ill-defined, usually starting in one quadrant of the mouth and often spreading across the midline to the opposite side. Frequently the pain changes location. The patient has often had many operations for the pain with little success. Many of these pains may be centralized due to wind up in the trigeminal caudalis nucleus of the brain stem. MRI of the face and skull is important to exclude a slow-growing cerebellar pontine angle tumor. Rarely a benign tumor of the trigeminal nerve or a meningioma causes facial pain.

TREATMENT D

Antidepressants. Tricyclic antidepressants should be the first tried with the newer serotonin in specific reuptake inhibitors used if the TCA's are ineffective.

Coping skills. Psychological counseling and coping skills training are important as many patients show signs of depression and have overwhelming stressors.

Anticonvulsants. Anticonvulsants used in the past have included carbamazepine, dilantin, and valproic acid. The newer anticonvulsants such as gabapentin might have a role to play as it has a lower side effect profile. Surgery and physical treatments for atypical facial pain are ineffective. Generally patients with unilateral atypical facial pain should not be offered surgical procedures.

TRIGEMINAL NEURALGIA (TIC DOULOUREUX)

Trigeminal neuralgia is characterized by electrical shocklike, stabbing pains usually unilateral during any one episode. There is an abrupt onset and termination of the pain. Between intervals the patient is pain-free. Non-noxious stimulation triggers the pain. The pain is usually restricted to the trigeminal nerve distribution.

TREATMENT E

Antidepressants. Tricyclic antidepressants should be trialed before the SSRIs.

Anticonvulsants. In particular dilantin and carbamazepine have been used successfully.

Baclofen. Baclofen has been reported to help in some patients.

PAIN SPECIALIST

If the above measures do not help the patient with the pain, referral to a pain specialist should be sought. The pain specialist may offer the following:

1. Medication optimization.
2. Further diagnosis or therapy, referral to a dentist, orofacial surgeon, or psychiatrist.
3. Sphenopalatine and stellate ganglion blocks to assess if sympathetic-mediated pain exists.
4. Gasserian ganglion neurolysis either by radiofrequency or by glycerol injection.Trigeminal neuralgia and intractable chronic cluster headaches have been successfully treated by this method.
5. Intravenous infusions such as phentolamine, lidocaine, or fentanyl may be used to assess the pathophysiology and help in treatment planning.
6. Multidisciplinary pain management program using a pain team, which enables the patients to take control of their pain and not allow the pain to control them.

CASE STUDY

Mrs. Y, a 31-year-old woman, complained of pain in her right jaw associated with occipital and temporal headaches. She thought the jaw pain may have been related to a car accident she had had several years earlier, although the pain had only started over the last year and had become worse over the last 2 months. She related the worsening of her jaw pain to a wide yawn some months earlier. At this time she had felt something click in her jaw. The pain caused disturbed sleep with early morning awakenings and was worse in the afternoon when she returned home from work. On a verbal analogue score her jaw pain was described as 85/100 going to 120/100 at times. The pain was worse on eating, but she had not lost weight. Dental examination revealed carious teeth requiring treatment. She had not followed the dentist's advice because of time constraints and finances. The headaches were described as 60/100. She worked as a cashier at a local supermarket and rated her job enjoyment as 2 on a scale of 0 (hated job) to 10 (best job imaginable). She was taking 500 mg acetaminophen tablets 10–12 per day. She smoked approximately 2 packs of cigarettes per day. She had started to drink about half a bottle of wine per evening. She stated this was to help calm her down after working with the pain.

On examination she appeared anxious but denied suicidal ideations. She had an interincisal (between teeth) gap of 40 mm when she opened her mouth. This created the pain over the right temporomandibular joint area. She was tender on palpation over the right temporomandibular joint area. Her bite pattern appeared normal. She had sensitivity on tapping the molar teeth. Putting an ice block on her teeth was exquisitely sensitive. The oral mucosa appeared to be normal, although she had poor dental hygiene and gingivitis. Her neck movements were restricted with pain on palpation particularly on the right side of the neck. She had trigger points in scalenes, sternocleidomastoid, temporalis and masseter muscles. Pressure on the greater occipital nerve area in the occiput recreated her headache.

Impression

1. Temporomandibular dysfunction with dental problems.
2. Environmental stressors (job dissatisfaction).
3. Excessive use of analgesics and increasing use of alcohol and cigarettes.
4. Possible depression as shown by early morning awakening and worsening of symptoms in the afternoon.

Plan

1. Decrease acetaminophen to a maximum of 4 g per day.
2. Referral to a dentist for treatment of dental caries.
3. Commence nortriptyline 25 mg at night increasing over the next 10 days to 100 mg at night.
4. To return after dental treatment.

The patient returned stating the dentist had had to fill four teeth. She had also seen an oral hygienist for teeth cleaning and instruction on dental hygiene and flossing. She was able to chew more comfortably on the right side, but the pain was still present. Her dentist had suggested a nighttime splint for her bruxism. Her sleep was still disturbed. Her medication included nortriptyline 100 mg q hs and acetaminophen 3 g per day. She had commenced taking over-the-counter nonsteroidal antiinflammatory drugs up to 10 tablets a day. She stated this took "the edge off her pain."

Plan

1. Blood level of nortriptyline to assess if it is in the therapeutic antidepressant range.
2. Discontinue the nonsteroidals, as they are usually ineffective in myofascial syndromes.
3. Tramadol 50 mg increasing from 1 to 2 tablets q 4 h to a maximum of 8 per day.
4. Physical therapy for neck mobilization.
5. Stretching exercises for masseters to increase jaw opening.
6. Consider trigger point therapy or massage therapy for her various trigger points.
7. Discuss the possibility of a job change and encourage her to examine her job options.

Her nortriptyline levels came back below the antidepressant therapeutic range. Nortriptyline was increased to 175 mg at night, which improved her sleep and her mood considerably. The pain was marginally controlled on tramadol and acetaminophen, but she continued to complain bitterly of pain. She requested an x-ray to identify damage that may have occurred at the time of the motor vehicle accident. It was explained that an x-ray was not indicated as (1) the x-ray appearance of the temporomandibular joint does not indicate pain even if grossly abnormal, and (2) it was unlikely that the pain was due to the accident because of the long time delay between accident and onset of pain. The click and jaw pain she had felt initially on yawning was probably due to a meniscal shift in the temporomandibular joint which in itself was not significant.

If excessive anxiety, overuse of medications, or depression continues, referral to a psychiatrist or psychologist would be appropriate.

Mrs. Y. was able to terminate her smoking and limited alcohol consumption to only social occasions. The increase of nortriptyline improved her sleep and her mood. Her pain, however, only improved significantly when she changed her job to a secretarial position and began dating steadily. Over time the tramadol was discontinued, and after 6 months the nortriptyline was also stopped. She still reported that she had relatively frequent headaches, but these were controlled on 500–1000 mg of acetaminophen. She was referred for 8 sessions of biofeedback, which significantly improved her headaches and relaxed her neck muscles.

SUGGESTED READINGS

Brown RS, Abramovitch K, Hinderstein B: Controversies of the diagnosis and treatment of temporomandibular disorders: An update and review of the literature. Texas Dent J Oct. 13–19, 1993

Sharav Y: Orofacial pain. pp. 563–582. In Melzack R, Wall PD (eds): Textbook of Pain. 3rd Ed. Churchill Livingstone, New York, 1994

Pediatric Pain Management

Chronic pain

Chronic pain is far less common in children than in adults. As a result, it is often inadequately recognized and treated. The pathophysiology of chronic pain is thought to be similar in both adults and children. There is usually a peripheral noxious event causing a central hyperexcitation within the dorsal horn cells. This leads to expanding receptive fields and a continued "wind-up" of central nociceptive neurons. This wind-up may cause the death of inhibitory neurons as well as a "rewiring" of interneurons (excitatotoxicity). Such central effects are thought to be the main driving force for the continued sensation of pain which is felt despite no continuing peripheral tissue damage. No medication as yet can reliably turn off this wind-up/hyperexcitatory phenomenon, but many centrally acting medications and psychotherapeutic techniques can modify it.

Recurrent abdominal pain, headaches, and limb pains occur in 5% to 10% of school children. Chronic continuous pain is less common and is usually associated with chronic conditions such as AIDS, cancer, sickle cell disease, arthritis, or neuropathic disorders. Many children presenting with chronic pain have other preexisting psychological disorders such as family dysfunction, post-traumatic stress syndrome, or eating disorders. A child psychologist is an important member of any team dealing with pain problems in this age group.

The treatment algorithm for chronic pain in children is presented in Figure 21-1.

NOCICEPTIVE PAIN

Diagnostic Criteria

1. The pain descriptors are varied.
2. If there is no repeated injury or inflammation, the pain intensity usually decreases over days to weeks.
3. The pain is generally relieved by opioids.
4. Nonsteroidal drugs are often effective.
5. An obvious cause for the pain such as fracture or cancer is apparent on careful examination.

The treatment is dependent on the cause of the pain. Some examples of nociceptive pain follow.

Bone pain. Severe bone pain relieved by nonsteroidals should be investigated by radiographic and other tests for cancer or infection. A history of trauma with continued pain should be another reason for radiographs.

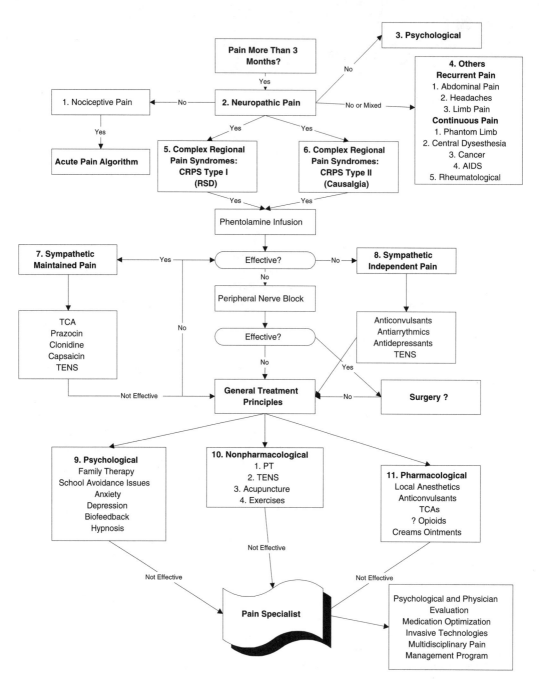

Fig. 21-1. Management of chronic pain in children. RSD, reflex sympathetic dystrophy; TCAs, tricyclic antidepressants; PT, physical therapy; TENS, transcutaneous electrical nerve stimulation.

Metabolic diseases. Diabetes and sickle cell crises can cause chronic pain with periodic acute exacerbations.

The arthritides. Juvenile rheumatoid arthritis is usually easy to diagnose clinically.

Myofascial pain. Children may have myofascial pain with trigger points, although this is less common than in adults.

Inflammation. Infection should be ruled out by careful history and examination.

TREATMENT

The acute pain algorithm (Fig. 7-1; also see Acute Pediatric Pain later in this chapter) can be followed. Pharmacologically, acetaminophen, nonsteroidal drugs, and opioids are usually the most useful. The methods of administration of opioids include transmucosal, nasal, continuous intravenous (IV), and patient-controlled analgesic devices (PCA). Intramuscular injections should be avoided.

Nonpharmacologic methods of treating acute pain are important. These include reassurance and honesty in describing potentially painful investigations and therapy. A calm, knowledgeable parent is a great advantage.

NEUROPATHIC PAIN

Diagnostic Criteria

1. Pain descriptors include burning, shooting, pins and needles, or strange feelings. Many other graphic pain descriptors may be used by children.
2. Allodynia (a normally nonpainful sensation is perceived as severe pain) may be present.
3. The pain persists or gets worse despite time.
4. The pain is often relieved partially by anticonvulsants or antidepressants. Large doses of opioids may be necessary, or the pain may be opioid-resistant.
5. The pain is rarely relieved by nonsteroidal drugs.
6. There is no obvious cause for the pain apparent on examination.

PSYCHOLOGICAL PAIN

Pain caused by psychological disturbances alone is rare in children, and its diagnosis should be one of exclusion. However, any pain syndrome can be affected by the child's secondary gain issues. The child may use his or her pain in an attempt to get love and attention in a dysfunctional family environment. Severely emotionally deprived children, depressed or anxious children, or those with overt psychopathologies should be evaluated by a child psychiatrist or psychologist. The child's emotional requirements should be examined as carefully as their physical needs.

OTHER GENERAL PAIN SITES

Recurrent Pain

Abdominal Pain

Recurrent cramping may be due to food allergies, especially lactose intolerance, infestations, toxins such as lead from environmental pollution, or constipation. Constipation may be pathologic due to a relatively atonic bowel because of deficits of the myenteric nerve plexus, or functional due to a low-roughage diet. Treatment depends on careful examination, the presence or absence of feces in the rectum, blood and stool tests, and other specialist investigations as indicated. (See Fig. 8-1 for the abdominal pain algorithm.)

Headaches

Depending on the age of the child, head circumference and growth parameters are important. Blood pressure should be measured. The skin should be closely examined for evidence of neurocutaneous disorders, such as von Recklinghausen disease. Sudden onset of severe headaches should raise the suspicion of an organic cause. Posterior fossa tumors, although uncommon, can occur with few neurologic signs. Childhood migraines can be treated similarly to those in adults. Nonpharmacologic methods should be emphasized as prophylaxis. The daily use of analgesics should be strongly discouraged. Prophylaxis for migraines may be necessary if the headaches are disrupting the normal life of the child. (See Fig. 15-2 for the headache algorithm.)

Limb Pain

The occurrence of limb pain, which causes the child to limp, should be carefully evaluated. The hips, knees, and ankles are common places for problems. These may be severe, as in slipped femoral epiphysis or tumors, or minor, as in traction apophysitis of the knee (Osgood-Schlatter) or achillocalcaneal junction (Severs). Treatment depends on the diagnosis.

Continuous Pain

Phantom Limb Pain

It is important to distinguish between the different types of pain associated with amputation. These would include stump pain and phantom limb sensation, as well as true phantom pain. Stump pain may be caused by an excitable neuroma, hematoma, or osteomyelitis. The indications for stump revision and search for neuromas are controversial and, unfortunately, surgery often has poor results. Children were widely regarded not to experience phantom limb pain. However, Krane and colleagues (1991), showed that the incidence of phantom pain in children was high, and the intensity of pain was often severe. Unfortunately, the pain was often ignored or disregarded by their health providers. Prevention of phantom limb pain includes having the amputation performed with an epidural-assisted general anesthetic and maintaining the epidural for 2 to 3 days postoperatively for pain relief. Early ambulation and physical therapy are also important. Established phantom limb pain is treated with transcutaneous electrical nerve stimulation (TENS), acupuncture, reassurance, tricyclics, and cognitive and behavioral techniques. Intravenous calcitonin has been found to be useful at the onset of phantom limb pain in adults. Now that it is available in nasal dosage form, it will be interesting to see if it has a similar efficacy.

Central Dysesthesia

Pain may occur after central nervous system lesions due to tumors or trauma. This "central dysesthetic pain" is often difficult to treat and requires centrally acting medications such as the anticonvulsants or sodium channel blockers. Unfortunately, it is often resistant to conventional therapies. (See Fig. 12-1 for the central pain algorithm.)

Cancer Pain

Procedure-related pain is often more common than tumor-related pain (for treatment, see the acute pain algorithm in Fig. 7-1). However, if tumor cells erode into nervous tissue, it gives rise to neuropathic pain. This pain is often severe and requires high doses of opioids to attempt to control it. Side effects may limit the amount of opioids that can be given. Methadone elixir is an effective and relatively inexpensive method to provide analgesia for children unable to swallow tablets. The required dose of opioid varies widely; the ideal is to have the pain controlled with a clear sensorium. If excessive somnolence is a problem, a tricyclic or ritalin may help. Changing the type of opioid may also prove effective. If there is good pain control with the opioids, but with excessive side effects, a PCA via a central line or a continuous subcutaneous infusion may be trialed. Occasionally an indwelling epidural or intrathecal catheter may be placed for continuous infusion of opioid with or without a low-dose local anesthetic. Other adjuvants include anticonvulsants, oral sodium channel blockers, and calcium channel blockers. Nonsteroidal drugs usually have a role to play as there is often a peripheral nociceptive element. (See cancer algorithm in Fig. 11-1.)

AIDS Pain

The pain associated with AIDS may be of central or peripheral origin. Abdominal pain, esophagitis, and pancreatitis are common. Opioids are among the most effective agents often combined with an anticonvulsant, especially if the pain has a sharp or lancinating component. (See Figs. 9-1 and 9-2 for the AIDS algorithm.)

Rheumatologic Disease

Children with arthritis, lupus, scleroderma, or mixed connective tissue disease may have pain due to joint deformation or ischemia. Aspirin and nonsteroidal drugs are the mainstay of treatment. Sympathectomy for ischemia is often only temporarily beneficial. Spinal cord stimulation may be appropriate in older children if ischemic pain is severe. TENS should be tried. Capsaicin cream 0.025% decreases joint swelling and pain, and it should be applied 3 to 4 times a day for 3 to 6 weeks over the inflamed joint before its usefulness can be assessed. (See the arthritis algorithm in Fig. 10-1.)

COMPLEX REGIONAL PAIN SYNDROME TYPE I (REFLEX SYMPATHETIC DYSTROPHY)

CRPS type I usually follows mild trauma and is not associated with significant nerve injury. It may follow a fracture, soft tissue injury, or prolonged bed rest. The distal aspect of the extremity is usually affected with proximal spread (glove and stocking distribution). The pain is usually burning and continuous and is exacerbated by movement and stimulation, especially cold. Allodynia, hyperalgesia, or both are present. Temperature asymmetry of more than 1 degree is present between the painful and nonpainful extremity. Three-phase bone scan shows subcutaneous blood pooling. Radiographs may show patchy demineralization.

Diagnostic Criteria

1. History of initiating injury or immobilization.
2. Continuing pain, allodynia, or hyperalgesia out of proportion to the initiating event.
3. Evidence at some time of edema, changes in skin blood flow, or abnormal pseudomotor activity in the painful area.
4. No other cause of the pain exists.

Criteria 2 to 4 must be satisfied.

COMPLEX REGIONAL PAIN SYNDROME TYPE II (CAUSALGIA)

CRPS type II onset usually occurs immediately after a partial nerve injury, but occasionally it may be delayed for months. Nerves most commonly affected are the median, ulnar, sciatic, and tibial.

Spontaneous burning pain is exacerbated by light touch, by temperature change, or with movement. Edema is usually present. Sympathetically maintained pain may be present. Atrophy of the skin and nails with loss of joint mobility may occur. Motor function is impaired. There is a temperature asymmetry between the affected and nonaffected side of more than 1.1°C. A three-phase bone scan shows periarticular uptake. Radiographs show patchy demineralization.

Diagnostic Criteria

1. Presence of continuing pain, allodynia, or hyperalgesia after nerve injury, not necessarily limited to the distribution of the nerve.
2. Evidence of edema, blood flow changes, or abnormal pseudomotor activity in the region of the pain.
3. Diagnosis excluded by other conditions that would cause a similar degree of pain and dysfunction.

All three criteria need to be satisfied.

Either type of CRPS may be sympathetic-maintained or sympathetic-independent. Differentiation is by sympathetic blockade, either by a stellate ganglion or lumbar sympathetic block or phentolamine infusion. The latter is less traumatic for a child. If the sympathetic block is successful (reduction of pain more than 75%), a medication trial of 4 to 6 weeks should be undertaken. Drugs such as the tricyclic antidepressants, prazocin, clonidine, capsaicin cream, other creams, lotions, or sprays, and opioids should be tried. TENS should also be trialed, avoiding placement of electrodes rods over the sensitive skin. (See the RSD algorithm, Fig. 26-1.)

All therapies are designed to diminish pain and allow active movement and physical therapy of the affected extremity. In children, there is often a very gratifying and rapid response to conservative therapy. The efficacy of invasive interventions such as spinal cord stimulation has not been reported in the therapy of sympathetic-maintained pain in children.

If sympathetic blockade is not effective, a diagnostic peripheral nerve block should be done. If a peripheral nerve block is successful, surgical opinion may be requested for freeing the entrapped nerve. A temporary catheter through which local anesthetics can be infused may be placed alongside the entrapped nerve in order to allow intensive physical therapy.

If sympathetic blockade is unsuccessful in diminishing the pain (sympathetic-independent pain), anticonvulsants, mexiletine, and tricyclic antidepressants should be trialed. TENS tends to be of less use in these situations but should be trialed for the myofascial component.

GENERAL TREATMENT PRINCIPLES

Psychological Therapy

The support of a child psychologist trained in pain management is important for supportive family therapy, biofeedback, hypnosis, and dealing with school avoidance. Anxiety symptoms should be treated, and depression should be looked for and treated vigorously. The therapist has to be empathetic as to the child's tolerance of various emotion-charged subjects. Starting the sessions with the child standing or sitting and not lying in bed maximizes his or her feelings of self-control. Psychosocial activities that are motivating for the child should be explored. These can include shopping, games, or sports. Biobehavioral techniques for controlling pain have been successfully taught in children from the age of 7 years.

Nonpharmacologic Therapy

Physical therapy. Physical therapy is important, and early return to school should be a high priority. Exercises and physical therapy should be coordinated with school activities so the least school time possible is lost. Ultrasound is contraindicated in children in whom the growth plates have not yet fused.

TENS. TENS should be trialed in all cases of chronic pain.

Acupuncture. Acupuncture is useful to trial, with some practitioners using "soft tissue" laser acupuncture instead of needles. Unfortunately, the literature on the efficacy of this form of therapy in children is lacking.

Pharmacologic Therapy

Drugs used for chronic pain include anticonvulsants, local anesthetics (such as mexiletine 10 mg/kg per day), baclofen for spasticity, opioids, prazocin (alpha-1 blocker), and clonidine (alpha-2 agonist). Most prescribing is based on extrapolation from adult treatments; little has been published prospectively on their use in children. Tricyclic antidepressants carry a small but significant risk of sudden cardiac events in children. If used, because of increased metabolism and excretion, they may have to be given twice daily. Doxepin (12.5–100 mg/kg per day) is available as an elixir and nortriptyline (1–3 mg/kg day) as a solution. Gabapentin, a new anticonvulsant (25 mg/kg per day maximum dosage), has proved very effective in adults with certain neuropathic pain syndromes. It probably can be tried as a first-line neuropathic pain agent in children.

PAIN SPECIALIST

The pain specialist(s) should ideally be working in a multidisciplinary environment. Both physical and psychological evaluations must be made so that a comprehensive treatment plan can be formulated. Medications should be optimized for the pain syndrome and diagnostic blocks done where necessary to identify the pathophysiology. The role of invasive technologies such as intrathecal pumps or spinal cord stimulators in intractable pain syndromes in children not responding to appropriate conservative therapy has not been clearly defined. A pain management program should incorporate all the different therapies outlined above and involve both child and parents in an intensive, educational, behavioral/operant program of teaching how to deal with chronic pain that is not responding to usual therapies.

CASE STUDY

A 5-year-old boy fell out of a tree and sustained a greenstick fracture of his left radius. He was evaluated, had a manipulation under anesthesia to straighten the bone and had a cast applied. There was no previous medical history of significance, and there was no neurologic deficit on examination.

He continued to complain of pain and was brought to the emergency room (ER) 2 days after the accident in severe pain, with the fingers and hand distal to the cast blue and swollen. The cast was removed, and the forearm alignment on repeat radiograph was satisfactory. There was mild pain over the site of the fracture, but the hand and fingers were exquisitely tender and swollen. He was given an intramuscular injection of morphine and phenergan, which appeared to settle him down. A back slab was applied, and he was discharged with acetaminophen elixir and a letter to follow up with his primary care physician the next day.

At the visit the following day he was still complaining of pain in his hand and was unwilling to have it examined. He appeared very subdued and somewhat withdrawn. His mother attributed this to a "talking to" his father had given him about being brave and not complaining. This had been precipitated by the child's continuing to cry after returning from the ER.

On examination the hand appeared slightly swollen and was very tender to touch. He was able to move all his fingers but not to make a fist.

Impression

1. Possibly recovering with swelling from too tight a cast.
2. Possibly early complex regional pain syndrome type I.

Plan

1. Ibuprofen 125 mg q 6 h for 3 days.
2. An arm sling was given to maintain the hand in an elevated position.
3. Instruction was given to the mother and the patient on icing and finger exercises.
4. See patient again in 3 days.

The patient did not return for follow-up until 10 weeks later. At this time his left hand was still swollen with his fingers very stiff and held in a "clawlike" manner. His wrist movement was minimal. He had been on vacation since his accident, which had occurred on the first day of school. His mother brought him back as she wondered if it was normal for a bone injury to take so long to heal. The ibuprofen had helped, and they continued to give it to him intermittently, although it did not appear to be as effective. He was sleeping poorly and was crying a lot.

On examination he appeared to be a very miserable child who held a baseball cap over his left hand. He was very noncommittal at first, and it later turned out he was terrified he might be given an injection for pain. He vividly remembered the "shot" he had been given in the ER. His hand was swollen with a shiny blue appearance to the skin. It was extremely tender to touch (allodynia) over the whole hand to just proximal to the wrist (glove distribution).

Impression   Complex regional pain syndrome type I.

Plan

1. Reassure the child that he will NOT be given any intramuscular injections.
2. Discuss with the mother and patient, in simple language, what the diagnosis might be and how important it will be for him to be followed up until the pain is under control. It is important the mother realize her son's discomfort is neither psychological nor a usual consequence of the initial injury.
3. Trial TENS.
4. Gabapentin 100 mg initially at night increasing to three times a day.
5. A codeine/acetaminophen combination (ideally codeine at 0.5 mg/kg, acetaminophen 15–20 mg/kg). The nearest nontriplicate medication for this child's weight (20 kg) was acetaminophen 300 mg with codeine 7.5 mg. This was prescribed for every 4 hours.
6. Consider referral to a pain specialist for a phentolamine infusion and possibly a child psychologist.
7. See patient in 1 week.

On follow-up 1 week later, the boy stated his pain was "better." Four poker chips were placed in front of him, and he was told each of them were "pieces of hurt." The first chip was "just a little hurt," the second and third were a "bit more hurt," and the fourth "the most hurt he could have." When asked how many "pieces of hurt" he had, the child pointed to two pieces. When asked how much it had hurt before starting treatment, he pointed to all four. His mother said he was now sleeping better and she had seen him begin to use the hand again by steadying objects held in his nonpainful hand. He had not used his left hand since the injury. His mother volunteered at this time that she was having marital problems and her husband was becoming physically abusive to her. He had not threatened the son, but had stated he thought the son was exaggerating his hand problem.

Plan

1. Continue gabapentin at 100 mg tid and the acetaminophen/codeine 300 mg/7.5 mg 4 to 5 times a day.
2. Continue the TENS, which was giving a good stimulation pattern on conventional, plus burst mode. He was wearing it most of the day and took it off at night.
3. Refer to a child psychologist with the parents for family therapy.
4. See patient weekly.

The boy's condition improved rapidly over the next 4 weeks. He was able to come off his analgesics, although the gabapentin was continued for another 4 weeks before tapering off. His TENS machine, looking much the worse for wear, was not required 6 weeks after commencing therapy. He continued for 10 sessions with a child psychologist, and his parents were reconciled after intensive family therapy. He required six sessions of physical therapy to encourage movement of his wrist and fingers, which returned to full and pain-free use.

Remarks Children often respond remarkably quickly to appropriate therapy with CRPS type I.

If his condition was not improving after one or two visits, an urgent referral to a pain specialist should be made. At that time, sympathetic blockade, possibly somatic blockade, and a psychological profile of child and family dynamics could be made. This would be followed by a treatment program as indicated by the evaluation.

Acute pain

NEONATES

Neonates do feel pain. Pain pathways are developed, although myelination is not complete by the 30th week after conception. Several studies have shown that inadequate perioperative analgesia in neonates resulted in a higher morbidity and probably mortality. The neonate (0–4 months) has different drug kinetics than the older child. They have a functionally immature liver and kidneys. This results in decreased conjugation (glucuronidation) and oxidation of drugs in the liver. By the end of the first month of life, liver enzymes reach adult functional capacity. The glomerular filtration rate in full-term infants is approximately 40% of adult function. This rapidly increases over the first 2 to 4 weeks of life. The blood-brain barrier is also immature in preterm and neonates, leading to higher central nervous system (CNS) drug levels. This, coupled with reduced ventilatory responses to hypoxemia and hypercapnia, results in a neonatal response to CNS depressants, such as opioids, which is difficult to predict.

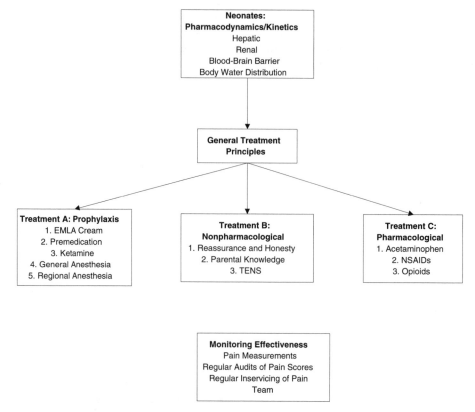

Fig. 21-2. Management of acute pain in children. NSAIDs, nonsteroidal anti-inflammatory drugs; TENS, transcutaneous electrical nerve stimulation.

GENERAL TREATMENT PRINCIPLES

Prophylaxis Before Surgery

TREATMENT A

EMLA cream. EMLA is a eutectic mixture of prilocaine and lidocaine. It can be placed as a thick layer over a proposed injection site a minimum of 1 hour before a procedure. This causes the skin to be anesthetic so that the child does not feel the injection.

Premedication. Premedication with an anxiolytic such as midazolam (0.5 mg/kg orally) may sufficiently sedate and calm the older child. An oral analgesic such as an opioid can be added if the procedure is going to be painful. Oral transmucosal fentanyl citrate (OTFC) is sucked like a lollipop. Its effect occurs within 10 to 30 minutes. It should be given 30 minutes before a painful procedure or surgery. Nausea is a major side effect. An oral nonsteroidal anti-inflammatory drug as a premedication is extremely useful. The potential problem of platelet aggregation inhibition does not appear to be of clinical significance perioperatively. All premedication can be given orally up to 2 hours before general anesthesia without increasing the risk of aspiration.

Ketamine. Ketamine (8–10 mg/kg) given intramuscularly tends to be painful; however, with adequate sedation, the child usually does not remember it. This gives a dissociative analgesia for a period of some 15 minutes, which may be all that is required for a procedure such as painful dressing changes. Atropine (orally) or glycopyrrolate (IV) needs to be given to decrease the excessive salivation that occurs with ketamine.

General anesthesia. A general anesthetic should be considered if the procedure is going to be repeated or is very painful.

Regional anesthesia. During anesthesia, or for repeated painful procedures, regional blockade, either single shots or a catheter, should be considered. Regional techniques include (1) caudal or epidural anesthesia; (2) peripheral nerve blocks; (3) interpleural blocks; (4) intercostal blocks [In children it is better to place a catheter for continuous infusion than to attempt repeated painful injections.]; (5) infiltration of the wound with bupivacaine or a ring block (e.g., for circumcision) during the procedure, can markedly decrease the child's pain and distress in the postoperative period.

Nonpharmacologic Therapy

TREATMENT B

Reassurance and honesty. It is important to reassure and to be honest with the child about the procedure and what is going to happen afterward. If a general anesthetic is involved, it is important the child be told he or she will wake up. Children often have unexpressed fears of going to sleep and not waking up.

Education. Parental knowledge is important in calming the child and not having him or her bombarded by irrational fears.

TENS. TENS can be used postoperatively in older children. Placing the electrodes proximal to the incision and getting a stimulation pattern over the wound can markedly reduce pain and may speed up healing.

Pharmacologic Therapy

TREATMENT C

Acetaminophen. The recommended dosage of acetaminophen is 10–15 mg/kg po, 4 hourly, or 20–25 mg/kg per rectum. However, infants have a greater volume of distribution, a greater clearance, and a slower elimination than adults. It has been shown that 25 mg/kg orally at 6- to 8-hour intervals gives effective therapeutic plasma levels below toxic levels in children. Acetaminophen also potentiates the effects of narcotics. It should be the primary choice of analgesia for most children, if there are no contraindications such as liver disease.

NSAIDs. Aspirin should be avoided because of the risk of Reye's syndrome (hepatic failure) in small children with a fever. Naprosyn (5 mg/kg 12 or 8 hourly), ibuprofen (10 mg/kg 6 hourly) have been used extensively for pediatric pain. They take up to 30 minutes to work when given orally. Their effect on platelet aggregation is not clinically important if the patient has normal platelets function initially. They should be given on a regular dose regimen for 2 to 3 days after the injury or surgery.

Opioids. Most authors recommend that children under 2 months should receive opioids only if monitored in an intensive or semiintensive care setting. This is due to hepatic immaturity, intrahepatic recirculation of the opioid, and blood-brain barrier immaturity, possibly leading to higher CNS concentrations and an increased risk of CNS depression. By 3 months of age, healthy infants have no greater risk of respiratory depression from opioids than adults. At this age, opioids can be given in the dosage (variable) that decreases the child's pain.

Codeine is available as an elixir and is probably the most commonly administered oral opioid in young children. Lipid-soluble narcotics are well absorbed by the nasal or buccal mucosa, for example, fentanyl, sufentanil, methadone, and buprenorphine (Stadol).

Table 21-1. Pain Measures in Children

Measure	Description	Indications for Use	Advantages	Disadvantages
Behavioral measures	Direct observation of overt behaviors, usually measured repeatedly at regular intervals, according to time or phase of procedure	Very young children; used with self-report; best reliability and validity are for short, sharp pain	Useful when child is unable to rate pain; less subject to bias than self-report	Not as well validated for longer lasting pain or for subtle behaviors (e.g., guarding wound); difficult to discriminate between pain and distress
Children's Hospital of Eastern Ontario pain scale (CHEOPS)[a]	Observed behaviors: crying, facial expression, verbal expression, torso position, and leg position	Originally used for postoperative pain and needle pain	Easy to learn and use; good reliability; validity	Insensitive to long-term pain
Faces scale[b]	Faces indicating intensity were derived from children's drawings	6–8 years	Strong agreement among children re: pain severity of faces and consistency of intervals; adequate test–retest reliability	Validity studies not yet completed
Visual Analogue Scale	Vertical or horizontal line with verbal, facial, or numerical anchors on a continuum of pain intensity	5 years and over	Reliable and valid: (e.g., child report correlates with behavioral measures and with parent, nurse, physician ratings); versatile (can rate different dimensions— pain and affect —on same scale)	Intervals on numerical scales may not be equal from a child's perspective

Measure	Description	Indications for Use	Advantages	Disadvantages
Oucher scale[c]	6 photos of children's faces indicating intensity; 100-point corresponding vertical scale	3–12 years	Reliable; adequate content validity; correlates with other VAS scales; presentation of both pictorial and numerical scales is applicable for broader age range	See VAS
Poker Chip Tool[d]	4 poker chips representing little hurt, a bit more hurt, more hurt, and most hurt; child chooses how many pieces of "hurt" he/she has	4–6 years	Reliable; well validated	See VAS

[a]From McGrath et al., 1985.
[b]From Bieri et al., 1990.
[c]From Beyer and Wells, 1989.
[d]From Hester, 1979.

199

Subcutaneous (less than 0.5–1 ml/h) infusion of opioids in cancer patients can be used if the oral route is not available.

Continuous IV infusion (0.025–0.03 mg/kg per hour morphine) has been used successfully in the postoperative period. An initial bolus of morphine 0.05–0.10 mg/kg should be given to ensure adequate analgesia before beginning the infusion. In infants less than 3 months of age, an infusion of 0.01–0.015 mg/kg per hour has been safely used.

Patient-controlled analgesic devices (PCA) can be used. Usually the child has to be older than 5 years of age. Morphine 0.02–0.03 mg/kg with a lockout time of 10 to 15 minutes can be used with or without a 0.01–0.02 mg/kg per hour basal rate. The initial dose is modified depending on the number of attempts and the occurrence of side effects.

Intramuscular injections should be avoided in young children. Surveys suggest that children will frequently deny pain in order to avoid an injection.

Monitoring Effectiveness of Treatment

Pain Measurements

Pain can be measured by what children say (self report), how their bodies react (biologic markers), or what they do (behavior markers). Self-report is probably the best but requires the child to have attained a certain cognitive development. Self-report may be strongly influenced with pain denial if there is fear of an injection following the response, if children do not trust the questioner, or if they feel they "have to be brave." For the younger or mentally impaired child, biologic and behavioral measures are used. See Table 21-1.

Biologic measures. While heart rate and oxygen saturation monitoring are easy valid measures of short, sharp pain, there are many other factors that influence both and decrease their efficacy as a longer-term guide.

Stress hormones released during painful procedures have an adverse effect on morbidity. Unfortunately, they also are poor monitors of continuing pain.

Behavioral measures. Several behavior measurement scales have been produced. The CHEOPS (Children's Hospital of Eastern Ontario Pain Scale) rates six behaviors. The Toddler Pre-School Postoperative Pain Scale has seven items on vocal, facial, and body expressions. The Postoperative Pain Score for infants (Table 21-2) has 10 behaviors.

Regular audits. The effectiveness of any pain measurement system is only as good as the conscientiousness of the measurer and the willingness of the physician to act upon it. As well as daily rounds, when pain scores should be assessed and medication changed accordingly, a formal collection of data should be made to assess the overall efficacy. Even if a formal collection is not made, regular meetings of the primary treating physicians should continually evaluate the efficacy of pain treatment regimens. Measurements are useless if there is no logical action based on their results.

PAIN SPECIALIST

The pain specialist should be part of a team that does not need to be a separate service. It can be nursing and pediatric unit-based. However, adequate measurement and treatment protocols need to be established, with ongoing inservicing. It is beholden to all care givers to practice good medicine. This includes adequate pain relief in the postoperative period and during acutely painful medical conditions. If further incentive is needed, several authorities have stated that clinicians who fail to provide a standard of pain management care may be liable for ethical or legal sanction.

Table 21-2. Postoperative Pain Score

	0	1	2
Sleep during preceding hour	None	Short naps; between 5 and 10 minutes	Longer naps; ≥10 minutes
Facial expression of pain	Marked, constant	Less marked, intermittent	Calm, relaxed
Quality of cry	Screaming, painful, high-pitched	Modulated, i.e., can be distracted by normal sound	No cry
Spontaneous motor activity	Thrashing around, incessant agitation	Moderate agitation	Normal
Spontaneous excitability and responsiveness to ambient stimulation	Tremulous, clonic movements, spontaneous Moro reflexes	Excessive reactivity (to any stimulation)	Quiet
Constant and excessive flexion of fingers and toes	Very pronounced, marked and constant	Less marked, intermittent	Absent
Sucking	Absent or disorganized sucking	Intermittent (3 or 4) and stops with crying	Strong, rhythmic with pacifying effect
Global evaluation of tone	Strong hypertonicity	Moderate hypertonicity	Normal for the age
Consolability	None after 2 minutes	Quiet after 1 minute or effort	Calm before 1 minute
Sociability (eye contact); response to voice, smile, real interest in face	Absent	Difficult to obtain	Easy and prolonged

SUGGESTED READINGS

Attia J, Amiel-Tison C, Mayer MN et al: Measurement of postoperative pain and narcotic administration in infants using a new clinical scoring system. Anesthesiology 66:A532, 1987

Beyer JE and Wells N: The assessment of pain in children. Pediatr Clin North Am 36:837, 1989

Bieri D, Reeve RA, Champion GD et al: Pain 41:139, 1990

Hester NO: Nurs Res 28:250, 1979

Houck CS, Troshyn SN, Berde CB: Treatment of pain in children. In Wall PD, Melzack R (eds): Textbook of Pain. Churchill Livingstone, New York, 1994

Krane EJ, Heller EB, Pomietto ML: Incidence of phantom sensation and pain in pediatric amputees. Anesthesiology 75:A69, 1991

McGrath P, Johnson GG, Goodman JT et al: J Adv Pain Res Ther 9:395, 1985

Chronic Perineal Pain

Although many causes of perineal pain are obvious on careful examination and their treatment is relatively straightforward, there are several less common pain presentations that create diagnostic and therapeutic difficulties.

Environmental stressors, poor coping strategies, and depression should be addressed early. Reassurance after appropriate investigations that there is no cancer is also important. Many of these patients are elderly and continue to complain of constant pain despite medications that may also have significant side effects. Early referral to a pain specialist may be appropriate to explore aspects of the physical and emotional nature of the pain, which may not be apparent on initial examination and treatment.

The treatment algorithm for perineal pain is given in Figure 22-1.

TREATMENT PLANS

Apparent on Examination

Many causes of chronic perineal pain are obvious on examination. These include disorders of the rectum and anus (hemorrhoids, fistulae, anorectal cancer) or the genitourinary system (infections, genitourinary cancer).

TREATMENT A

Referral. Referral to a specialist such as a surgeon or urologist may be indicated.

Antibiotics. Urinary infections require urinalysis. Antibiotics should be started after the urine has been sent for culture and sensitivity. Specific causes of urethritis such as sexually transmitted diseases must also be considered.

Surgery. Surgery may be necessary for perineal cancer with or without radiation of pain.

Previous Surgery

Phantom Anus

Chronic pain may develop following surgery to the perineum. Phantom anus pain has been estimated to occur in approximately 23% of patients following anal excision. The late onset of pain is associated with a 25% tumor recurrence rate.

Pudendal nerve damage. Trauma to the pudendal nerve may follow operations to the pelvic viscera, lumbar spine, or anal canal. The pudendal nerve contains autonomic afferents and efferents. Damage may give rise to a sympathetically maintained burning pain. (See Ch. 26, complex regional pain syndrome type II, causalgia.)

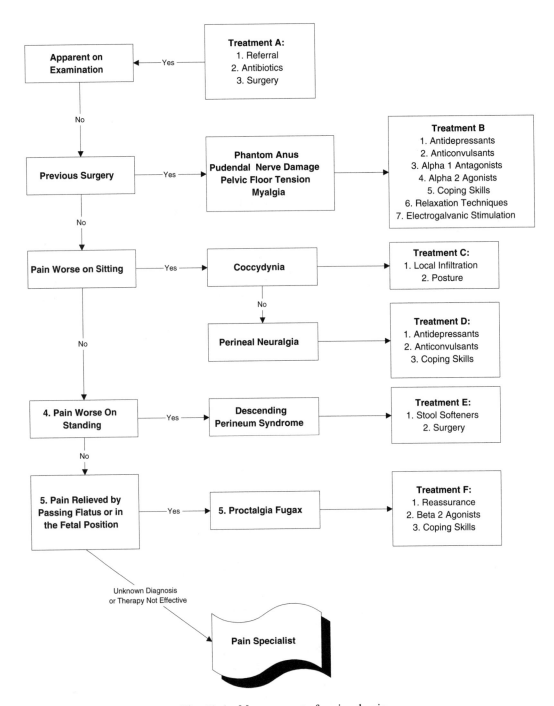

Fig. 22-1. Management of perineal pain.

Pelvic Floor Tension Myalgia

Pain in the pelvic floor muscles and their attachments may also occur following surgery.

TREATMENT B

Antidepressants. Tricyclic antidepressants should be tried with increasing doses until antidepressant level is reached. If sleep is a problem, a more sedating anticyclic can be trialed.

Anticonvulsants. Anticonvulsants such as gabapentin, carbamazepine, and phenytoin should be trialed. Gabapentin has the lowest side effects profile and probably should be trialed first.

Alpha-1 blockers. If there is a sympathetically maintained component, which usually presents as allodynia, an alpha-1 blocking agent can be trialed. Prazocin up to 6 mg per day, or phenoxybenzamine up to 40 mg per day can be trialed.

Alpha-2 agonists. Clonidine is an alpha-2 agonist which may have a beneficial effect in neuropathic and sympathetically maintained pain syndromes. It enhances central inhibition pathways and decreases norepinephrine release peripherally.

Coping skills. If the patient appears to be coping badly with the pain and various life stressors, a referral to a psychologist for coping skill training is appropriate.

Relaxation techniques. Relaxation is particularly useful in pelvic floor tension myalgia.

Electrogalvanic stimulation. Electrogalvanic stimulation may be effective in pelvic floor tension myalgia.

Pain Worse on Sitting

Coccydynia

Coccdynia is pain around the coccyx radiating into the sacrum, adjacent muscles, and soft tissues. It may be associated with anorectal discomfort, and pain is made worse by sitting or defecation. The most common causes are falling from a chair, and childbirth. The coccyx is usually extremely tender to palpation. Mobilization of the coccyx via the anus recreates the pain.

Perineal Neuralgia

Perineal neuralgia occurs almost exclusively in women over the age of 60. Patients present with a well-localized, burning pain in the anus, which may radiate to the sacrum, thighs, lower abdomen, or perineum. Pain is usually aggravated by sitting and relieved by lying down or standing. Trauma to the pudendal nerves may be a precipitating factor. The patient often has major environmental stressors and poor coping skills.

TREATMENT C

Local anesthetic infiltration. For coccydynia local infiltration of the sacrococcygeal ligament with local anesthetic and steroid may have a long-lasting effect.

Posture. Sitting correctly and using appropriate cushioning or a donut ring can decrease the pain of coccydynia significantly.

TREATMENT D

Antidepressants. Initially tricyclics or, if these are unsuccessful, other newer serotonin-specific reuptake inhibitors should be trialed up to antidepressant doses. Suicidal ideation must be inquired about, and referral to a psychiatrist is important if a firm plan of suicide is present.

Anticonvulsants. Gabapentin, carbamazepine, phenytoin, or valproic acid can be trialed. Improvement should be noticed in 2 to 3 weeks. If there is no improvement over this period of time, the medication should be changed.

Coping skills. Patients with these syndromes often have extremely poor coping skills and may have a dysfunctional environment. They should be referred to a psychologist for evaluation and therapy.

Pain Worse on Standing

Descending Perineum Syndrome

Descending perineum syndrome is more common in women and presents with a dull aching pain in the posterior perineum and anal canal. Pain is prominent after defecation, or prolonged standing, and is relieved by lying down. Pain is associated with abdominal descent during straining, defecation, and standing. Careful examination usually reveals the perineum descending below the plane of the ischial tuberosity on straining.

TREATMENT E

Stool softening. Stool softeners, and advice regarding avoidance of straining, should be given.

Surgery. Surgery is often necessary for pelvic floor repair.

Pain Relieved by Flatus and Fetal Position

Proctalgia Fugax

Proctalgia fugax syndrome occurs more commonly in men, usually beginning in early adult life and ceasing spontaneously in late middle age. Pain is felt in the upper anal canal and usually lasts at least 30 minutes. It can occur suddenly and is particularly common at night. The pain is usually relieved by flexing at the hips into a fetal position, or by passing flatus. There is a high incidence of irritable bowel syndrome. A genetic predisposition has been suggested.

TREATMENT F

Reassurance. Giving the patient a diagnosis and assuring them it does not indicate cancer or other serious disease, and informing them of the expected "cure" with time, will often allow the patient to come to terms with the discomfort.

Coping skills. Proctalgia fugax is a syndrome that is extremely difficult to treat and usually spontaneously remits with time. A psychological evaluation is extremely useful to help the patient cope with excessive stressors.

Beta-2 agonists. Sabutamol or other beta-2 agonists have been successfully prescribed in some patients with this syndrome.

PAIN SPECIALIST

If treatment at a primary level fails to significantly resolve the pain, a referral to a pain specialist should be made. The pain specialist may suggest the following.

Medication optimization. If various medications have not be trialed they can be started. Other medications, including narcotics, should be withdrawn if they have been ineffective.

Sympathetic blocks. Several of the perineal pain syndromes have possible sympathetic components. Blocking the sympathetic efferents to the perineum is done by an injection into the ganglion of Walther (ganglion impar) located at the anterior surface of the sacral coccygeal junction. If a local anesthetic block removes the pain, a neurolytic block with phenol can be considered.

Pudendal nerve block. The pudendal nerve can be blocked both via the perineum or, in females, via the vagina. If this removes the pain, pudendal neuralgia is a probable diagnosis. If there is a possibility of scar tissue, a surgical referral may be appropriate.

Caudal analgesia. A caudal injection of local anesthetic may decrease the pain of coccydynia or several of the perineal pain syndromes. If successful, this could be followed by selective sacral root blocks and potentially radiofrequency ablation or neuritic destruction.

A differential spinal or epidural. A spinal or an epidural local anesthetic block can be performed to help differentiate between pain of central or peripheral origin.

Infusions. Intravenous infusions of lidocaine, phentolamine, or opioids may indicate effective pharmacologic therapies for the various syndromes.

Multidisciplinary pain management. A pain team involving psychologists, physicians, physical therapists, occupational therapists, and possibly vocational counselors can be very effective in helping the patient deal with the pain syndrome. Many of the perineal pain syndromes are not amenable to conventional treatment. Invasive technology such as spinal cord stimulators are also not particularly effective in these syndromes.

CASE STUDY

Mrs. C., a 65-year-old woman, presented with a long history of pain in the anus referred, on occasions, to the thighs and perineum. In the last 3 months the pain had been getting worse and was described as a burning sensation. On a verbal analog score the patient's pain on average was at 60/100 and when at its worst, 100/100. There was no history of any precipitating events. She had had six children, all of whom had been delivered vaginally. The youngest was now 24 years old. She stated that the pain was worsened by sitting and was somewhat eased by lying down or standing. When she walked or strained she got a feeling of discomfort in the perineal region and worried about wetting herself. There was no history of incontinence of feces or urine. She stated that she had firm bowel movements every 2 to 3 days. Straining the stool made the pain worse. There was no history of operations in the past 10 years. The pain was not improved by passing flatus or bending her knees to the chest. On examination there was no obvious cause of her pain. There were no hemorrhoids, and rectal examination was normal. Examination of the vagina revealed mild candidiasis of the cervix. On straining there was no obvious perineal floor descent. Examination of the anus and vagina increased her pain.

Impression Perineal myalgia.

Plan

1. Nortriptyline initially 10 mg q hs, increasing by 10 mg every 3 nights until 40 mg is reached. If the patient is tolerating the medication well, and has no reduction in symptoms, the dosage may be raised by 25 mg every 3 nights, until 100 mg dosage is reached. At this time a blood test can be done to see if this is within therapeutic antidepressant range. The nortriptyline dosage can be revised until antidepressant dosage levels are reached. Care must be taken in the elderly when using tricyclics. Hypotension is a potentially dangerous side effect.

2. Referral to a gynecologist. The gynecologist reported no pathology and a Pap smear was normal. He did not recommend any further investigations at this stage. He blocked the pudendal nerve with no improvement in her symptoms.

The patient returned after 3 weeks stating that she was sleeping better but her pain was unchanged.

Plan

1. Continue nortriptyline until 100 mg q hs is reached.
2. Trial gabapentin 100 mg initially building up slowly as tolerated until 600 mg three times a day.
3. The patient at this time admitted to having significant problems with her grandchildren. The grandchildren were apparently involved in a bitter dispute between the parents. A counselor was suggested to her, and a name of a marriage counselor was given to her to give to her children.

The patient returned in 3 weeks stating that her pain was improved but she was becoming confused. The dosage of nortriptyline at this stage was 75 mg at night and gabapentin 300 mg three times a day. Confusion and sedation appeared once she had increased gabapentin. She stated that the pain was still 60/100. However, it did not go up to the severe 100/100 as previously.

Plan

1. Decrease gabapentin dosage to decrease confusion and sedation. After a period of 2 weeks, the confusion usually eases and sedation often improves, allowing the dosage to be increased again.

After this stage a referral to a pain specialist should be considered. A ganglion impar block, differential spinal, diagnostic infusions, and psychological evaluation may be considered.

Postmastectomy and Post-Breast-Surgery Pain

One in eight women will develop breast cancer, of which roughly 60% will be treated with mastectomy, with or without reconstruction. While cure of disease is of most importance, some of these women, once surgically treated, are left with ill-defined postmastectomy or postreconstruction pain syndromes. The incidence of postmastectomy pain (PMP) may be as high as 28%. The onset of pain ranges from 2 weeks to 6 months. The pain described ranges from mild to intractable and disabling. Most women report abnormal sensation in the axilla and medial aspect of the arm after mastectomy. About 10–64% of women will report phantom breast sensation, of which 80% are painful. If premastectomy pain is present, there is a higher incidence of phantom breast pain.

There are many causes of PMP. The most common explanation is injury to the intercostobrachial nerve after axillary dissection. This results in neuropathic pain in the distribution of this nerve (axilla and medial aspect of arm). Other nerves such as the thoracodorsal, pectoral nerves, and long thoracic nerve may be injured, which may result in neuropathic or myofascial pain because they innervate musculature of the thoracic wall. Nonsurgical causes of nerve injury and pain also exist, such as radiation and metastasis. Cancer metastasis to the ribs should be ruled out if the pain location is on the chest wall.

Chronic pain after breast reconstruction is poorly reported. Women who have breast reconstruction suffer all of the consequences of the postmastectomy patient and may also suffer from the consequences of the reconstruction. It appears that the incidence of pain after reconstruction with autologous tissue is no different than mastectomy without reconstruction. When using implants, however, the incidence of pain may increase. There are many methods of breast reconstruction, which range from reconstruction without the use of implants to tissue expansion and implant use.

Second to arm pain, the most common cause of pain with autologous breast reconstruction without implants is abdominal pain. This is most likely caused by damage to the intercostal nerves that innervate the flap. Patients who report pain after reconstruction with implants usually describe it as sharp pain around the area of the implant. This pain may be due to the fibrosis around the implant with resultant nerve compression. All members of the health care team who treat breast cancer patients must understand the importance of breast reconstruction in the management of breast cancer. The disfigurement of a mastectomy can be devastating to many women, and breast reconstruction can restore body image. Instead of viewing pain as a hindrance to breast reconstruction, medical professionals should investigate the causes of the pain and strive to learn how to better manage the pain by improving the surgical techniques and medical management.

POSTMASTECTOMY PAIN

Postmastectomy pain management is shown in Figure 23-1.

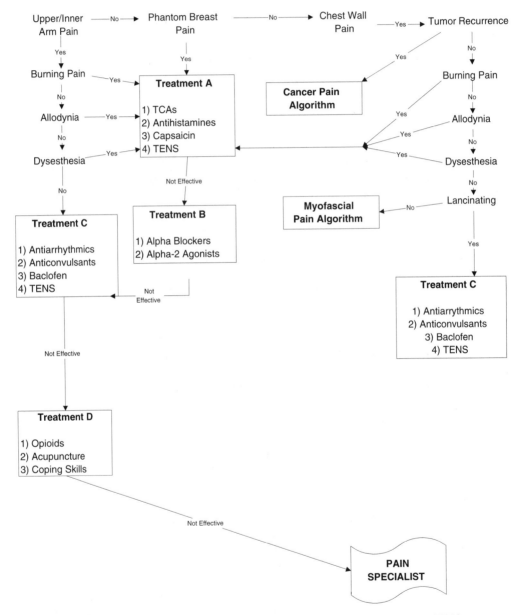

Fig. 23-1. Postmastectomy pain management. TCAs, tricyclic antidepressants; TENS, transcutaneous electrical nerve stimulation.

TREATMENT A

1. Tricyclic Antidepressants (TCAs): Antidepressants may be beneficial in PMP; TCAs are the treatment of choice. Treatment should not be limited to TCAs, as newer antidepressants may be beneficial. The choice of antidepressant depends on the patient's sleep pattern and tolerance. If the patient has disturbed sleep, a more sedating antidepressant such as amitriptyline should be chosen. If no sleep disturbance is present, a less sedating antidepressant such as nortriptyline may be beneficial. Doses up to 150 mg/24 hr have been reported effective. A combination of amitriptyline and fluphenazine may be tried if a TCA alone is ineffective. A 4-week trial of therapy should be attempted before it is determined to be ineffective.
2. Antihistamines: The addition of hydroxyzine at bedtime may improve the patient's symptoms as well as sleep patterns.
3. Capsaicin: Capsaicin cream may be helpful in PMP. Initially, 0.025% capsaicin should be tried. If this dose is unsuccessful, a 0.075% cream can be tried. Initially, this cream may burn after application; however, this symptom will disappear with continued use. As significant depletion of substance P from the peripheral nerve terminals can take up to 3 weeks, treatment must be continued for this minimum period of time before efficacy can be gauged. The patient must use this cream three to four times a day for it to be effective.
4. TENS: A transcutaneous electrical nerve stimulator (TENS) may improve PMP. If no benefit is seen after a week of using different frequencies on a set regimen, it is doubtful that it will be of long-term benefit. (See Fig. 33-1.)

TREATMENT B

1. Alpha-1 blockers: PMP may result from sympathetic instability and may be maintained by the sympathetic nervous system. Because of this, the alpha blockers may be beneficial. The drugs of choice are prazosin, phenoxybenzamine, or terazosin titrated to effect. Significant improvement should be noticed within 2 weeks if this regimen is effective.
2. Alpha-2 agonists: Clonidine may improve PMP by preventing the release of norepinephrine peripherally and inhibiting central pain pathways. Clonidine may be administered orally or by transdermal patch. Significant improvement should be noted within 1 to 2 weeks if this regimen is effective.

TREATMENT C

1. Antiarrhythmics: Mexiletine may be effective in PMP. This drug can be titrated up to a maximum of 10 mg/kg per day. Another antiarrhythmic that may be effective is tocainide. Significant improvement should be noted within 1 to 2 weeks if this drug is effective.
2. Anticonvulsants: Carbamazepine is the current anticonvulsant of choice; however, gabapentin may be a worthwhile first-line drug, as it has a very low side effect profile. Others that may be effective include phenytoin, valproic acid, and clonazepam. Significant improvement should be noted within 1 to 2 weeks if these drugs are effective.
3. Baclofen: Baclofen is an antispasmodic that may be beneficial in neuropathic pain. This drug can be titrated to effect. Significant improvement should be noted within 1 to 2 weeks if the drug is effective.
4. TENS: TENS may improve PMP. If no benefit is seen after a week of using different frequencies on a set regimen, it is doubtful that it will be of long-term benefit. (See Fig. 33-1.)

TREATMENT D

1. Opioids: If the above treatment regimens fail, a trial of low-dose opioids may be beneficial. Neuropathic pain syndromes such as PMP are less responsive to opioid therapy. If

a reasonable dose of opioids is not effective in pain treatment, referral to a pain specialist should be considered.

2. Acupuncture: By central neuromodulation and decreasing local muscle spasm, acupuncture should logically help in PMP. Unfortunately, there are no controlled studies that demonstrate its efficacy.

3. Coping Skills: Inquiry should be made into mood and suicidal ideation. Patients with overt depression or active suicidal thoughts should be referred to a psychiatrist for therapy in conjunction with other therapies. Simple coping skills should be taught and family support encouraged in all instances where they are lacking.

POST-BREAST-RECONSTRUCTION PAIN

Management of pain after breast reconstruction (PBRP) is shown in Figure 23-2.

TREATMENT A

1. Antidepressants: Antidepressants may be beneficial in PBRP; TCAs are the treatment of choice. Treatment should not be limited to the TCAs, as newer antidepressants may be beneficial. The choice of antidepressant depends on the patient's sleep pattern and tolerance. If the patient has disturbed sleep, a more sedating antidepressant such as amitriptyline should be chosen. If no sleep disturbance is present, a less sedating antidepressant such as nortriptyline may be beneficial. Doses up to 150 mg/24 hr have been reported effective. A combination of amitriptyline and fluphenazine may be tried if a TCA alone is ineffective. A 2- to 4-week trial of therapy should be attempted before deciding that it is ineffective.

2. Antihistamines: The addition of hydroxyzine at bedtime may improve the patient's symptoms as well as sleep patterns.

3. Capsaicin: Capsaicin cream may be helpful in PBRP. Initially, 0.025% capsaicin should be tried. If this dose is unsuccessful, a 0.075% cream can be tried. Initially, this cream may burn after application; however, this symptom will disappear with continued use. As significant depletion of substance P from the peripheral nerve terminals can take up to 3 weeks. Treatment must be continued for this minimum period of time before efficacy can be gauged. The patient must use this cream three to four times a day for it to be effective.

4. TENS: TENS may improve PMP. If no benefit is seen after a week of using different frequencies on a set regimen, it is doubtful that it will be of long-term benefit. (See Fig. 33-1.)

TREATMENT B

1. Alpha-1 blockers: PBRP may result from sympathetic instability and may be maintained by the sympathetic nervous system. Because of this, the alpha blockers may be beneficial. The drugs of choice are prazosin, phenoxybenzamine, or terazosin titrated to effect. Significant improvement should be noted within 1 to 2 weeks if this regimen is effective.

2. Alpha-2 agonists: Clonidine may improve PBRP by preventing the release of norepinephrine peripherally and inhibiting central pain pathways. Clonidine may be administered orally or by transdermal patch. Significant improvement should be noted within 1 to 2 weeks if the drug is effective.

TREATMENT C

1. Antiarrhythmics: Mexiletine may be effective in PBRP. This drug can be titrated up to a maximum of 10 mg/kg per day. Another antiarrhythmic that may be effective is tocainide. Significant improvement should be noted within 1 to 2 weeks if this regimen is effective.

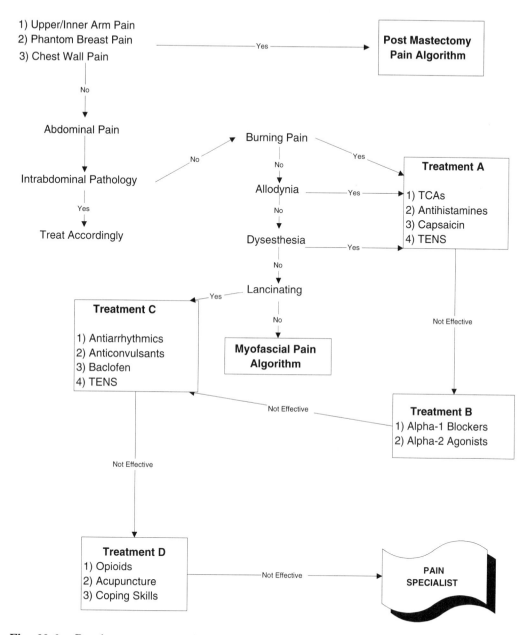

Fig. 23-2. Post-breast-reconstruction pain management. TENS, transcutaneous electrical nerve stimulation.

2. Anticonvulsants: Carbamazepine is the current anticonvulsant of choice; however, gabapentin may be a worthwhile first-line drug, as it has a very low side effect profile. Others that may be effective include phenytoin, valproic acid, and eclonazepam. Significant improvement should be noted within 1 to 2 weeks if the drug is effective.

3. Baclofen: Baclofen is an antispasmodic that may be beneficial in neuropathic pain. This drug can be titrated to effect. Significant improvement should be noted within 1 to 2 weeks if effective.

4. TENS: TENS may improve PBRP. If no benefit is seen after a week of using different frequencies on a set regimen, it is doubtful that it will be of long-term benefit. (See Fig. 33-1.)

TREATMENT D

1. Opioids: If the above treatment regimens fail, a trial of low-dose opioids may be beneficial. Neuropathic pain syndromes such as PBRP are less responsive to opioid therapy. If a reasonable dose of opioids is not effective in pain treatment, referral to a pain specialist should be considered.

2. Acupuncture: By central neuromodulation and decreasing local muscle spasm acupuncture should logically help in PBRP. Unfortunately, there are no controlled studies that demonstrate its efficacy.

3. Coping Skills: Inquiry should be made into mood and suicidal ideation. Patients with overt depression or active suicidal thoughts should be referred to a psychiatrist for therapy in conjunction with other therapies. Simple coping skills should be taught and family support encouraged in all instances where they are lacking.

PAIN SPECIALIST

If pain persists despite the above regimen, a referral to a pain specialist is indicated. The pain specialist should evaluate the patient both physically and psychologically. Therapies may include:

1. Medication optimization or withdrawal. Frequently, the pain specialist will optimize medications by adjusting doses or trying different combinations. In cases where the excessive or improper use of medications interferes with the patient's ability to function, the pain specialist may withdraw the medications.

2. Diagnostic blocks to evaluate the pain mechanism. Because of the frequent involvement of the various nerves that supply the breast area (or abdominal area in cases of postreconstruction pain), diagnostic nerve blocks may be performed to locate the injured nerve causing the pain. These may include blockade of the intercostobrachial nerve or long thoracic nerve. Sympathetic blockade may be performed to rule out sympathetically mediated pain.

3. Intravenous drug infusions. Pain specialists frequently use intravenous drug infusions to evaluate the response of the pain to various classes of drugs. These include lidocaine, phentolamine, or opioid infusions. These infusions provide the pain specialist with information about the physiologic aspects of the pain and will guide therapy.

4. Stimulatory techniques. If a specific nerve can be identified as the cause of the pain, peripheral nerve stimulation may be beneficial.

5. Multidisciplinary pain management program. This approach involves a group of specialists trained in pain management. Each member of the team addresses specific problems the patient faces. The team usually includes a pain physician, psychologist or psychiatrist, and physical therapist. Other members may include a social worker and vocational rehabilitation counselor. The objectives are to rationalize medication, teach

coping skills, educate, and give vocational guidance where appropriate. The long-term objective is to allow individuals to control their pain and not let the pain control them.

CASE STUDY

Mrs. X is a 45-year-old woman who had a modified radical mastectomy with immediate breast reconstruction for intraductal breast cancer. The reconstruction was performed with a free rectus abdominis flap. The patient had an uneventful surgery and postoperative course. Her skin incisions healed well, and she was extremely happy with her cosmetic result. As the patient recovered from the surgery, she noticed numbness in her axilla and medial aspect of her arm on the side of the operation. Approximately 2 months after surgery, she began noticing pain in this area, which she described as a constant burning pain. The pain increased to the point where even the presence of loose clothing over the painful area increased her pain. The patient also reported intermittent, sharp, shooting pains in an area just above her umbilicus. Although she noticed this pain, it was much less distressing than the pain in her axilla and medial arm. The average visual analog pain score (VAS) was 60/100. The VAS was from 0 (no pain) to 100 (worst pain imaginable). The pain interfered with her sleep. Medications included ibuprofen, 400 mg every 6 hours, and hydrocodone, 5 mg, with acetaminophen, 500 mg every 4 hours, with minimal pain relief. On examination she was mentally alert and in no obvious distress. Light touch in the axilla and medial arm caused severe pain, which lasted for 2 to 3 minutes. Sensory examination of this area showed a decreased sensation to touch, temperature, and pinprick. Palpation of the area above the umbilicus showed sharp pain. Sensory examination was normal.

Impression

1. Postmastectomy pain secondary to intercostobrachial nerve injury.
2. Postreconstruction pain secondary to intercostal neuroma in abdomen.

Plan

1. Increase the hydrocodone to 7.5 mg with acetaminophen and continue on an as-needed basis.
2. Discontinue ibuprofen; it has little efficacy in neuropathic pain.
3. The patient has both an allodynia and lancinating pain. Start a tricyclic antidepressant. If the TCA is not too sedating and the patient continues to complain of pain, add hydroxyzine at bedtime.
4. Start an anticonvulsant such as gabapentin for the lancinating pain.
5. See patient in 10 days.

The patient returned stating that the lancinating and allodynia pain was improved. She still suffered from considerable discomfort in the axillary region. She also stated that her sleep was much improved.

Plan

1. Continue the TCA.
2. Capsaicin cream 0.025% rubbed on the area three times a day for 3 weeks should be tried.
3. TENS unit.
4. See patient in 4 weeks.

The patient returned with no improvement in allodynia. The TENS trial was unsuccessful.

Plan

1. Discontinue the capsaicin.
2. Add prazosin.
3. See patient in 2 weeks.

The patient returned with no improvement in allodynia.

Plan

1. Discontinue the hydrocodone and give a trial of a stronger opioid such as sustained-release morphine, methadone, or fentanyl patch.
2. Start a bowel maintenance regimen.

The above measures should be instituted on a primary care level. If they fail to produce relief, a consultation with a pain specialist should be considered. Early referral is recommended when the usual treatment modalities as outlined above are inadequate.

SUGGESTED READING

Wallace AM, Dobke M, Wallace MS. Breast Pain. In Anesthesia: Biologic Foundations. 1995 (in press)

Wallace MS, Wallace AM, Lee J, Dobke M. Pain after breast surgery: a review of 288 cases. Pain, 1995 (in press)

Post-Thoracotomy Pain

Post-thoracotomy pain (PTP) is a common pain syndrome that occurs after major thoracic surgery. In the immediate postoperative period after thoracic surgery, the pain can be severe but usually resolves in the majority of the patients. However, a significant number will experience long-term post-thoracotomy pain. Reports on the incidence of chronic post-thoracotomy pain at 6 months range from 26% to 67%. Of the patients with persistent pain, 9% to 66% will require medical intervention, and many will be refractory to therapy.

Although the causes of post-thoractomy pain are usually identifiable, treatment can be difficult. The most common cause of pain results from surgical trauma to the intercostal nerve during rib retraction. In most cases, this nerve trauma is unavoidable, as the surgeon requires adequate exposure to perform the surgery. Other causes of pain include scar pain, myofascial pain of the chest wall, and tumor recurrence.

Post-thoracotomy pain that results from intercostal nerve injury is characterized by a burning pain, dysesthesias, and allodynia along the scar. There may also be intermittent lancinating pain. If this characteristic pain is absent, the patient may be suffering from myofascial pain, which is often a dull, deep ache in the chest wall. The surgical scar may develop small neuromas. These neuromas can be located by gently tapping along the scar. When the neuroma is gently tapped, a sharp localized pain will result. Since the majority of thoracotomies are performed for the removal of lung cancer, tumor recurrence should always be ruled out as the cause of the pain.

Management of post-thoracotomy pain is given in Figure 24-1.

TREATMENT PLANS

TREATMENT A

Antidepressants. Antidepressants may be beneficial in PTP; the tricyclic antidepressants (TCAs) are the drugs of choice, but treatment should not be limited to the TCAs, as the newer antidepressants may prove to be advantageous. The choice of antidepressant will depend on the patient's sleep pattern and tolerance. If the patient has disturbed sleep, a more sedating antidepressant such as amitriptyline should be chosen. If no sleep disturbance is present, then a less sedating antidepressant such as nortriptyline may be beneficial. Doses up to 150 mg per 24 hours have been reported effective. A combination of amitriptyline and fluphenazine may be tried if a TCA alone is ineffective. A 2- to 4-week trial of therapy should be attempted before the decision is made that it will be ineffective.

Antihistamines. The addition of hydroxyzine at bedtime may improve the patient's symptoms and also improve sleep.

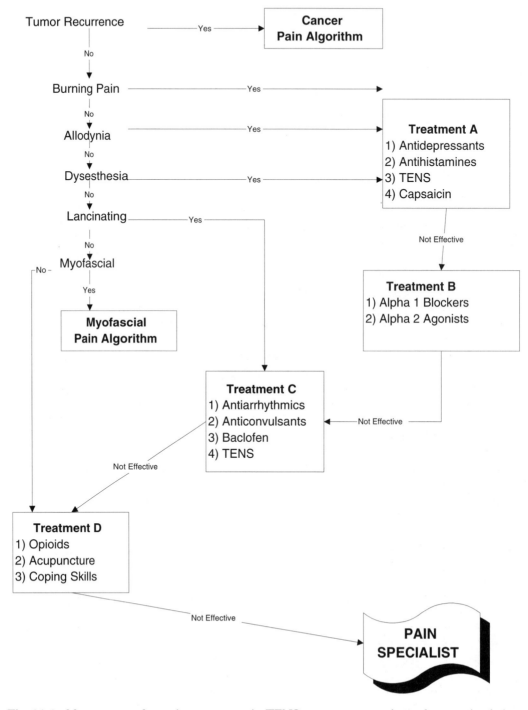

Fig. 24-1. Management of post-thoracotomy pain. TENS, transcutaneous electrcal nerve stimulation.

TENS. A transcutaneous electrical nerve stimulator (TENS) may improve PTP. If no benefit is seen after a week of using different frequencies on a set regimen, it is doubtful that it will be of long-term benefit.

Capsaicin. Capsaicin cream may be helpful in PTP. It is suggested that initially 0.025% capsaicin be tried. If this is unsuccessful, then a 0.075% cream can be tried. After the first applications, this cream may burn, but this will disappear with continued use. As significant depletion of substance P from the peripheral nerve terminals takes up to 3 weeks, treatment must be continued for this minimum period of time before efficacy can be gauged. The patient must use this cream 3 to 4 times per day for it to be effective.

TREATMENT B

Alpha-1 blocker. PTP may result from sympathetic instability and may be fed by the sympathetic nervous system. Because of this, the alpha blockers may be beneficial. The drugs of choice are prazosin, phenoxybenzamine, or terazosin titrated to effect. Significant improvement should be noticed within 1 to 2 weeks if effective.

Alpha-2 agonists. Clonidine may improve PTP by preventing the release of norepinephrine peripherally and central inhibition of pain pathways. Clonidine may be administered via the oral route or transdermal patch. Significant improvement should be noticed within 1 to 2 weeks if effective.

TREATMENT C

Antiarrhythmic agents. Mexiletine may be effective in PTP; it can be titrated up to a maximum of 10 mg/kg per day. Tocanide is another antiarrhythmic drug that may be effective. Significant improvement should be noticed within 1 to 2 weeks if these agents are effective.

Anticonvulsants. Carbamazepine is the current anticonvulsant of choice; however, gabapentin may be a worthwhile first-line drug, as it has a very low side effect profile. Others that may be effective are phenytoin, valproic acid, and clonazepam. Significant improvement should be noticed within 1 to 2 weeks if these drugs are effective.

Baclofen. Baclofen is an antispasmodic agent that may be of benefit in neuropathic pain. This drug can be titrated to effect, and significant improvement should be noticed within 1 to 2 weeks.

TENS. TENS may improve PTP. If no benefit is seen after a week of using different frequencies on a set regimen, it is doubtful that it will be of long-term benefit.

TREATMENT D

Opioids. If the above treatment regimens fail, then a trial of low-dose opioids may be of benefit. Unfortunately, neuropathic pain syndromes such as PTP are less responsive to opioid therapy. If a reasonable dose of opioids is not effective in pain treatment, then a referral to a pain specialist should be considered.

Acupuncture. By central neuromodulation and decreasing local muscle spasm, acupuncture should logically help in PTP. Unfortunately, there are no controlled studies showing it to be effective.

Coping skills. Inquiry should be made into mood and suicidal ideation. Patients with overt depression or active suicidal thoughts should be referred to a psychiatrist for therapy to run in conjunction with other therapies. Simple coping skills should be taught and family support encouraged in all instances where these are found to be lacking.

PAIN SPECIALIST

If pain persists despite the above regimen, referral to a pain specialist is indicated. The pain specialist should evaluate the patient both physically and psychologically. Therapies may include the following:

Medication optimization or withdrawal. Frequently, the pain specialist will optimize medications by adjusting doses or trying different combinations. In cases where the excessive or improper use of medications interferes with the patient's ability to function, the pain specialist may withdraw the medications.

Diagnostic blocks to evaluate the pain mechanism. Due to the frequent involvement of the intercostal nerve, a diagnostic intercostal nerve block may be performed to locate the injured nerve causing the pain. A long thoracic nerve block may also be performed to rule out involvement of this nerve. Neurolysis may be done if a single nerve is shown to be involved. Sympathetic blockade may be performed to rule out sympathetically mediated pain.

Intravenous drug infusions. Pain specialists frequently use intravenous drug infusions to evaluate the response of the pain to various classes of drugs, including lidocaine, phentolamine, or opioid infusions. These infusions will give the pain specialist information on the physiologic aspects of the pain and will guide therapy.

Stimulatory techniques. Spinal cord stimulation may be beneficial. If a specific nerve can be identified as the cause of the pain, peripheral nerve stimulation may be beneficial. Also, dorsal column nerve stimulation may be beneficial.

A multidisciplinary pain management program. The multidisciplinary approach involves a group of specialists trained in pain management. Each member of the team addresses specific problems the patient faces. The team usually includes a pain physician, psychologist or psychiatrist, and physical therapist. Other members may include a social worker, vocational rehabilitation counselor, and others. The objectives are to rationalize medication, teach coping skills, educate, and give vocational guidance where appropriate. The long-term objective is to allow the individuals to control their pain and not let the pain control them.

CASE STUDY

Mr. X, 60 years old, was diagnosed with adenocarcinoma of his right lung 6 months previously. He underwent a right upper lobectomy for removal of this cancer. He recovered well from his surgery, but approximately 2 months later, he developed chest wall pain around his surgical incision. He had a bone scan that was negative. He presented with continued pain around the surgical incision. He described the pain as constant with intermittent lancinating pain. The skin was very sensitive to touch, and he stated that just the presence of clothing over this area caused pain. On examination, the patient had obvious allodynia around the surgical incision. He had decreased sensation to touch, pinprick, and temperature around the scar. Tapping along the scar produced a lancinating pain that shot around to the front of his chest. He had tried hydrocodone tablets for the pain without any relief. He was presently taking extra strength acetaminophen.

Impression Post-thoractomy pain.

Plan

1. If the acetaminophen is helping the patient, this may be continued on a prn basis.
2. Start a tricyclic antidepressant. If the TCA is not too sedating and the patient continues to complain of pain, add hydroxyzine at bedtime.

3. Start an anticonvulsant such as gabapentin for the lancinating pain.
4. See patient in 10 days.

The patient returned and stated that the lancinating pain was much improved, but the burning pain is persisting. He was unable to increase the TCA beyond 25 mg because of urinary retention.

Plan

1. Try a TCA with less anticholinergic effect, for example, nortriptyline.
2. Capsaicin cream 0.025% rubbed on the area qid for 3 weeks should be tried.
3. Trial a TENS unit.
4. See patient in 10 days and again in 3 weeks.

The patient returns stating that the urinary retention had resolved, and he was able to increase the nortriptyline up to 100 mg. Although his sleeping had improved, he still has considerable burning pain. TENS had not helped.

Plan

1. Discontinue the capsaicin and the TENS. If the TCA is helping the patient sleep, this may be continued even if it is not providing pain relief.
2. Choose one of the following: prazosin, phenoxybenzamine, terazosin, or clonidine.
3. See patient in 10 days.

The patient returned and stated that the pain was much improved, but he still continued to have daily episodes of severe pain.

Plan

1. Add tramadol.

The above measures should be instituted on a primary care level. If they fail to produce relief, a consultation with a pain specialist should be considered. Early referral is recommended when the usual treatment modalities as outlined above are proving inadequate.

SUGGESTED READINGS

Loeser JD: Peripheral nerve disorder (peripheral neuropathies). pp. 211–219. In Bonica JJ (ed): The Management of Pain. Lea & Febiger, Philadelphia, 1990

Wynn-Parry CB, Withrington R: The management of painful peripheral nerve disorders. pp. 395–401. In Melzack R, Wall PD (eds): Textbook of Pain. Churchill Livingstone, New York, 1984

25 | Pregnancy and Chronic Pain

The pregnant chronic pain patient presents a medication management problem because of the drugs the embryo and fetus may be exposed to during treatment. Pregnant patients may suffer from any of the pain problems discussed in this book; however, the management of this patient group is different.

When treating the pregnant chronic pain patient, an emphasis on nonpharmacologic methods of pain control should be tried before resorting to pharmacologic therapy. Please review the chapter on nonpharmacologic therapies when treating the pregnant patient with chronic pain. The algorithms presented in this book can be used for the pregnant pain patient; however, the nonpharmacologic methods presented should be tried first (e.g., physical therapy, TENS, acupuncture, massage). When using transcutaneous electrical nerve stimulation (TENS) therapy, the electrodes should not be placed on the trunk or abdomen, as the effects of electrical stimulation on the fetus is unknown. Table 25-1 lists the drugs used in chronic pain management and the Federal Drug Administration (FDA) recommendations on their use.

Only when the benefits of the drug justify the potential risk to the fetus should pharmacologic therapy be used. Most of the drugs used in chronic pain have no demonstrated teratogenic effect in clinical doses, but some of the drugs have implications for the fetus (Table 25-2).

The nursing mother also presents problems because administered drugs are excreted in the milk and passed to the baby. If medications must be used to control pain, the mother should be advised not to breast feed her child.

Pain management in the pregnant patient is shown in Figure 25-1.

TREATMENT A

If the pain is located on the trunk, TENS therapy should be avoided, as the effects of electrical stimulation of the fetus are unknown. However, other nonpharmacologic methods of pain control may be effective. When using acupuncture, the acupuncturist must avoid electrical stimulation of the needles if they are placed on the trunk. Physical therapy, massage, and psychological counseling may be beneficial.

TREATMENT B

If the pain is located on the head or extremities, TENS therapy may be used if electrode placement is limited to these locations. See Treatment A.

TREATMENT C

If a drug is available in category A of the FDA recommendations for drugs used in pregnancy, this drug should be tried.

Table 25-1. FDA Recommendations for Use in Pregnancy

A	B	C	D	E
None	Meprotaline Cyclobenzamine	Opioids NSAIDS Acetaminophen Tramadol Tricyclics SSRIs Trazadone Venlafaxine Tegretol Phenytoin Clonazepam Gabapentin Mexiletine Tocainide Prazosin Phenoxybenzamine Terazosin Clonidine Hydroxizine Baclofen Dantrolene Carisoprodal Cyclobenzamine Methocarbamol Orphenadrine Fluphenazine Haloperidol Steroids Dextroamphetamine Methylphenidate Sumatriptan Propranolol	Valproic acid	Ergotamine

A. Controlled studies show no risk. Adequate, well-controlled studies in pregnant women have failed to demonstrate risk to the fetus.

B. No evidence of risk in humans. Either animal findings show risk but human findings do not, or, if no adequate human studies have been done, animal findings are negative.

C. Risk cannot be ruled out. Human studies are lacking, and animal studies are either positive for fetal risk or lacking. However, potential benefits may justify the potential risk.

D. Positive evidence of risk. Investigational or postmarketing data show risk to the fetus. Nevertheless, potential benefits may outweigh the potential risk.

E. Contraindicated in pregnancy. Studies in animals or humans, or investigational or postmarketing reports, have shown fetal risk outweighs any possible benefit to the patient.

Table 25-2. Drugs with Special Considerations

Drugs	Precaution
Opioids	Babies born to women on chronic opioid therapy may show withdrawal symptoms shortly after birth.
NSAIDs	NSAIDs should be avoided in late pregnancy because of possible closure of the ductus arteriosus. Also, NSAIDs may increase the incidence of dystocia and delayed parturition.
Steroids	Babies born to women on chronic steroid therapy may show signs of hypoadrenalism.

TREATMENTS D AND E

If a drug from category A fails or is not available, only after the risks/benefits are weighed should a drug in category B or C be used in the pregnant patient. The patient should be educated on the potential risk of the drug to the fetus.

PAIN SPECIALIST

If pain persists despite the above regimen, a referral to a pain specialist is indicated. The pain specialist will evaluate the patient both physically and psychologically. Therapies may include:

1. Medication optimization or withdrawal. Frequently, the pain specialist will optimize medications by adjusting doses or trying different combinations. In cases where the excessive or improper use of medications interferes with the patient's ability to function, the pain specialist may withdraw the medications.
2. Diagnostic nerve blocks to evaluate the pain mechanism.
3. Sympathetic blockade. If the patient responds to sympathetic blockade, a series of blocks may be performed. If pain relief is consistent but short lived, a neurolytic procedure of the sympathetic chain may be performed.
4. Epidural Steroid Injection. If the patient suffers from radicular pain, an epidural steroid series may be helpful. Many women with a pre-existing radiculopathy have worsening of symptoms with pregnancy. An epidural steroid injection series may be a better option than systemic medication therapy and may provide long-term relief until the baby can be delivered. There is a systemic effect of epidural steroids but, since this is short term, there is a negligible effect on the fetus.
5. Differential spinal or epidural injection. If the patient suffers from pain in the trunk or lower extremity, a spinal or epidural injection of local anesthetic can provide information about the pain pathways. If a sensory and motor block does not relieve the patient's pain, the pain is considered centralized.
6. Intraspinal drug therapy. Infusion of opioids, baclofen, or local anesthetics into the intrathecal or epidural space may provide excellent pain relief in selected cases. Intraspinal clonidine holds promise for the treatment of reflex sympathetic dystrophy (RSD). Internalized systems can provide long-term drug therapy with low maternal blood levels. However, there are no reports of the use of intraspinal drug therapy in the pregnant patient.
7. A multidisciplinary pain management program. This approach involves a group of specialists trained in pain management. Each member of the team addresses specific patient problems. The team usually includes a pain physician, psychologist or psychiatrist, and physical therapist. Other members may include a social worker and vocational rehabilitation counselor. The objectives are to rationalize medication, teach coping skills, educate, and give vocational guidance where appropriate. The long-term objective is to allow individuals to control their pain and not let the pain control them.

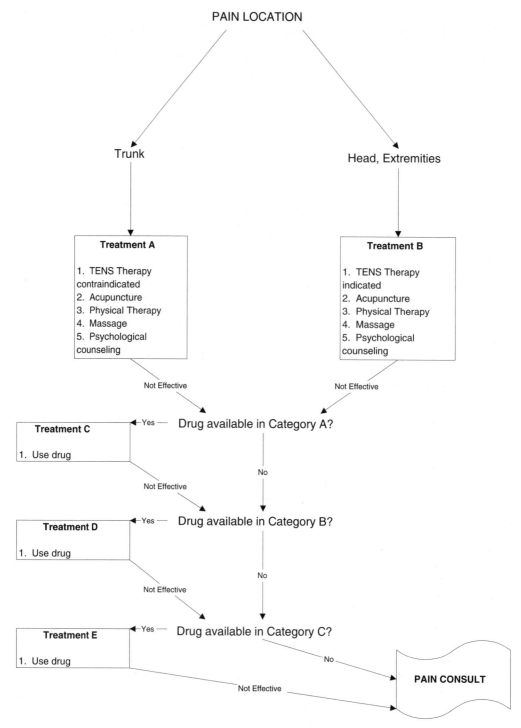

Fig. 25-1. Pain management in the pregnant patient. TENS, transcutaneous electrical nerve stimulation.

CASE STUDY

Mrs. X is a 33-year-old G1P0 who is 8 weeks pregnant. She has suffered from a long history of headaches for which she takes nonsteroidal anti-inflammatory drugs (NSAIDs) and propranolol. On discovery of her pregnancy at 4 weeks, she ceased taking the NSAIDs and propranolol and has since suffered from almost daily headaches. There is no pattern to the headaches, which may occur either day or night. She rates them on a verbal analog score of 70 out of 100 at their worst. There is no aura, flashing lights, or nausea. She has a supportive husband who states that he is occasionally awakened at night by her crying because of the severity of the pain. On examination, multiple trigger points are noted in the muscles at the base of her skull and the temporalis muscles.

Impression   Daily tension-type headache.

Plan

1. TENS therapy to the upper neck and temporalis muscles.
2. Referral to a physical therapist for massage and head and stretching exercises of the neck musculature.

The patient returns to the clinic and states that the headaches have decreased in frequency, but she still suffers from extremely severe episodes approximately twice a week.

Plan

1. Refer for biofeedback therapy.

The patient was taught biofeedback techniques, which helped tremendously. She still suffered from occasional severe exacerbations, which were not relieved with any of the current techniques. Although these episodes were infrequent, she feared them daily and felt helpless because they did not respond to treatment. A physician located near the clinic is trained in acupuncture.

Plan

1. For the severe episode unresponsive to the current techniques, instruct the patient to undergo acupuncture therapy.
2. If the severe episodes occur on the weekends or after clinic hours, instruct the patient to take acetaminophen as needed for the pain on a limited basis.

The patient received acupuncture treatment, which relieved her pain. The patient reported that 500 mg acetaminophen was adequate in relieving the severe episodes when acupuncture was unavailable. She required this dose approximately once per week.

SUGGESTED READING

Physician's desk reference. 48th Ed. Medical Economics, Montvale, NJ, 1995

Reflex Sympathetic Dystrophy

COMPLEX REGIONAL PAIN SYNDROMES I AND II

Reflex sympathetic dystrophy (RSD) is a complex pain syndrome characterized by continuous pain in all or a portion of an extremity that does not involve a major nerve. Causalgia is defined as a burning pain, allodynia, and hyperpathia of the extremity that involves a major nerve. These syndromes usually occur after trauma, but there is no relationship between the severity of the trauma and the development of RSD or causalgia. The syndromes are usually associated with sympathetic hyperactivity, but blockade of the sympathetic nervous system does not always relieve the pain. If sympathetic blockade relieves the pain, the syndrome is termed sympathetically maintained pain (SMP). If sympathetic blockade does not relieve the pain, the syndrome is termed sympathetically independent pain (SIP).

Because of the recognized complexity of this syndrome, the International Association for the Study of Pain has adopted a new classification. Complex regional pain syndrome I (CRPS I) is a pain syndrome as described above that does not involve a nerve injury, and complex regional pain syndrome II (CRPS II) involves a nerve injury. Nerves most commonly affected in CRPS II are the median, ulnar, sciatic, and tibial nerve. Both CRPS I and II can be sympathetically maintained, sympathetic-independent, or a combination of both. Table 26-1 summarizes the diagnostic criteria for this pain syndrome.

Laboratory findings in RSD are inconsistent and depend on the stage of the syndrome. Stage I occurs within the first 2 to 6 months and is characterized by a warm painful area. A bone scan shows increased uptake, and plain films are normal. Stage II occurs within 6 months to a year and is characterized by a painful area that looks fairly normal on physical examination. A bone scan will be normal, and plain films show normal to slight demineralization. Stage III occurs after 1 year and is characterized by a painful cold extremity with severe atrophic changes. The bone scan demonstrates decreased uptake, and a plain film shows severe demineralization.

Due to the complexity of this syndrome, treatment can prove very difficult. If the patient does not respond rapidly to the algorithm presented in this chapter, a pain specialist referral is indicated. Delay in referral can prove detrimental to the long-term outcome.

Management of reflex sympathetic dystrophy pain is shown in Figure 26-1.

TREATMENT PLANS

TREATMENT A

Tricyclic antidepressants. The antidepressants have been demonstrated to be effective for RSD in clinical trials with the tricyclic antidepressants (TCAs) the agents of choice.

Table 26-1. Diagnostic Criteria for Complex Regional Pain Syndrome

Complex regional pain syndrome I (RSD)
  1. History of initiating injury or immobilization
  2. Continuing pain, allodynia, or hyperalgesia out of proportion to the initiating event.
  3. Evidence at some time of edema, changes in skin blood flow or abnormal pseudomotor activity in the painful area.
  4. No other cause of the pain exists.
  Criteria 2 to 4 must *be satisfied.*

Complex regional pain syndrome II (causalgia)
  1. Presence of continuing pain, allodynia, or hyperalgesia after nerve injury, not necessarily limited to the distribution of the nerve.
  2. Evidence of edema, blood flow changes, or abnormal pseudomotor activity in the region of the pain.
  3. Diagnosis excluded by other conditions that would cause similar degree of pain and dysfunction.
  All 3 criteria must be satisfied.

Although the TCAs have been proven effective in clinical trials, treatment should not be limited to these as the newer antidepressants may prove to be beneficial. The choice of the antidepressant will depend on the patient's sleep pattern and tolerance. If the patient has disturbed sleep, a more sedating antidepressant such as amitriptyline should be chosen. If no sleep disturbance is present, then a less sedating antidepressant such as nortriptyline may be beneficial. Doses up to 150 mg per 24 hours have been reported effective. A combination of amitriptyline and fluphenazine may be tried if a TCA alone is ineffective. A 4-week trial of therapy should be attempted before the decision is made that it will be ineffective.

Antihistamines. The addition of hydroxyzine at bedtime may improve the patient's symptoms and also improve sleep.

TENS. A transcutaneous electrical nerve stimulator (TENS) may improve the pain of RSD, but this method will worsen the symptoms if placed over the areas of allodynia. If the patient suffers from a severe sensory deficit, more proximal placement may prove helpful. If no benefit is seen after a week of using different frequencies on a set regimen, it is doubtful that it will be of long-term benefit.

Capsaicin. Capsaicin cream may be helpful in RSD. It is suggested that initially 0.025% capsaicin be tried. If this is tolerated, then a 0.075% cream can be tried. Initially, this cream may burn after application; however, this will usually disappear with continued use. As significant depletion of substance P from the peripheral nerve terminals takes up to 3 weeks, treatment must be continued for this minimum period of time before efficacy can be gauged. The patient must use this cream 3 to 4 times per day in order to be effective.

Physical therapy. The objective of therapy in RSD is to maintain a level of comfort for the patient so that he or she can commence exercising the affected part. Exercising the tissue appears to diminish the pain syndrome, sometimes to extinction. Physical therapy (PT) should therefore be used early in the treatment of RSD. The patient's pain is often exacerbated with movement; therefore, he or she will limit movement to protect the limb and decrease the pain. This limited movement may result in joint, ligament, and tendon contractures. The patient must be educated on the importance of exercise and informed that hurt does not mean harm. Initially, the exercises will be painful but as the therapy pro-

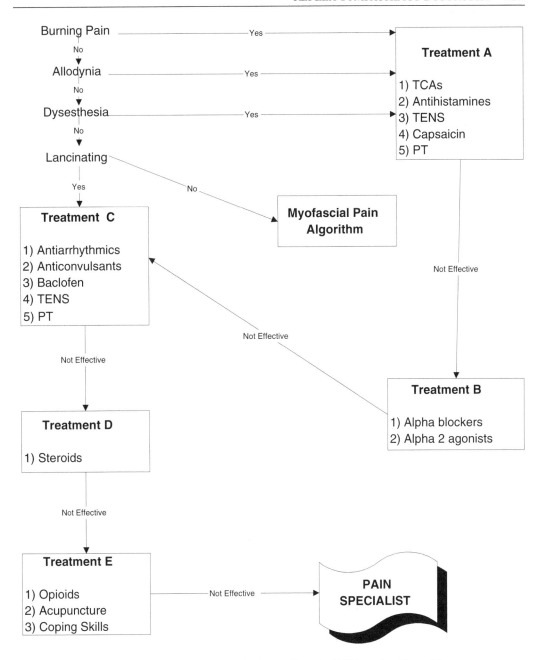

Fig. 26-1. Management of reflex sympathetic dystrophy pain. TCAs, tricyclic antidepressants; TENS, transcutaneous electrical nerve stimulator; PT, physical therapy.

gresses, the pain should decrease. A simple method of exercise is to instruct the patient to use a scrubbing brush in the affected hand. The brush should be held in the hand and the brush placed on a low, flat surface. Keeping the elbow straight and putting pressure on the brush by leaning over it, the patient should "scrub" the surface lightly for 1 minute twice a day, the first day. This should increase by 1 minute a session to 5 minutes twice a day. The hand will swell, and the pain initially will get worse. If the patient can tolerate it (daily encouragement should be given), by day 10 the patient may remark that he or she is sleeping better and the pain is not as bad. At this stage, the patient should continue to "scrub" daily but add carrying a bag in that hand for as long as tolerated. This may be a plastic bag, initially with minimal weight, but the weight should be increased as tolerated. This stressing of the tissue by compression (scrubbing) and distraction (carrying a bag) after 3 to 4 weeks will allow more specific physical therapy of the hand to be carried out successfully. If therapy is severely limited secondary to the pain, a referral to a pain specialist should be made to discuss the possibility of performing nerve blocks (continuous by a catheter or intermittently) in conjunction with PT.

TREATMENT B

Alpha-1 blockers. RSD often results from sympathetic instability and may be sustained by the sympathetic nervous system. Because of this, the alpha blockers may be beneficial. The drugs of choice are prazosin, phenoxybenzamine, or terazosin titrated to effect. Significant improvement should be noticed within 1 to 2 weeks if the drug is effective.

Alpha-2 agonists. Clonidine may improve the pain of RSD but by a different action from the alpha blockers. Prazosin and phenoxybenzamine block the action of norepinephrine on peripheral nerves, and clonidine prevents the release of norepinephrine peripherally and acts on the inhibitory pathway centrally. Clonidine may be administered orally or transdermally. Significant improvement should be noticed within 1 to 2 weeks if the drug is effective. Clonidine is ineffective in the presence of a TCA.

TREATMENT C

Antiarrythmic agents. Mexiletine may be effective for RSD. This drug can be titrated up to a maximum of 10 mg/kg per day. Tocanide is another antiarrhythmic drug that may be effective. Significant improvement should be noticed within 1 to 2 weeks if these agents are effective.

Anticonvulsants. Carbamazepine is currently the anticonvulsant of choice. However, the newer anticonvulsant gabapentin may prove more effective, as it lacks many of the side effects of the older drugs. Phenytoin and valproic acid may also be effective. Clonazepam has also been used with some success for neuropathic pain. Significant improvement should be noticed within 1 to 2 weeks if these agents are effective.

Baclofen. Baclofen is an antispasmodic agent that may be of benefit in neuropathic pain. This drug can be titrated to effect. Significant improvement should be noticed within 1 to 2 weeks if it is effective.

TENS. TENS may improve the pain of RSD, but this method will worsen the symptoms if placed over the areas of allodynia. If the patient suffers from a severe sensory deficit, more proximal placement may prove helpful. If no benefit is seen after a week of using different frequencies on a set regimen, it is doubtful that it will be of long-term benefit.

PT. PT should be used early in the treatment of RSD. The patient's pain is often exacerbated with movement; therefore, he or she will limit movement to protect the limb and decrease the pain. This limited movement may result in joint, ligament, and tendon contractures. The patient must be educated on the importance of PT and informed that hurt does not mean harm. Initially, the PT will be painful but as the therapy progresses, the pain should decrease. If therapy is severely limited secondary to the pain, a referral to a pain specialist should be made to discuss the possibility of performing nerve blocks (continuous by a catheter or intermittently) in conjunction with PT.

TREATMENT D

Steroids. The use of steroids in the treatment of RSD is controversial. A short course of steroids may prove beneficial in an acute exacerbation of the pain.

TREATMENT E

Opioids. If the above treatment regimens fail, a trial of low-dose opioids may be of benefit. Keep in mind that neuropathic pain syndromes such as RSD are less responsive to opioid therapy. If a reasonable dose of opioids is not effective in pain treatment, a referral to a pain specialist should be considered.

Acupuncture. By central neuromodulation and decreasing local muscle spasm, acupuncture should logically help in CRPS I. Unfortunately, there are no controlled studies showing it to be effective.

Coping skills. Inquiry should be made into mood and suicidal ideation. Patients with overt depression or active suicidal thoughts should be referred to a psychiatrist for therapy to run in conjunction with other therapies. Simple coping skills should be taught and family support encouraged in all instances where these are found to be lacking.

PAIN SPECIALIST

If pain persists despite the above regimen, a referral to a pain specialist is indicated. The pain specialist will evaluate the patient both physically and psychologically. Therapies may include the following.

Medication optimization or withdrawal. Frequently, the pain specialist will optimize medications by adjusting doses or trying different combinations. In cases where the excessive or improper use of medications interferes with the patient's ability to function, the pain specialist may withdraw the medications.

Diagnostic nerve blocks to evaluate the pain mechanism. Peripheral nerve blocks can be very helpful in differentiating CRPS I and CRPS II. Response to peripheral nerve block is also helpful in predicting response to peripheral nerve stimulation.

Sympathetic blockade. A sympathetic block is routine in the diagnosis of RSD. If the patient responds to sympathetic blockade, then a series of blocks may be performed. If pain relief is consistent but short-lived, a neurolytic procedure of the sympathetic chain may be performed.

Intravenous drug infusions. Pain specialists frequently use intravenous drug infusions to determine what type of drug the pain responds to. These infusions include lidocaine, phentolamine, or opioids. These infusions will give the pain specialist information on the physiologic aspects of the pain and will guide therapy.

Differential spinal or epidural block. If the patient suffers from pain in the trunk or lower extremity, a spinal or epidural injection of local anesthetic can provide information on the pain pathways. If a sensory and motor block results in the painful area without relieving the patient's pain, the pain is considered centralized.

Peripheral nerve stimulation. If conservative therapies have failed and the patient has at least a 75% reduction in pain with a peripheral nerve block, a peripheral nerve stimulator may be effective.

Spinal cord stimulation. Patients who suffer from pain in the extremities may benefit from spinal cord stimulation. If the pain responds to a single peripheral nerve block (CRPS type II), a peripheral nerve stimulator is probably more appropriate.

Intraspinal drug therapy. Infusion of opioids, baclofen, or local anesthetics into the intrathecal or epidural space may provide excellent pain relief in selected cases. Intraspinal clonidine holds promise for the treatment of CPRS I&II. Internalized systems can provide long-term drug therapy.

A multidisciplinary pain management program. The multidisciplinary approach involves a group of specialists trained in pain management. Each member of the team addresses specific problems the patient faces. The team usually includes a pain physician, psychologist or psychiatrist, and physical therapist. Other members may include a social worker, vocational rehabilitation counselor, and others. The objectives are to rationalize medication, teach coping skills, educate, and give vocational guidance where appropriate. The long-term objective is to allow the individuals to control their pain and not let the pain control them.

CASE STUDY

A 35-year-old male construction worker sustained an injury to his right foot as the result of a pneumatic sand blaster striking the foot. The injury resulted in multiple fractures of the metatarsals requiring surgical repair, which was performed uneventfully. Two months later, the patient complained of a continuous burning pain in the entire foot. He stated that light touch was extremely painful and refused to wear a sock or shoe on the foot. Examination revealed a well-healed surgical scar and a warm, swollen foot. There is no evidence of infection. The patient was concerned about his job and was considering suing the company for negligence. He was currently taking ibuprofen and 10 to 12 hydrocodone tablets with acetaminophen a day.

Impression   Possible complex regional pain syndrome type I.

Plan

1. Stop the ibuprofen, as NSAIDs have little efficacy.
2. Start a tricyclic antidepressant. If the TCA is not too sedating and the patient continues to complain of pain, instruct the patient to add hydroxyzine at bedtime.
3. Instruct the patient to try and decrease the opioid and acetaminophen to no more than 8 per day.
4. Refer for physical therapy.

Patient returns and states that he has noticed some decrease in his pain but still requires some more pain relief. He is continuing to take 10 to 12 of the opioid/acetaminophen preparation per day. He did not follow up with the physical therapy because the first session was too painful.

Plan

1. Continue the above medications.
2. Consider referring to a pain specialist for nerve blocks to be performed in conjunction with physical therapy.
3. Add an alpha blocker or clonidine.
4. Trial of capsaicin cream 0.025% rubbed on the area qid for 3 weeks should be tried.
5. Trial a TENS unit.

Patient returns and states that 3 weeks of capsaicin cream therapy has not proved effective. He is continuing to use the TENS unit with some success. He was referred to a pain specialist who performed a sympathetic block, which enabled him to tolerate physical therapy. He noticed some improvement with the clonidine; however, he continues to take 10 to 12 of the opioid preparation a day. He states that his employer is pressuring him to return to work, and he has decided to pursue litigation against the company.

Plan

1. Discontinue the capsaicin.
2. Continue the TENS.
3. Consider replacing the hydrocodone/acetaminophen preparation with a longer acting opioid such as sustained release morphine or methadone.
4. Remember that the patient may have secondary gain with the pending litigation. However, this should not hinder treatment. At this point, a referral to a psychologist may be necessary to help the patient cope with the pain and his anger.

The patient was referred to a local psychologist who taught him coping skills and relaxation techniques. The patient stated that his burning pain was decreased, but he was developing dysesthesias in the area. He was on a stable dose of methadone and had actually decreased the dose from the previous visit.

Plan

1. Continue treatment as is.
2. Add gabapentin.

The above measures should be instituted on a primary care level. If they fail to produce relief, a consultation with a pain specialist should be considered. As a general rule, results of therapy are much poorer for any chronic pain condition that lasts longer than 6 months before adequate therapy is instituted. Early referral is therefore recommended.

SUGGESTED READINGS

Bonica JJ: Causalgia and other reflex sympathetic dystrophies. pp. 220–243. In: The Management of Pain. Lea & Febiger, Philadelphia, 1990

Campbell JN, Raja SN, Selig AJ, Belzberg AJ, Meyer RA: Diagnosis and management of sympathetically maintained pain. Prog Pain Res Manage 1:85–100, 1994

Sickle Cell Anemia

Sickle cell anemia is an inherited disorder characterized by the presence of hemoglobin S, which causes red blood cell sickling in the presence of decreased oxygen tension. The sickled red blood cells cause sludging within the microcirculation, which leads to vaso-occlusive disorders that can cause severe pain at multiple sites within the body (sickle cell crisis).

Sickle cell anemia is most prevalent among African-Americans (1 in 400 to 600) and Hispanics (1 in 1,500 to 2,000). Homozygotes for hemoglobin S will manifest clinical sickle cell anemia. Causes of sickle cell crisis include hypothermia, dehydration, exertion, hypoxemia, acidosis, and bacterial or viral infections. However, it is difficult to predict when a sickle cell crisis will occur.

Sickle cell patients manifest both acute and chronic pain. The acute pain occurs with each sickle cell crisis and is located in virtually any site of the body. The acute painful episodes of sickle cell crisis may vary greatly in severity and duration and may last from a few hours to 3 to 5 days. The most common sites of the pain are the abdomen, low back, and extremities (mainly the joints). The pain may be associated with redness and swelling of the joints.

Chronic pain may also accompany the thrombotic infarctions that may occur with each sickle cell crisis. These infarctions affect visceral organs, vertebrae, and the femoral head, which may lead to chronic abdominal pain, vertebral compression fracture causing low back pain, or aseptic necrosis of the femoral head causing hip pain. Chronic hemolysis may also lead to pigmented gallstones and chronic cholecystitis.

Unfortunately, the frequent medical attention that these patients require may result in misunderstandings between the medical system and the patients. These patients may be mistaken for malingerers and drug seekers and are sometimes inadequately treated. Their disease often results in psychological problems that should be identified and addressed, but should not be a reason for withholding pain management.

In the past, most cases of sickle cell crisis have been managed in a hospital environment. However, with the advent of home health care, it is now possible to manage this problem in the patient's home. Every effort should be made to manage the crisis in the patient's home if skilled nursing is available. The management of sickle cell anemia is presented in Figure 27-1.

TREATMENT PLANS

TREATMENT A

Hydration. Adequate hydration should always be instituted in sickle cell crisis. The route of hydration will depend on the severity of the crisis. In mild crises, oral hydration should be adequate. However, in severe crises, intravenous hydration should be used. Adequate hydration creates hemodilution to reverse vascular sludging and protects the kidneys against hemolysis.

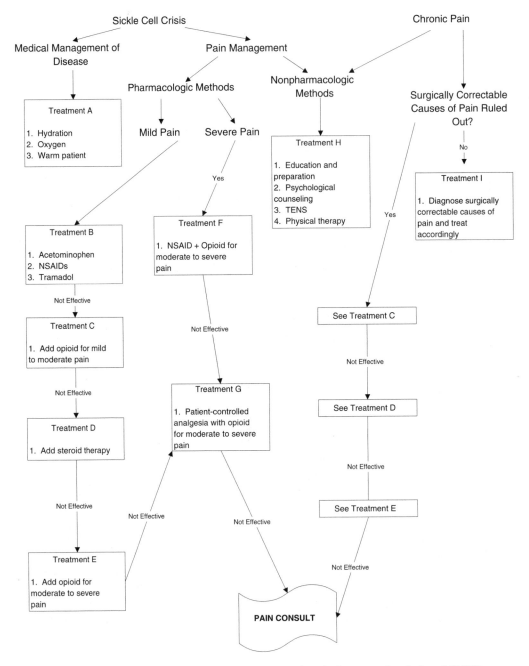

Fig. 27-1. Sickle cell anemia. TENS, transcutaneous electrical nerve stimulation; NSAIDs, nonsteroidal anti-inflammatory drugs.

Oxygen. The severity of the crisis will determine whether supplemental oxygen is indicated. It is controversial whether supplemental oxygen is useful in the absence of hypoxemia. However, in severe cases, it is useful and indicated.

Warmth. Peripheral hypothermia (i.e., in the extremities) causes vasoconstriction and lower affinity of hemoglobin for oxygen, which can lead to further sickling. Therefore, the patient with sickle cell crisis should be kept warm.

TREATMENT B

Analgesics. The pain of sickle cell crisis is nociceptive in origin and therefore should be sensitive to opioid and nonopioid analgesics. Acetaminophen and nonsteroidal anti-inflammatory drugs (NSAIDs) are clearly the agents of choice in mild to moderate sickle cell crisis. The newer analgesic, tramadol, may also prove very useful for sickle cell crisis. Keep in mind that patients with sickle cell disease may have underlying renal impairment and caution should be excercised when using the NSAIDs. If these agents are not enough for adequate pain relief, ketorolac 15–30 mg, IV or IM, may be added every 6 hours.

TREATMENT C

Opioids. If treatments A and B are not effective, then the addition of an opioid for mild to moderate pain should be added, for example, codeine, hydrocodone, or oxycodone preparations.

TREATMENT D

Corticosteroids. There have been reports that the use of systemic steroids are beneficial in the treatment of sickle cell crisis. These should be administered during the crisis and then tapered off.

TREATMENT E

Opioids. If treatments A and B are not effective, the weak opioid should be replaced with an opioid for moderate to severe pain. A long-acting opioid should be used on a time-contingent basis with a short-acting opioid used for breakthrough pain.

TREATMENT F

NSAIDs plus opioids. Severe pain in sickle cell crisis should be aggressively managed with the NSAIDs plus a strong opioid.

TREATMENT G

Patient-controlled analgesia. If the above measures fail, the patient may be a candidate for patient-controlled analgesia (PCA). This can be achieved using either an intravenous or subcutaneous method of delivery (see Ch. 3 on opioids). This method can be instituted in the patient's home with the help of a home health care agency.

TREATMENT H

Education. With any chronic or recurring pain condition, patient education can be very effective. The patients should be educated about their disease, prevention of crises, the drugs used for pain management, and proper utilization of the drugs.

Coping skills. Since stress can lead to a sickle cell crisis, psychological counseling can be very effective in pain management. The psychologist can teach coping skills, relaxation, and biofeedback techniques.

TENS. Transcutaneous electrical nerve stimulation (TENS) has proved very useful in acute sickle cell crises localized to a specific area—for example, a joint. However, due to the multiple anatomic sites of the pain in sickle cell crisis, TENS may be of little benefit.

Physical therapy. Physical therapy for sickle cell crisis differs from traditional techniques used for chronic pain syndromes. The use of passive techniques such as mild excercise, splinting, and the local application of heat may be useful.

TREATMENT I

Chronic pain resulting from sickle cell anemia frequently has surgically correctable causes, such as chronic cholecystitis, aseptic femoral necrosis, and fractures. Therefore, when the sickle cell patient complains of pain in the absence of sickle cell crisis, a workup should be performed to rule out these causes. Once these causes have been ruled out, pain management is similiar to the treatment of the acute episodes.

PAIN SPECIALIST

If pain persists despite the above regimen, a referral to a pain specialist is indicated. The pain specialist will evaluate the patient both physically and psychologically. Therapies may include the following:

Medication optimization or withdrawal. Frequently, the pain specialist will optimize medications by adjusting doses or trying different combinations. In cases where the excessive or improper use of medications interferes with the patient's ability to function, the pain specialist may withdraw the medications.

Regional blockade techniques. The use of regional anesthesia in sickle cell crisis has not been extensively studied, although it has a theoretical advantage. The use of epidural anesthesia for back and lower extremity pain may be useful. If a lumbar sympathetic block with local anesthetic is successful in relieving pain, the patient may be a candidate for neurolysis.

A multidisciplinary pain management program. The multidisciplinary approach involves a group of specialists trained in pain management. Each member of the team addresses specific problems the patient faces. The team usually includes a pain physician, psychologist or psychiatrist, and physical therapist. Other members may include a social worker, vocational rehabilitation counselor, and others. The objectives are to rationalize medication, teach coping skills, educate, and give vocational guidance where appropriate. The long-term objective is to allow the individuals to control their pain and not let the pain control them.

CASE STUDY

The patient is an 8-year-old black boy who presented complaining of low back, abdominal, and bilateral knee pain. He was in the office 1 week earlier complaining of nasal congestion, sore throat, and a cough. At that time he was diagnosed with an upper respiratory infection and had no signs of sickle cell crisis. He was sent home on decongestants and ordered to drink a lot of fluids. His temperature was 101.5°F. He rated his pain as a 40 of 100. His mother had given him acetaminophen for the pain, which was ineffective.

Impression   Sickle cell crisis.

Plan

1. Since the acetaminophen was ineffective, start an NSAID.
2. Since the patient is capable of taking oral fluids, continue to hydrate orally.

3. If the NSAIDs are inadequate, instruct the patient to add tramadol every 6 hours as needed.
4. Educate the patient about the disease and the causes and plans for managing the pain.

The patient returned the following day stating that his pain had increased to a 50–60 of 100. He noticed an improvement in the pain with each NSAID taken, but the pain relief was inadequate. He did not notice any improvement with the tramadol. He was capable of drinking plenty of fluids and was urinating well.

Plan

1. Discontinue the tramadol.
2. Continue the NSAIDs.
3. Add an opioid for mild to moderate pain to be taken as needed for inadequate pain relief.

The patient's mother called the office and stated that her son's pain was worsening. He was afebrile and still continued to drink plenty of fluids with no problem.

Plan

1. Add a steroid.

The patient recovered from this episode of sickle cell crisis. Over the next 5 years the patient had approximately five crises per year, with a couple of them requiring home intravenous PCA therapy and one hospital admission for dehydration. With each crisis, the patient continued to complain of increasing abdominal pain, which did not resolve with the resolution of the crisis. The mother was concerned that it was becoming more and more difficult to wean the patient off the opioids with each crisis due to the pain.

Plan

1. Surgical consultation.
2. Continue the patient on the opioids until surgically correctable causes of the pain can be ruled out.

The surgeon determined that the patient had an enlarged tender spleen possibly as a result of recurrent splenic infarcts. He recommended that the patient have his spleen removed. After the spleen was removed, the abdominal pain resolved. The patient continued to have recurrent sickle cell crisis, with most of them being managed at home. Because of concerns over the development of poor coping skills, the patient and his family were referred to a psychologist, who worked with the patient and his family. The patient was taught coping skills and relaxation techniques, and the family underwent counseling to improve their understanding of what the patient was experiencing. He eventually joined a sickle cell anemia support group.

SUGGESTED READINGS

Lewis MS, Stratton Hill C, Warfield CA: Medical disease causing pain. pp. 329–342. In Raj PP (ed): Practical Management of Pain. Mosby Year Book, St. Louis, 1992
Weisman SJ, Schechter NL: Sickle cell anemia: pain management. pp. 508–516. In Sinatra RS, Hord AH, Ginsberg B, Preble LM (eds): Acute Pain Mechanisms and Management. Mosby Year Book, St. Louis, 1992

Spasticity

Spasticity is defined as a disorder of motor control caused in part by a reduction in cortical influences on the spinal cord. It is characterized by weakness, impaired coordination, increased motor tone, increased tendon jerks, and release of cutaneomuscular reflexes such as the Babinski response. It is a syndrome, not a disease, and its features may not be the same even if the underlying cause appears to be identical.

When examining muscle tone, the patient should be placed in a supine, comfortable position for 5 to 10 minutes. This makes it easier to determine the extent of muscle tightness, spontaneous spasms, and involuntary movement.

Simple scales can be used to document muscle tone, spasms, and hygiene score (Tables 28-1 to 28-3).

Painful spasticity may occur secondary to injuries of the central nervous system (CNS) (e.g., multiple sclerosis, stroke, spinal cord trauma, and head injury). Although some degree of spasticity may be utilized by paraplegics for most activities of daily living, uncontrolled spasms often interfere with their functioning. Patients with spinal cord injury may develop adductor spasms, which interfere with their toiletry.

The treatment algorithm for spasticity is shown in Figure 28-1.

INTERFERING WITH ACTIVITIES OF DAILY LIVING

TREATMENT A

1. Coping skills. The patient with a significant spinal cord injury often has much anger and resentment. Specially trained social workers and psychologists are important in enabling the individual to cope with self-esteem, affect, mood, and sexual dysfunction. The period of adjustment from being active and healthy to inactive and dependent is often difficult and requires intensive psychotherapy.

Table 28-1. Ashworth Score (1984): Muscle Tone

0	No increase in tone.
1	Slight increase in tone, gives a "catch" when muscle flexed or extended.
2	More marked increase in tone but muscle easily flexed.
3	Considerable increase in tone, passive movement difficult.
4	Affected part rigid in flexion or extension.

Table 28-2. Penn (1981) Score: Muscle Spasms

0	No spasms.
1	Spasms increased by stimulation.
2	Infrequent spasms, less than 1 an hour.
3	Spasms more than 1 an hour.
4	Spasms more than 10 an hour.

2. Environmental modification. Modifications may have to be made to the patient's dwelling place or, in severe cases, the individual may have to be cared for in a specialized institution. Various state agencies and funds can help with these modifications. A center specializing in spinal cord injuries usually has a list of available community services.
3. Orthotics. Various braces and aids are important to help the individual with his or her spasticity problems. An occupational therapist and a trained prosthetist often work closely together to individualize the orthotics for the person. Prolonged sustained stretching of muscles is achieved with splints, serial casting, or orthotic devices.
4. Physical methods.
   a. Repetitive daily passive stretching and range of movement exercises are important.
   b. Relaxation and volitional slow movement performed frequently with or without biofeedback. These use residual segmental reflexes.
   c. Standing with support diminishes early contractions and the stretch reflex excitability.
   d. Various body and head positions in supine, sitting, and standing postures modify muscle hypertonia.
   e. Cooling the muscle may diminish spasticity for several hours.
   f. Twenty minute occlusion of the arterial supply by an external cuff may diminish muscle hypertonia.
5 . Manual or electronic aids. There are many electronic aids and devices including motorized wheelchairs to help the individual become more independent. Computers have been effective in helping the individual get back into successful functioning in society. Computer training may play an important role in rehabilitation.

FIXED JOINT DEFORMITY

In a fixed joint deformity, the joint cannot be straightened even after a motor block with local anesthetic. If the deformity interferes with activities of daily living, especially toiletry, a surgical opinion may be sought and tendolysis of the tendons attaching the muscles or even osteotomies may be necessary.

TREATMENT B

1. Quinine. Mild spasms or cramps especially of the calf muscles, which occur at night, may be effectively treated with quinine, 200 to 300 mg at bedtime.

Table 28-3. Hygiene Score (Adductor Score)

0	Independent with self-care.
1	One person able to clean and catheterize with ease.
2	One person able to clean and catheterize with effort.
3	One person able to clean and catheterize only with major difficulty.
4	Two people able to clean and catheterize easily.
5	Two people able to clean and catheterize with difficulty.

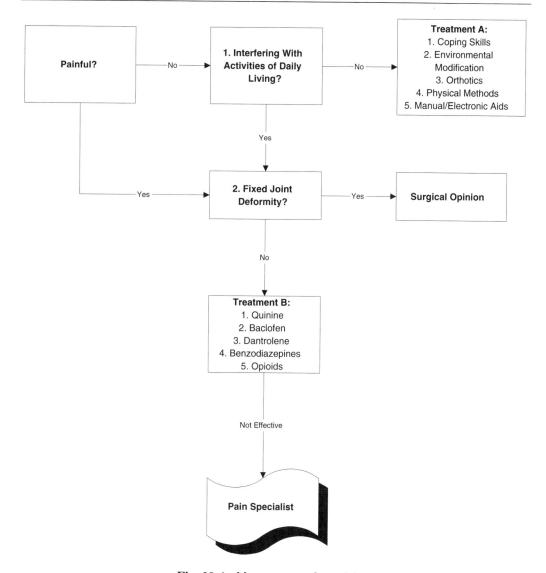

Fig. 28-1. Management of spasticity.

2. Baclofen. Baclofen is only minimally metabolized and is excreted unchanged by the kidneys. The biologic half-life in most patients is 3 to 4 hours. Baclofen acts on both presynaptic and postsynaptic receptors within the CNS. It crosses into the CNS poorly when taken orally, but in some patients it can produce marked alleviation of spasm without generalized muscle weakness. An initial dose of 5 mg twice a day can be increased to 5 mg every 3 days, to a maximum of 20 mg every 6 hours. In many patients, a low dose of 5 to 10 mg four times a day is adequate. Abrupt withdrawal of medication should be avoided, as it may cause a temporary rebound. Discontinuation should be over a period of 2 weeks. Baclofen use is often limited by side effects that include severe drowsiness, insomnia, dizziness, weakness, mental confusion, and gastrointestinal distress.

3. Dantrolene. Dantrolene's main effect is peripheral. It produces generalized muscle weakness. Medication begins with 25 mg a day, increasing cautiously up to 50 mg twice a day. If no benefit is demonstrated within 6 weeks, therapy should be stopped. Major side effects include hepatotoxicity, which should be carefully monitored with regular liver function tests.

4. Benzodiazepines. Diazepam (Valium) is as effective a muscle relaxant as both dantrolene and baclofen. However, its marked side effects of generalized weakness and somnolence limit its usefulness. Many pain practitioners feel that benzodiazepines are contraindicated in the treatment of chronic pain. They may increase pain perception and are highly addictive. Benzodiazepines should probably not be given for chronic spastic disorders, especially those associated with pain, except in small amounts and for short periods of time.

5. Opioids. Severe pain caused by muscle spasms may be ameliorated by use of opioids. Opioids decrease both the incidence of spasms and the pain associated with them.

PAIN SPECIALIST

The pain specialist may try to decrease the muscle spasm by motor blocks with either phenol or botulinum toxin. There is little reported evidence that botulinum toxin, which is extremely expensive, gives longer results than the older and cheaper phenol. It is less painful, however, and does not need as precise a localization of the motor point. Therefore, it is much more convenient for the therapist, especially when dealing with children. If botulinum toxin is used, the dose should be low (< 300 to 350 units) and should not be given more than every 3 months to prevent antibody formation, which lessens its effectiveness. Neurolytic peripheral nerve blocks and intrathecal blocks with phenol and alcohol have also been used with great effectiveness. The effect of the blocks is usually temporary, although with intrathecal blocks it may be permanent. The risk of incontinence with intrathecal blocks must be pointed out to the patient before the procedures are attempted.

Intrathecal catheters infusing baclofen or morphine have been effective in dealing with spasticity of the lower extremities. The implantable pumps infusing the medication may be programmed to increase or decrease the drug. This allows the individual to use the spasticity for functioning during the day and to markedly decrease the spasticity at night to allow a good night's sleep. Spinal cord stimulation may also modify motor control in some patients.

CASE STUDY 1

G.M. was a 3-year-old girl with cerebral palsy (CP) whose parents had recently moved into the area. The child's physical development landmarks had been delayed, but mentally she appeared to have normal intelligence. She was having difficulty standing and sitting upright because of hamstring and calf shortening. Recently, increasing adductor spasm had begun to make changing her diaper difficult. Her mother appeared to be well informed and concerned. One reason she had chosen the new area to live in was because of a local school that catered to children with CP. She was doing passive stretching exercises with the child daily.

Impression   Child with CP. Ashworth Scale 3 of the hamstrings and calves, 4 of the adductors. Penn muscle spasm score 0, hygiene score 2+.

Plan

1. Referral to a physical therapist who works at the CP school for exercises, walking skills, instruction of the mother and father, and advice on orthotics.

2. Social worker referral for exploration of the facilities available for the child and wheelchair possibility at a later stage.

3. School referral for peer group support.
4. Referral to pain center for possible motor point blocks or obturator nerve (adductor muscles) and tibial nerve (calf muscles) phenol block. This to occur once the child is undergoing active physical therapy.

Children with CP require a great deal of aggressive therapy during their early years to allow them to fulfill their potential. This requires expertise that is usually found only in the environs of a CP center or school. The parents are an important factor in motivating and helping these children achieve their goals. Older children with severe spasticity of the lower limbs may be candidates for intrathecal baclofen pumps.

CASE STUDY 2

Mr. C was a 34-year-old paraplegic with a complete lesion at T4. His paraplegia had occurred after a motor vehicle accident 5 years ago. He was fully mobile in a wheelchair and modified van and was working as a computer programmer. One year after his accident, he began to experience a burning pain over his abdomen. With time, this pain progressed to involve the right leg, with severe lancinating pains that caused involuntary spasm, bringing his right leg up toward his chest. These spasms lasted several seconds, occurring several times an hour. They occurred spontaneously and were interfering with his sleep. He had tried over-the-counter anti-inflammatory drugs and had been given an opioid acetaminophen preparation by a friend. The anti-inflammatory drugs were ineffective, but the opioid acetaminophen preparation had helped slightly. In his recent history, he had undergone operations for kidney stones. He had undergone a urinary tract diversion operation and practiced self-catheterization and enema bowel washouts. He was on no medications for pain. On examination, he had a flaccid paraparesis and was insensate below T4. During the history and examination, he had several episodes when his leg flexed at the hip and knee and he was in obviously severe pain for several seconds.

Impression Central dysesthetic pain secondary to muscle spasms. Ashworth Score 1, Penn score 3+, Hygiene Score 0.

Plan

1. Baclofen, 5 mg twice a day, increasing every 3 days by 5 mg every 6 hours, until 20 mg every 6 hours or until significant side effects (usually somnolence) are reached.
2. Tell patient to modify his bed so the foot of the bed is slightly raised. This may diminish autonomic disturbances caused by postural changes.
3. See patient in 3 weeks.

The patient returned and reported that his spasms had decreased in frequency, but he could not take more than 5 mg of baclofen every 6 hours because dizziness and drowsiness interfered with his work. His sleep was still disturbed.

Plan

1. Maintain baclofen at 5 mg every 6 hours.
2. Add 24-hour acetaminophen-opioid combination, increasing to a maximum dose of acetaminophen of 4 g/day.
3. Trial transcutaneous eletrical nerve stimulation (TENS) for his abdominal pain; he should avoid placing the electrodes on the insensate skin.

The patient returned stating the TENS at almost full intensity over his back at the T3-4 level had improved his abdominal pain by 50%. His spasms occurred approximately one to three times an hour and were no longer as painful. His sleep had improved, but he was still frequently awakened with the pain. He still complained of drowsiness, which he considered to be due to the baclofen. He had had to increase his laxatives since starting the opioid-acetaminophen combination.

Plan

1. Stop the acetaminophen-opioid combination medicine, which was at the maximum recommended dosage. As the opioid appeared to be helping, he was started on methadone, 10 mg twice a day, increasing to 20 mg three times a day over the next few weeks. He signed an "opioid contract" before beginning the methadone.

His spasms were controlled to three to four a day on methadone and baclofen for approximately 1 year. Gradually, the combination appeared to be less effective. The baclofen was unable to be increased above 30 mg a day because of excessive drowsiness. Gabapentin, 300 mg three times a day, improved the burning pain over his abdomen but did not help his spasms.

He was referred to a pain specialist and, after successful trialing, had an intrathecal pump placed, which delivered 100 µg of baclofen intrathecally a day. His spasms were well controlled; he had no drowsiness, and he was weaned off his methadone and oral baclofen. The pump was refilled every 3 months and over the next few years, as tolerance occurred, his daily baclofen dose increased to 500 µg/day.

SUGGESTED READING

Bishop B: Spasticity: its physiology and management. Phys Ther 57:371, 1977
Nash J, Nielson PD, Odwyer NJ. Reducing spasticity to control muscle contracture of children with cerebral palsy. Dev Med Child Neurol 31:471, 1980

SECTION III

Psychological aspects of pain management and the difficult pain patient

Psychology of Chronic Pain

Diane M. Novy
David V. Nelson

The most tenable theories for understanding chronic pain acknowledge the role of psychological components (namely, affective, behavioral, and cognitive), not as purely secondary reactions to sensory-physical ones, but as integral parts in the experience of chronic pain (for detailed review of theories of chronic pain see Novy et al., 1995). It follows that potential maladaptive tendencies implicating affect, behavior, and cognition (i.e., thought patterns having to do with appraisals, attitudes, beliefs, and expectancies), in the face of sensory-physical pain, frequently require multidisciplinary treatment. The overall aim of this treatment is improvement of the quality of life, despite pain. This aim is achieved by facilitating adaptive feelings, behaviors, and thoughts about a person's pain.

This chapter discusses potential maladaptive tendencies associated with chronic pain and highlights some treatment strategies, many of which are based on psychological theoretical underpinnings, to target these tendencies. It is hoped that primary care physicians can use implications for their treatment of chronic pain sufferers from our presentation of some treatment strategies. In this chapter we also provide suggestions for the initiation of a referral to a patient for an evaluation and possibly treatment by a pain psychologist/psychiatrist or for a multidisciplinary pain clinic involving these disciplines.

POTENTIAL MALADAPTIVE TENDENCIES ASSOCIATED WITH CHRONIC PAIN

Chronic pain can be associated with negative-affect, pain-related behaviors, and inaccurate cognitions, all of which seem intricately interwoven within the person suffering from pain and also between the person suffering with pain and others in his or her environment. For example, the affective experience can involve loss of control, loss of pleasant activities and sources of self-esteem, and anxieties and anger about further deterioration and loss. Some of these symptoms, which can worsen the perception of pain, are actually criteria of depression (Williams, 1993).

Persons suffering with chronic pain may present with certain pain-related behaviors including excessive rest; disrupted daily activity patterns, characterized either by a general reduction or by recurrent large fluctuations; disrupted social, marital, employment, and recreational activities; overuse of analgesics and of psychotropic drugs; and repeated seeking of medical help even when appropriate modes of treatment have been exhausted (Williams, 1993). These behaviors may become reinforced by environmental contingencies (i.e., association with particular consequences), such as having someone relieve the person in pain of certain chores around the house or of going to work. Also, when a person has a painful condition that flares up in certain circumstances, such as when lifting heavy objects, he or she may begin to avoid these activities. Reactions from others (e.g., in some cases, being highly solicitous of pain behavior without encouraging other behaviors, particularly those that allow the person to become increasingly active) may unwittingly reinforce less adaptive behaviors, which over time become part of the person's typical behavior pattern. Indeed, the person may even begin to describe the pain as having "taken over," such that behavior is governed by the intention of avoiding increased pain. These difficulties often are compounded by the attempt to explain all the behaviors by reference to the original trauma or demonstrable pathology; when this fails, it is not unusual for the patient's distress and distorted behavioral patterns to be attributed (particularly by others) to psychological factors, such as personality or psychopathology, for which the equivalent lay model is that it is "all in the mind" (Williams, 1993). These explanations risk undermining further the person's self-esteem and sense of control. A sense of control may be further eroded by certain cognitive distortions, such as catastrophizing, contemplation of a bleak future, and rumination about the cause of pain. These cognitive distortions can be intricately interwoven with the person's negative affective state and pain-related behaviors.

Alterations in the person's lifestyle, employment status, and family life typically parallel the aforementioned affective, behavioral, and cognitive changes. The following excerpt of a letter from a wife to her husband's psychologist elaborates some of these alterations, particularly his maladaptive attitude:

Whether or not I will be able to visit you again because of my working nights, I don't know but that perhaps if I could explain my husband's attitudes it might help you understand his problems... the questionnaire you gave him to complete and send back became a tremendous ordeal for him. Why, I'll never know, because the questions were simple, but in the state of mind he is in, everything gets to be a chore... since his back operation five years ago he has become increasingly impatient and progressively slower with no ambition at all to even try to help himself. He had made himself an invalid and it has become very difficult for me or my family to tolerate his constant complaining. He blames me, blames our two sons, who he says don't help him around the house when in fact he does little or nothing to help himself. He does exactly the same things day after day with projects he starts and never completes and always because of his health... to dwell on his illness is what he wants and only that he will do, believe me. (Flor and Turk, 1985, p. 268).

PSYCHOLOGICAL STRATEGIES FOR TARGETING MALADAPTIVE TENDENCIES

Obviously, the informed consent of a person needing treatment is required before any treatment can occur. In order to improve the quality of life of a person with chronic pain certain concrete aims must be accomplished. These include increasing physical activity; withdrawing unnecessary medications; decreasing pain-related maladaptive behaviors; increasing well behaviors; and teaching skills for monitoring, challenging, and changing maladaptive thoughts and feelings. Multiple disciplines employing various strategies, many of them psychologically based, for targeting maladaptive tendencies may be needed to carry out these concrete aims of treatments. A few of the commonly used strategies follow; they are summarized in Table 29-1.

Support

It seems likely that any person who is concerned about his or her physical problems along with pain, and who is distressed by disability and its consequences, may be helped by receiving psychological support. Support does not have to come only from psychologists; in

Table 29-1. Psychological Strategies for Targeting Maladaptive Tendencies

Strategy	Purpose Served
Support	Patient feels accepted
Establishing new contingencies	Breaks up maladaptive contingencies
Shaping	Reinforces approximation to desired behavior
Modeling	Provides examples of adaptive behaviors
Relaxation and biofeedback	Helps to reduce overall level of anxiety and pain (directly or indirectly depending on training strategy used)

fact, members of other disciplines typically incorporate support routinely in their overall treatment regime.

Support involves accepting a person, his or her complaints, and the seriousness of his or her condition. It also means recognizing and appreciating the abilities, motivation, and strengths of a person coming for assistance. Support requires providing an explanation for the suffering experienced and offering encouragement. The usual notion of support involves the idea that a person's defenses will not be challenged (Merskey, 1986). However, in working with persons suffering with chronic pain, supportive challenging, in addition to other typical kinds of support, is often needed to facilitate greater adaptation to chronic pain. Thus, we recommend incorporating support in the implementation of the more challenging strategies that follow.

Establishing New Contingencies

Strategies from a psychological theory of learning and behavior (namely, operant-behavior theory as described in Fordyce, 1976) can be useful for establishing new contingencies between physical activities and rest. The typical contingency is usually created unwittingly either by the person suffering with pain and/or by encouragement from others by having the person engage in physical activity (exercise) until he or she reaches a high enough degree of pain or fatigue to require stopping and resting. This cycle of activity/exercise leading to an increase in pain or fatigue and requiring rest only serves to confirm feelings of failure in the person. This pattern also may confirm for the person the dangers of unaccustomed movement and effort, thereby making physical activity an undesirable behavior. The person then tends to avoid the activity completely or forces him or her to endure it for as long as possible.

Our recommendations for an activity regime follow those suggested by Fordyce (1976) and incorporate the fact that a person in pain is likely inactive and easily fatigued. We employ rest as a reinforcement to reward the completion of physical activities. This is done by determining a comfortable baseline of physical activity (a description of the physical activities is given in Ch. 32) in the first 2 days of treatment, and reducing the baseline by 20 to 50% (in some cases the reduction may exceed this) to provide a realistic starting point. This is followed by increases (i.e., new quotas) in the amount of activities or exercise to be done each day. In this way, rest is used as a reinforcement for physical activity, allowing the person to perform the activity we want to decrease (rest) as a reinforcement for the behaviors we wish to increase (physical activity) (Roberts, 1986; Williams, 1993). The benefits (e.g., improved physical conditioning, greater flexibility, and enhanced self-esteem) derived from physical activity provide important evidence against commonly held beliefs that all sensory-physical sensations are unpleasant or signal danger of further physical damage. Obviously, these benefits are reinforcers also, which together with a graded and gradual activity regime change the activity–pain symptoms–rest contingencies to activity–rest, without the symptoms of unduly increased pain.

A related target for a new contingency is the tendency for persons in pain to overdo physical activities periodically and then have subsequent exacerbations of pain and demoralization. To facilitate appropriate pacing (i.e., doing an amount of activity that can be adequately managed), a modest baseline of activity is used at the outset, followed by gradual increases in time and/or difficulty of activity. In this way, activity is time-contingent, rather than pain-contingent. Gains tend to be steady and linked to the person's increasing fitness, strength, and mobility.

Medication usage is another area that has utility for a new contingency. Large numbers of persons suffering with chronic pain take medications (e.g., analgesics, antidepressants, and hypnotics/tranquilizers) according to their perception of pain. Indeed, a large majority of patients seen in multidisciplinary pain centers take opiate analgesics, many in combination with benzodiazepines (prescribed as hypnotics, anxiolytics, or as an attempt to relieve muscle spasms). It is not unusual for these persons to rely highly on these medications, even though they continue to report high levels of pain with concomitant medication side effects such as oversedation or cognitive (reversible) impairment.

Most persons suffering with chronic pain will adhere to a progressive withdrawal schedule for unnecessary drugs, if the schedule is slow enough to minimize withdrawal symptoms. As the unnecessary medications are gradually withdrawn, plain aspirin or plain acetaminophen may be gradually added to the regimen of necessary medications on a time-contingent (i.e., prearranged and regularly scheduled time intervals) rather than a pain-contingent basis (i.e., as-needed or according to the person's perception of pain). Change to a time-contingent schedule breaks up the contingency between pain and medication. When the medications are given on a time-contingent basis, the medication becomes less of an issue, thereby affording the person the opportunity to use and assess his or her own coping skills. Pain reduction can then be attributed to self-made adjustments such as stretching or improved pacing rather than the medication (Roberts, 1986).

Shaping and Modeling

Desired behaviors (e.g., physical activation) can be divided into successive gradual steps that can be taught sequentially. Praise and attention can be used to reward each of these steps so that a person can move on to the next step after he or she has completed the previous one. This type of behavior modification is referred to as shaping and is associated with a new behavior being learned slowly as a person comes closer and closer to approximating the desired level of that behavior (activation) (Roberts, 1986).

A person's environment typically has "models" for adaptive behavior. It is often useful to direct attention to such models. For example, in our pain center, we have an employee who suffers from a chronic pain condition. This employee is able to function well because of his adherence to an exercise program. When this information is shared with patients, the employee serves as a model for adaptive behavior.

Relaxation and Biofeedback

Because of the connection between stress and physiologic processes in producing pain, relaxation and biofeedback often are used to help a person deal with his or her pain. However, rarely is the connection between stress and physiologic processes straightforward; often, antecedent and concurrent cognitions (e.g., attitudes, beliefs, expectancies) play a role. In these cases, identification of the cognitive components must occur so that they may be incorporated into treatment. Having noted this, relaxation has the potential for direct muscular relaxation effects, for reducing generalized arousal, and for utility as a distraction or attention diversion strategy. One particular type of relaxation, progressive muscle relaxation, has achieved popularity for persons suffering with pain. This technique requires the focus of a person's attention on specific muscle groups while alternately tightening and relaxing these muscles. Practice with progressive muscle relaxation and frequent utilization of it have shown promise for reducing overall feelings of stress and anxiety. Additional potential benefits of relaxation are reduction of pain perception and enhancement of sleep (often much needed). Biofeedback procedures are used to teach voluntary control over a bodily function, such as muscle tension, by monitoring its status with information from electronic devices. Biofeedfback and relaxation are often used together so as to enhance the potential benefits.

Cognitive-Behavioral Techniques

Cognitive-behavioral treatment techniques consist of a wide range of strategies and proce-dures designed to bring about alterations in pain sufferers' perceptions about their situa-tions and their ability to execute self-control over their lives. These techniques include cog-nitive distraction or attention diversion and cognitive coping strategy training or restructuring. Exposure to these techniques typically encompasses an educational component, training in the new skill, practice with the new skill, and transfer of the new skill to various settings and situations (Holzman et al., 1986). Education serves dual purposes: first, to convey informa-tional content and answer questions; second, to credit the person with the capacity to understand and use the information.

As was said earlier, persons in pain are often preoccupied with their pain and physical symptomatology in general. It is not unusual for them to be highly focused on internal cues and to perceive new physical sensations as causes for alarm. If distractions from these sen-sations and also pain are not possible, these persons may benefit from exposure to individ-ualized cognitive distraction training. In this training, a distraction that is credible for a particular person is recommended as a focus for a particular time. As an example, for a low back pain sufferer who typically is focused on his pain when driving to work, listening to a stimulating and engaging talk show may serve as a more effective distraction than the music he is accustomed to hearing. Of course, for another person music may be both soothing and distracting. Guided imagery is a related cognitive distraction technique whereby the person tries to alleviate discomfort by conjuring up a mental scene that is incompatible with the pain.

Cognitive restructuring refers to the process of reconceptualization that is often needed to help a person alter negative thoughts and feelings. A person is not told to stop negative thinking, but rather is asked to evaluate the evidence for such thoughts. Often when evi-dence is evaluated, the reality of the situation makes it apparent that the negative thoughts are inaccurate or out of proportion to what they should be. For example, it is not unusual for a person with chronic pain with no evidence of progressive deterioration in physical status to fear ongoing tissue damage. This concern must, of course, be acknowledged; the evidence for the concern, however, also must be evaluated. In so doing, the likely unfounded and illogical concern can be replaced by alternative, realistic thoughts. The person can even be helped to generate a list of accurate statements about his or her condition. With enough rehearsal, practice, and role playing, statements on the accurate list can replace negative thoughts (Holzman, 1986).

AN ILLUSTRATIVE EXAMPLE UTILIZING PSYCHOLOGICAL STRATEGIES FOR TARGETING MALADAPTIVE TENDENCIES

A 30-year-old man was enrolled in our outpatient, 3-week intensive pain management program. He suffered low back pain secondary to a work-related accident which occurred approximately two years ago. He had two lumbar surgeries and passive physical therapy as previous treatments. The patient had been relying on opioid medication among a large array of other medications for pain relief; nonetheless, he reported his pain to be a constant 70 on a 0 to 100 pain scale. The patient presented as excessively deconditioned, anxious, and depressed. He had been unemployed since the accident, and his financial status was a major concern for him and his family. He felt hopeless about returning to work as a truck driver; he had never considered any other type of employment.

At the outset of the program, a great deal of explanation was provided to the patient about our program and about our view of his condition. As a result, he understood his diagnosis and could be active in formulating goals for treatment. He also felt supported and understood, as well as confident and comfortable with us. His goals included greater mobility, reduced anxiety, depression, and hopelessness, and preparation for return to the workforce.

Upon being evaluated by the physical therapist, a comfortable baseline of physical activities was established for the patient. His baseline was reduced by 20% and gradual incremental quotas were set as goals. By so doing, rest was used as a reinforcement for physical activity. The resulting greater flexibility and enhanced self-esteem derived from physical activity provided the patient important evidence against his beliefs that all sensory-physical sensations are unpleasant and associated with an exacerbation of pain. He even vowed to model the example set by certain staff members who walked in a nearby park for half of their lunch hour.

The patient also was receptive to the idea about being tapered off unnecessary medications via a "pain cocktail" (see Chemical Dependence in Ch. 30) (Fordyce, 1976). Although he could have had information about the exact contents of the cocktail, he decided to let us deal with the intricacies of the contents, thereby giving him one less thing to worry about. Over the course of 2 weeks, his opioid and benzodiazepine medications were withdrawn. He remained on 25 mg of amitriptyline at bedtime and one plain aspirin twice daily. Any success he attained in physical therapy and with decreased pain perception, now 40 on a 0 to 100 scale, was credited by the patient to his own efforts and not the medications. Thus, he began to feel better about himself, less depressed, more active and ready to think about employment.

Vocation counseling with the patient resulted in his pursuing employment as a truck dispatcher with his previous employer. His financial concerns were somewhat alleviated, which served to reduce his overall anxiety level. Also useful in regard to his overall level of anxiety were the relaxation skills and training from biofeedback that were part of his intensive pain management treatment.

While this illustrative example may have fallen in place much easier than some other patients with chronic pain dysfunction, the utility of the strategies are the point of emphasis. Clearly, not all patients will respond identically; modifications and adjustments in treatment strategies must be individually tailored.

SUGGESTIONS FOR INITIATING A REFERRAL TO A PAIN PSYCHOLOGIST OR PSYCHIATRIST

The initiation of a referral to a pain psychologist or psychiatrist or a multidisciplinary pain center employing such professionals may be warranted if a person is excessively disabled by pain (e.g., deactivated and demoralized) and has not responded well to primary care treatment. Such a referral can be specifically for treatment recommendations and/or actual treatment. It is important to keep in mind that a person in pain may be very defensive and sensitive to such a referral. Indeed, it frequently happens that a person misconstrues the referral to mean that his or her pain is "all in the mind." It is necessary, therefore, to correct any misconceptions and also to convey the reasons for the referral directly and positively. For example, a frequent reason for a referral is that pain psychologists and psychiatrists have specific expertise in helping a person make important adjustments so that the quality of life can be improved. As can be gathered from this chapter, it takes remarkable abilities, courage, motivation, and resiliency for a person to adapt to a chronic pain condition. A referral to a professional who will utilize and foster these strengths might actually be a tribute to the sufferer of pain.

SUGGESTED READINGS

Flor H, Turk DC: Chronic illness in an adult family member: pain as a prototype.

Fordyce WE: Behavioral Methods for Chronic Pain and Illness. Mosby, St. Louis, MO, 1976

Holzman AD, Turk DC, Kerns RD: The cognitve-behavioral approach to the management of chronic pain. pp. 31–50. In Holzman AD, Turk DC (eds): Pain Management: A Handbook of Psychological Treatment Approaches. Pergamon Press, New York, 1986

Merskey H: Traditional individual psychotherapy and psychopharmacotherapy. pp. 51–70}. In Holzman AD, Turk DC (eds): Pain Management: A Handbook of Psychological Treatment Approaches. Pergamon Press, New York, 1986

Novy DM, Nelson DV, Francis DJ, Turk DC: Perspectives of chronic pain: an evaluative comparison of restrictive and comprehensive models. Psychol Bull 118:238–247, 1995

Roberts AH: The operant approach to the management of pain and excess disability. pp. 10–30. In Holzman AD, Turk DC (eds): Pain Management: A Handbook of Psychological Treatment Approaches. Pergamon Press, New York, 1986

Turk DC, Kerns RD: Health, Illness, and Families: A Lifespan Perspective. Wiley, New York, 1985

Williams AC: In-patient management of chronic pain. pp. 114–139. In Hodes M, Moorey S (eds): Psychological Treatment in Disease and Illness. Gaskell and The Society for Psychosomatic Research, London, 1993

30 | The Difficult Pain Patient

David V. Nelson
Diane M. Novy
Hugh G. Gallagher

Pain patients and the extent to which their symptoms are accompanied by complicating psychological features present in virtually unlimited ways. This chapter addresses some of the most common, challenging, and also vexing problems primary care physicians will need to appreciate to optimally address the needs of their diverse patients with pain. Given that primary care physicians are involved in the long-term maintenance of well-being for pain patients, sensitivity to psychological matters and psychiatric disorders is essential. Whether the primary care physician is seeing the patient at the outset of the pain complaints or taking back the responsibility for implementing a treatment plan begun at a tertiary care pain center, astuteness in discerning patients' needs and appropriate flexibility in implementing psychologically based interventions are required.

This chapter first addresses the most common associations of psychological syndromes and psychiatric disorders seen with pain. It then reviews basic psychological styles or types that the busy practitioner is likely to encounter, as well as strategies for dealing with the individual cases. Finally, the chapter focuses on one particularly problematic area, chemical dependence. In this manner, the astute and sensitive clinician can appreciate how better to target management of the patient with pain. Pain patients present along the full continuum from optimal adjustment (i.e., dealing with pain adequately despite serious challenges) to the most debilitated and decompensated. Our focus is primarily on helping the primary care physician understand the more challenging psychological issues that arise.

Psychiatric disorders and chronic pain

David V. Nelson
Diane M. Novy

Conventional wisdom maintains that, as pain persists, the psychological cost to the individual increases, affective distress evolves from a predominantly anxious to more depressed presentation, and other psychological dysfunctions (e.g., disability, family strains) progressively compound their adverse impact. Recent research, however, has begun to challenge these traditional assumptions. At least in acute and chronic low back pain conditions, systematic and objective comparisons now suggest that there is more variability in psychological responses within each group (acute and chronic) and more overlap between groups than previously suspected. Anxiety and depression, along with anger, frustration, and irritability, are perhaps the most common affective responses seen in conjunction with pain conditions. It is important for the practicing primary care physician to appreciate these emotional features, along with their behavioral, cognitive, and social correlates, to adequately address and manage the full range of psychological disturbances associated with pain problems.

While there have been some attempts to identify a "pain-prone" personality, the literature to support this theory has been substantially flawed. Pain potentially afflicts all segments of the general population, without discriminating according to sociocultural, demographic, or other artificial distinctions, although variations in the manifestations of pain exist in various subgroups. For example, certain categories of people (e.g., injured workers) in certain settings (e.g., tertiary pain centers) may predominate, and ethnic variations in the expression of pain have long been acknowledged. Likewise, the different psychological syndromes and psychiatric disorders afflict all segments of the population, occasionally with differentially disproportionate representation in one subgroup or another (e.g., chronic schizophrenia more so in lower socioeconomic strata). Nonetheless, the combination of these two facts (the ubiquity of pain and of psychological symptomatology/psychiatric disorders) leads to the inescapable conclusion that pain conditions can present with virtually all combinations of one or more psychiatric symptoms or disorders. Such symptom patterns or disorders may be simply coexistent with, reactive to, or contributory to the particular pain problem.

PSYCHOLOGICAL SYMPTOMATOLOGY AND PSYCHIATRIC DISORDERS THAT MOST COMMONLY PRESENT WITH CHRONIC PAIN

Depression

Significant depressive symptomatology has been reported in widely varying prevalence rates, ranging from approximately 10% to 80% of chronic pain patients. In general, substantially higher proportions of depressed individuals are found in persons with chronic pain than in the general population. Although estimates vary, perhaps as many as 10% to 25% meet diagnostic criteria for major depressive disorder. Other diagnoses also may be applied such as adjustment disorders with depressive symptomatology. In addition, the denial of depressed and other negative affect is common in a subset of chronic pain patients, although many of these individuals manifest many of the constellation of symptomatology typically associated with depression. These include vegetative disturbances accompanied by excessive self-devaluation, pessimism, cognitive processing inefficiencies, crying spells, decreased interest in and pleasure derived from everyday activities, and irritability. Depressed psychiatric patients commonly report a disproportionately higher amount of pain complaints. High, albeit widely varying, prevalence rates of pain symptoms in 27% to 100% of clinically depressed patients have been reported. Hence, regardless of which is first manifested or primary, pain or depression, once depression has set in, a vicious cycle may be perpetuated unless there is specific intervention.

For depressed chronic pain patients, treatment of the depression per se is as necessary as any other component of the pain experience. This may sometimes be accomplished by any of the standard therapies available, including behavioral activation, cognitive or other psychotherapies, and antidepressant medication. Medication often only partially improves depressive symptomatology, and other aspects must also be targeted for optimal response (e.g., psychotherapy addressing dysfunctional attitudes and beliefs about pain and disability). Suicidal ideation, innuendo, or threat should be treated as truly life-threatening until thorough assessment proves the risk otherwise; even then, one must be on the alert for deteriorations in mood or communications about suicide. There must be no hesitation about questioning to unambiguous clarity the frequency of ideation, the extent of discouragement and pessimism, the lethality of proposed suicidal means, the reasons for living or lack thereof, and the willingness to cooperate in reducing risks (e.g., removing guns from the home, picking up tricyclic prescriptions on a weekly or, if necessary, daily basis). If there is any remaining or unsettled question in the physician's mind or any lack of cooperation on the part of the patient, referral to appropriate resources is indicated, such as urgent referral to a psychologist or psychiatrist, preferably one skilled in dealing with pain patients, or, in extreme cases, to the police, emergency room, or local mental health crisis evaluation team. If the risk of suicide is imminent, all other concerns become secondary until the crisis is addressed.

Anxiety

Heightened arousal and anxiety are normal initial responses to the threat of pain. Evidence suggests that under some circumstances anxious individuals experience heightened pain and that anxiety may be associated with increased muscle tension and other physiologic processes potentially augmenting the experience of pain. In addition, the relation is curvilinear. Both very low and very high arousal are related to a relative absence of pain, and intermediate arousal and above average anxiety are related to increased or more apparent pain than would otherwise be the case. Furthermore, denial of anxiety in very defensive terms by a pain patient is cause to investigate the reason for that denial because the anxiety in such a patient may be finding expression in other forms not immediately apparent to the individual.

It has been estimated that as high as 30% of chronic pain patients have a diagnosable anxiety disorder; generalized anxiety and panic are common among these. More than 50% of diagnosable anxiety patients have comorbid psychiatric disorders such as depression and substance abuse. Many chronic pain patients with anxiety may suffer from these coexistent psychiatric disorders as well. Fortunately, anxiety disorders are among the most treatable mental disorders, with substantial numbers often responding to specifically targeted psychotherapies (such as cognitive-behavioral therapy for panic) and carefully selected medications. In this regard, poorly targeted (and ill-advised) prescription of anxiolytics and related sedative-hypnotic drugs is known to cause as many or more problems in chronic pain patients than to help. If medications are tried, judicious use of antidepressants may be as or more efficacious in many patients.

Somatization and Related Somatoform Disorders

The essential distinguishing aspect of the somatoform disorders is the presence of physical symptoms suggesting a medical condition despite the lack of any organic or physical findings. These symptoms cause clinically significant distress or impairment in social, occupational, or other areas of functioning. Further, they do not appear to be under voluntary control. On the other hand, the most confusing aspect in pain conditions is that a sizeable number of pain patients manifest very high levels of somatic preoccupation and disease conviction (the hallmarks of hysteria and hypochondriasis) sometimes quite disproportionate to any demonstrable physical pathology. However, given the current state of incomplete knowledge about the physical bases of pain conditions, and the fact that many pain conditions present with subtle or insufficiently recognized physical causes, it is hazardous to diagnose a psychiatric somatoform disorder simply in the absence of demonstrable physical disease or physical findings on physical examination. For example, there are now good reasons for supposing that nondermatomal sensory abnormalities in myofascial and complex regional (e.g., "reflex sympathetic dystrophy") syndromes have true physiologic bases. That is, individual nociceptive cells in the dorsal horn respond to stimulation from receptor fields that are much wider than a single dermatome, and there is a certain plasticity in the nervous system that can result in alteration in the presence of persistent pain. Similarly, the "giveway weakness" often associated with conversion hysteria may be mistakenly labeled when the actual problem is "pain inhibition" that occurs either voluntarily or involuntarily when a patient is pressed to perform a particularly painful maneuver on physical examination and knows that doing so will cause pain. Indeed, the absoluteness of physical findings as the *sine qua non* of legitimate pain is difficult to support among chronic pain patients. The diagnoses of conversion or other somatoform disorders based on *Diagnostic and Statistical Manual of Mental Disorders*, 4th edition (DSM-IV) criteria must be used with great caution.

Hysterical and hypochondriacal features in chronic pain patients may be better understood in this fashion. Hysteria in such patients may actually reflect an unconscious increase in existing symptoms for a wide variety of motives, some of which may be understood in behavioral reinforcement contingencies, family systems issues, psychodynamic formulations, and others. Rarely, however, does pain exist solely as a solution to some unconscious conflict. Still, a variety of factors can operate in a person's life that might lead to some increase in perceived discomfort without being fully aware of how this process operates. On the other hand, the element of strong disease conviction in the minds of many pain patients is very common and is routinely observed in tertiary pain centers and other settings in which patients have demonstrable physical pathology. The important mechanism here is likely to be cognitive misinterpretation of mild body sensations, hence leading to what appears in the eyes of others as unjustified somatic symptom magnification. This is also closely allied with the coexisting experience of anxiety in many pain patients, given that many of the symptoms of anxiety have a physiologic basis or are perceived in such terms (e.g., racing heart, sweating, hot and cold flashes, shortness of breath, nausea, chest and other pains). Again, the important mechanism of cognitive misinterpretation is salient. Also, as mentioned previously, clinically depressed patients often report at a high frequency somatic symptoms, including pain, which can be mistakenly confused as a primary somatization disorder.

All that having been said, there may occasionally be a place for the diagnosis of a somatoform disorder or somatoform features in extreme cases of pain, particularly in the primary care setting where primary care physicians routinely are asked to assess and treat conditions that have no obviously identifiable organic cause (e.g., some headaches). Primary care physicians are often the first professional sought out when patients experience physical discomforts, regardless of how compelling the psychological contribution actually is. The following disorders may occur with pain in their symptom constellation.

Somatization Disorder

Somatization is a polysymptom disorder involving multiple organ systems and often accompanied by a belief that one is sickly. It may extend over several years, with symptoms that are not adequately explained by physical disease or injury, or attributable to medications, drugs, alcohol, or another primary psychiatric disorder (e.g., chest pains during panic attacks). Less fully florid presentations may be more common. Such patients typically relate their concerns in intensely or overly dramatic (i.e., histrionic) tones; but they are vague, imprecise, or even inconsistent historians and resent the implication that their obviously intense emotional distress may be anything other than an understandable reaction to such serious illness.

Treatment of somatization disorder or its variants is best managed by primary care physicians who see patients on a regularly scheduled appointment basis (e.g., every 4 to 6 weeks), prevent unnecessary or dangerous procedures and hospitalizations, and supportively inquire about areas of stress in the patient's life without implying that "it's all in your head." Inquiry must be done not by implying that the "real" cause of the patient's somatic complaints is psychosocial in nature, but rather by helping the patient cope with, not eliminate, symptoms. Palliation then becomes the primary therapeutic orientation, and medications are generally not helpful unless there is a clinically detectable level of depression or anxiety (e.g., panic disorder). Such an approach in a randomized controlled trial led to substantial reductions in health care utilization in the intervention group, largely through decreases in hospitalization rates, and without adverse impact on health status or patients' reported satisfaction with care.

Conversion Disorder

Pain, numbness, and weakness are the "conversion triad in the pain clinic" (Bouckoms and Hackett, p. 49). A temporal relation between a psychosocial stressor and the onset of symptoms, as well as an apparent unconscious conflict or motivation, must be discerned. Conversion disorder cannot be diagnosed in the presence of pain only. At least one other unexplained symptom must be present and some gain apparent, although the symptoms are not produced in a consciously voluntary manner. A primary recommended treatment strategy is to suggest that the conversion symptom(s) will improve, that diagnostic tests of the presumably affected area show no damage, and that recovery will be gradual, with specific suggestions such as weight bearing despite pain at first, then ambulating with the assistance of a walker. Phrasing of suggestions can be somewhat of an art. Examples are available in references, but, at a minimum, confident expressions of optimism about recovery by the physician are likely to be helpful. Confrontation is generally ill-advised. Psychologically based treatment may have to be recommended in refractory cases, but it may be resisted. It is important to keep in mind, as well, that as many as 13% to 30% of patients initially diagnosed with conversion symptoms later developed a diagnosable physical disorder that in retrospect would have included the initial symptom manifestation. As with all somatoform disorders, great caution is advised in applying such labels, although related mechanisms may confuse the clinician.

Somatoform Pain Disorder

Somatoform pain is certainly one of the most confused and confusing disorders in psychiatric nomenclature. The diagnosis has made the transition in the official DSM from one of pain of inadequately explained origin on a physical basis to now (DSM-IV) potentially include virtually all clinical presentations in which pain is the predominant focus; where it is of sufficient severity to warrant clinical attention; causes clinically significant distress or impairment in social, occupational, or other important spheres of functioning; and in which psychological factors are judged to have an important role in the onset, severity, exacerbation, or maintenance of the pain. It is hard to imagine any pain disorder associated with any significant distress or impairment that would not fit that categorization. Treatment recommendations then would vary widely according to the idiosyncracies of the case.

Hypochondriasis

Hypochondriasis is characterized by the preoccupation of fear of having, or the idea that one has, a serious disease based on misinterpretation of bodily symptoms or bodily functions. Such preoccupation and fears persist despite appropriate medical evaluation and reassurance and result in significant distress or impairment in social, occupational, or other important areas of functioning. Unfortunately, it is difficult to discern when excessive concern about one's health (a common phenomenon, particularly in physically stressed and diseased individuals) crosses into becoming a psychiatric disorder. Management is similar to somatization disorder: provide a long-term relationship with the patient on a regularly scheduled basis; avoid unnecessary diagnostic and overly aggressive medical interventions; recommend simple, modest, and relatively benign measures to enhance comfort by attention from the physician (e.g., application of heat, ointments, vitamins); and focus on helping the patient to cope with and tolerate a certain level of somatic symptomatology without being able to have it cured (i.e., palliation). The physician might best cope by remembering that no medical cure presently exists for the need to be sick.

Factitious Disorders

The essential feature of a factitious disorder with physical symptoms is the intentional production or faking of physical symptoms, as opposed to the somatoform disorders where the element of voluntary intention is lacking. Self-inflicted injuries, intriguingly and elaborately detailed symptom recitals but difficulty tracking down actual records, multiple hospitalizations over a lengthy course, inconclusive investigations and operations, narcotics seeking, poor access by the health care team to family members, running away in response to confrontation, and often ambivalence manifested toward health care professionals are all sometimes associated with the disorder. Such a profound need to assume the sick role has defied effective treatment formulations, although it is presumed that psychotherapy would be indicated if such patients "would just stay around" (Bouckoms and Hackett, p. 51).

Malingering

Malingering is the intentional production of false or grossly exaggerated physical symptoms, motivated by external incentives such as financial compensation, avoiding work, evading prosecution, or obtaining drugs. It is much akin to lying and is often episodically used as a poor means to deal with stress. Malingering is distinguished from factitious disorders by the clear pretense undertaken for an obvious external incentive rather than a need to assume the sick role for its own inherent value where external incentives are lacking. No effective treatments are known, although confrontation sometimes brings the immediate pretense to a halt.

Psychosis

While schizophrenia, psychotic depression, organic psychoses, and dementias can all present with the symptom of pain, schizophrenia more commonly is associated with a reduction in the subjective complaints of pain. Indeed, schizophrenia appears to be associated with the lowest complaints of physical or psychological pain of any of the psychiatric disorders, as manifested in the higher incidence of diseases progressing to dangerous and even life-threatening stages before they are detected (e.g., ruptured appendices, silent myocardial infarctions, bleeding ulcers). In a small number of individuals, however, delusions may be fixed around somatic dysfunction (particularly monosymptomatic hypochondriacal psychosis), may be quite bizarre, and/or may be particularly linked to persecutory ideation. Some dementias may also present with pain, as if the language to describe discomforts of all kinds has found expression in the language of pain. Rare as they are, psychotic patients with such pains may not seem eager to be cured of their discomforts and may resist the idea that it is possible to do so.

Drug Addiction

Drug addiction, distinguished from simple physiologic drug dependence (see Chemical Dependence for a fuller discussion of these issues) is probably more common in patients who are given opiates and sedative-hypnotics and who have coexisting personality disorders, particularly passive-dependent personalities. Treatment must address the addiction component as directly as other aspects of the pain experience in comprehensive management.

Personality Disorders

Passive-dependent personalities may be at higher risk for developing addictions in the course of their pain conditions, particularly when they are prescribed opiates. There is also some weak evidence that individuals with premorbid introverted/obsessoid characteristics are more likely to suffer at heightened levels of depression, anxiety, and irritability in conjunction with their pain conditions, once afflicted, although they are not the only ones who will develop such mood disturbances. In general, however, personality disorders or personality traits of a very ingrained nature are more likely to color the expression of the pain experience and determine somewhat the degree to which management difficulties arise than to explain the etiology of specific pain complaints. For example, patients may run quite different courses depending on the extent to which they manifest antisocial, avoidant, borderline, histrionic, passive-dependent, passive-aggressive, or isolated schizoid features. Appropriate management depends on the recognition of these features and adjustment by the physician of his or her responses in light of them.

SUGGESTED READING

American Psychiatric Association: Diagnostic and Statistical Manual of Mental Disorders. 4th Ed. American Psychiatric Association, Washington, DC, 1994

Bouckoms A, Hackett TP: The pain patient: evaluation and treatment. pp. 39–68. In Cassem NH (ed): Massachusetts General Hospital Handbook of General Hospital Psychiatry. 3rd Ed. Mosby–Year Book, St Louis, 1991

Hadjistavropoulos HD, Craig KD: Acute and chronic low back pain: cognitive, affective, and behavioral dimensions. J Consult Clin Psychol 62:341–349, 1994

Merskey H, Chandarana P: Chronic pain problems and psychiatry. pp. 45–56. In Tyrer SP (ed): Psychology, Psychiatry and Chronic Pain. Butterworth-Heinemann, Oxford, 1992

Philips HC, Grant L: The evolution of chronic back pain problems: a longitudinal study. Behav Res Ther 29:435–441, 1991

Reich J, Tupin J, Abramowitz S: Psychiatric diagnosis of chronic pain patients. Am J Psychiatry 140:1495–1498, 1983

Romano JM, Turner JA: Chronic pain and depression: does the evidence support a relationship? Psychol Bull 97:18–34, 1985

Smith GR Jr, Monson RA, Ray DC: Psychiatric consultation in somatization disorder. N Engl J Med 314:1407–1413, 1986

Sternbach RA: Pain Patients: Traits and Treatment. Academic Press, New York, 1974

Turk DC, Salovey P: Chronic pain as a variant of depressive disease: a critical reappraisal. J Nerv Ment Dis 172:398–404, 1984

Managing difficult personality styles

David V. Nelson

Diane M. Novy

No one knows better than the primary care physician that people adopt a great diversity of styles of functioning in everyday living. Each individual's personality is unique, but certain commonalities seem to cut across groups. It is helpful to be able to systematize these observations to identify various general styles of responding to management techniques, particularly if a "difficult" patient is encountered. Personality in this context is understood to refer to a person's characteristic patterns of thought, behavior, and feelings. Under stress, such as in chronic disease states, an individual's typical personality traits may become more inflexible and maladaptive. By understanding basic personality types, the primary care physician can understand better the meaning of illness for a patient and his or her performance in the role of a patient. In a classic work on biopsychosocial dimensions of the patient in medical practice, Leigh and Reiser (1992) set forth a modified and expanded version of a typology originally described by Kahana and Bibring (1964). We now modify and expand on their descriptions with an eye toward placing them within the context of the primary care management of pain patients.

By identifying personality types, there is no presumption that individual patients will fit neatly into one category. Rather, certain key features of a patient's style might indicate a strong tendency to involve some of the attributes discussed in each of one or more categories. Management of any difficulties would require the application of a certain amount of clinical judgment as to the extent of the relevance of these characterizations for guiding intervention in a particular case. Also, the physician's own personality might have some of the attributes of one or more of these types, and unless recognized in oneself, one's own personality might unwittingly interact (or even conflict) with a patient's personality in a less than optimal manner.

PERSONALITY TYPES: CHARACTERISTICS AND MANAGEMENT STRATEGIES

Various personality types are characterized and management strategies suggested. Do not confuse the labels for these with specific diagnosable psychiatric syndromes because such a full syndrome may or may not actually be present (Table 30-1).

Taking Care of the Hateful Patient

In a classic 1978 article in the *New England Journal of Medicine*, Groves provided a conceptualization of some of the most difficult patients seen in medical practice (Table 30-2), those who engender "aversion, fear, despair or even downright malice in their doctors" (Groves, p. 883). While a natural inclination might include a wish to transfer these patients to someone else's care, the primary care physician cannot often practically do so. Further, transfer is usually not helpful to the patient. It is better to recognize the feelings engendered by such patients and use these feelings as cues to guide appropriate management responses.

Table 30-1. Characteristics and Management Strategies for Various Personality Types

Personality Types	Characteristics	Management Strategies
Dependent, demanding	Need a lot of reassurance Want special attention Become dependent on physicians and other health care providers Frequent, inappropriate, "urgent" calls Feel angry and rejected when demands not met May provoke hostility and conflict in physicians and other health care providers May be viewed as "enjoying" the sick role	Provide warm support and reassurance Firm limits on excessive neediness and manipulativeness
Orderly, controlling (obsessive-compulsive)	Relatively little outward emotional expressiveness Do not show feelings much Complete, precise, and nonemotional symptom descriptions Sick role difficult to assume Feel out of control when sick and under physician's care Can become complaining, contentious, and accusatory Extremely focused on precise attention to details of care (e.g., punctuality) Angry and/or critical if expectations not met Do not accept blanket reassurances (will question physician's competence)	Enlist patient as part of health care team Enlist in clinically relevant diary recording Give detailed explanations compatible with patient's educational background Help patient cooperate by giving sense of control
Dramatizing, emotional (histrionic)	Initially charming, fun to talk to Dramatic, impressionistic, diffuse vs precise descriptions Sometimes sexual overtones and may be overtly seductive "Special" relationship to physician Polarizes feelings of staff Need to be attractive, desirable Sick role may or may not be compatible: opportunity to "flirt" safely, or situation may feel overly restricted	Show some warmth and concern Set boundaries/limits Repeatedly reassure Reconcile staff splitting

Continues

Table 30-1. *Continued*

Personality Types	Characteristics	Management Strategies
Long-suffering, self-sacrificing (masochistic)	Often wailing, complaining with long list of hard luck and disasters (e.g., complications after surgeries, side-effects, and new complaints instead of relief) Endure protracted pain and suffering—"born to suffer" Often pride in taking care of someone else ("altruism") despite own suffering Guilt feelings do not allow enjoyment of life Appear as if exhibiting misfortunes, suffering and "altruism" Pain and suffering a lifestyle to maintain interpersonal relationships React negatively to reassurance Very frustrating to physicians and guilt-inducing Physicians may unwittingly perpetuate patient's misfortunes by rejecting patient	Give "credit" to suffering Express appreciation for courage and perseverance in suffering Accept limited goals for treatment Express some degree of pessimism regarding cure vs. management or palliation Emphasize symptom improvement to facilitate patient's "altruism" Differentiate from cynicism and suffering due to actual medical complications (not just "refusal to improve")
Guarded, suspicious (paranoid)	Vigilant regarding possibility of harm (intentionally or unintentionally) Overly sensitive to possibility of criticism Misinterprets motive, actions, and words of others Misreads symptoms or information as ominous threats Blames others for illness Does not enjoy sick role - increased sense of vulnerability Difficulty trusting physicians sufficiently to cooperate fully	Assume relatively neutral attitude Label suspiciousness as "sensitivity" Help direct blame to more impersonal things like institutional or insurance regulations Provide consistency and reasonably detailed information
Superior, special (narcissistic)	Behave like VIPs even if they are not Snobbish, sometimes grandiose Often proud of their bodies and physical abilities Sometimes mask with exaggerated, artificial humility Often arrogance and disdain toward others Air of tentativeness when provided information	Tolerate a certain amount of arrogance and allow patient to boast of strengths Maintain attitude of professional competence and not obeisance to patient

Continues

Table 30-1. *Continued*

Personality Types	Characteristics	Management Strategies
	"Name dropping" Sick role disagreeable and threat to integrity of body image Find faults and weaknesses in physicians to retain a sense of superiority Engender resentments and counterattacks by physicians	
Seclusive, aloof (schizoid)	Remote, detached, as if not in need of interpersonal contact Extreme preference for privacy Minimally communicative Shyness, aloofness, lack of personal response may be mistaken as depression instead of personal eccentricities Sick role a threat to isolation and self-absorption Submit to treatment without signs of affective involvement Occasionally, however, illness used as an excuse for interpersonal relationships without true intimacy	Recognize and respect need for privacy One or two staff members may help to "translate" for others
Impulsive, acting out tendencies	Spur of the moment, without deliberation Lack tolerance for sustained thinking or frustration Remorse after the fact but with repetition of maladaptive cycles May have very significant history of interpersonal and legal difficulties Seek rather immediate relief of even minor discomforts Have difficulty tolerating any treatment process that is protracted or involves discomfort May have history of significant aggression toward health care personnel or facilities, particularly when immediate relief is not forthcoming Intensely disliked and seen as defective and childish by medical personnel	Adopt an attitude similar to any other organic defect (in this case, a possible defect in the integrative functions of the brain) To the extent possible, prevent situations in which the defect would result in major unfortunate consequences Firm limits on acting out behavior in absence of internal controls (may be quite reassuring to patients) Mobilize friends and relative to serve as external controls and support

Continues

Table 30-1. *Continued*

Personality Types	Characteristics	Management Strategies
Mood swings (cyclothymic)	Exaggerated "ups and downs" Reaction to illness and sick role depends on phase of swing, exaggerating presentation either overly optimistically or pessimistically Heightened risk for developing major depression with the stress of illness Must rule out bipolar disorder	Recognize style to identify potential for exaggerations Refer as needed for further evaluation and treatment of affective symptomatology
Intense, unstable relationships (borderline personality)	Polarize staff members and characterize them in extreme "all good" or "all bad" terms Confused and confusing at times Unstable, often stormy interpersonal relationships Affective instability and unpredictability Changeable unpredictably regarding attitudes and demeanor Sometimes manipulative (as well as fully intended) suicidal acts Can regress rapidly and experience transient psychotic episodes Sick role useful and/or stressful	Caring, consistent approach with clearly explicit expectations and limit setting Reconcile staff splitting May require long-term psychotherapy for any effective or enduring change Exercise great caution in applying the label "borderline" (which is a highly charged term and will potentially brand the patient indefinitely and may compromise any actually needed care)

(Adapted from Leigh and Reiser, 1992, and Kahana and Bibring, 1964, with permission.)

In a number of aspects, Groves' conceptualization overlaps with the personality types sketched by Leigh and Reiser. However, they bear mentioning specifically because the astute clinician can often identify aspects of these more specific trait combinations and guide his or her management accordingly.

In general, it is not how one feels but how one behaves toward such individuals that matters. Having an understanding of the negative emotions that are inevitably stirred up by "hateful" patients can help the primary care physician sustain a helping and helpful relationship by using such feelings to cue more appropriate behaviors on his or her part. Attempts at disavowal of such negative feelings may only result in a higher frequency of errors of diagnosis and treatment. Admittedly, "Disavowal of hateful feelings requires less effort than bearing them. But such disavowal wastes clinical data that may be helpful in treating the 'hateful patient'" (Groves, p. 886). The challenge, then, is to integrate the understanding of the patient's psychology with reasonable, and still compassionate, care, even if the goals are actually limited accordingly.

**Table 30-2. Groves' Conceptualization of the
Characteristics and Management of Difficult Patients**

Hateful Patient	Clinical Characteristics	Negative Emotions Engendered	Management Strategy
Dependent clingers	Escalating requests for reassurance Extreme attention seeking Overly needy; bottomless pit Physician presumed inexhaustible	Power and specialness change to exhausted stamina Weariness Frustration Aversion	Limit setting on expectations, intensity of relationship, time, availability
Entitled demanders	Devalue and intimidate staff Constantly threatening (e.g., litigation, punishment)	Fear and shame Guilt and depression Counterattack	Support the entitlement ("right" to first rate medical care) but rechannel its direction Avoid complicated logical (or illogical) debates Limit unreasonable demands
Manipulative help-rejecters	"Crocks"—symptom replacement "Nothing helps" Pessimistic Seemingly masochistic Lurking, disguised depression Self-defeating manipulativeness	Anxiety Irritation Depression Self-doubt	"Share" the pessimism Regularly scheduled follow up visits for "maintenance" of modest gains Limits on unrealistic expectations Limits on demanding hostility Appeal to sense of entitlement
Self-destructive deniers	"Glory" in own destruction Profoundly dependent at base but relentlessly defeating of physician's attempts to preserve their lives May be chronically suicidal in some form	Dread Self-blame Heroic rescue vs bland hopelessness (or even wish that patient would die)	Referral for evaluation of potentially treatable depression Adopt attitude of compassion as if "terminal illness" Curb desire to abandon Continue to attempt to preserve life despite odds

SUGGESTED READING

Groves JE: Taking care of the hateful patient. N Engl J Med 298:883–887, 1978

Kahana R, Bibring G: Personality types in medical management. pp. 108–123. In Zinberg N (ed): Psychiatry and Medical Practice in a General Hospital. International Universities Press, New York, 1964

Leigh H, Reiser MF: The Patient: Biological, Psychological, and Social Dimensions of Medical Practice. 3rd Ed. Plenum Medical Book Company, New York, 1992

Chemical dependence

Hugh G. Gallagher
David V. Nelson
Diane M. Novy

There is little in the literature to help direct the management of the addicted pain patient. Patients with either chronic pain or addiction can be difficult to treat, and the complexities of therapy increase when a patient presents with both. Pain can inhibit the patient seeking recovery from addiction, and addiction may be an undesired sequela of chronic pain treatment. Drugs of addiction among chronic pain patients include opioids, benzodiazepines, barbiturate combinations, and muscle relaxants. Clinicians must recognize the coexistence of addiction and understand its significance when evaluating a patient with a pain problem. They should also be alert, when prescribing potentially dependency-producing medications to recovering alcoholics and drug addicts, to the risks of using otherwise effective medications. Multidisciplinary pain centers have the necessary expertise to deal with the problems encountered when dealing with the addicted patient.

There are many parallels between addiction and chronic pain. Both can be disabling, chronic, and/or relapsing problems, and they each have behavioral manifestations with pronounced psychological and social consequences (Table 30-3). Patients presenting with either problem may find it difficult to obtain effective, compassionate care, and cure is rare.

TERMINOLOGY

Addictive Disease A condition that inclines the individual toward the use of a substance or substances in an uncontrolled, compulsive, and potentially harmful way. This state is characterized by concentration on obtaining or using the substance, loss of control over its use, and continued use despite negative consequences. Some substances produce pleasant or euphoric effects, which makes them reinforcing agents and potential objects of addiction. However, the actual determination of addiction rests with the user, not the substance.

Chemical Dependency A spectrum of conditions ranging from simple physical dependence to self-destructive abuse of drugs and/or alcohol.

Physical Dependence Development of withdrawal symptoms after abrupt withdrawal of the drug or administration of an antagonist. It occurs with prolonged use and can be accompanied by tolerance to its pharmacologic effects.

Tolerance Occurs when increasing doses are required to elicit the same initial effect.

Abstinence A state of abstaining from a substance on which one is dependent, without necessarily developing effective means of coping with pain and stress.

Recovery A conscious process through which psychological and physical well-being are cultivated.

CAUSATIVE FACTORS

Addictive disease develops because of a combination of psychosocial and environmental factors, biological predisposition, and exposure to specific chemical agents. The course of the disease varies widely; an individual may use the agent in a nonaddictive way for a prolonged period and

**Table 30-3. A Comparison of DSM-IV Criteria for Drug Dependence
Applied to Opioid Abusers and Nonaddicted Chronic Pain Patients**

Diagnostic Criterion	Pain Patient	Opioid Abuser
Opioids often taken in larger amounts or over a longer time than the person intended	Able to maintain medication schedule between physician visits	Unable to ration use over days or weeks
Persistent desire or one or more unsuccessful efforts to cut down or control opioid use	May want to decrease use, but when pain becomes worse, reluctantly agrees to continue medication	Relapses to drug use after detoxification
A great deal of time spent in activities necessary to acquire opioids, taking opioids, or recovering from their effects	May spend a lot of time in physician visits. He is generally cooperative with physicians about nonopioid analgesic strategies. Is more disabled without medication.	Time is spent acquiring money to buy drugs, using drugs and drug related activities. Most free time spent with other users
Frequent intoxication or withdrawal symptoms present when expected to fulfill major role obligations at work, home, or school	Occurs rarely, if ever	Common
Important social, occupational or recreational activities given up or reduced because of opioid use	Activities given up primarily because of pain. May be more active on opioids	Activities not related to drug use cease to be interesting or important
Continued opioid use despite knowledge of having a recurrent social, psychological, or physical problem	May continue medication despite concerns about addiction expressed by family or friends	Drug use continues despite arrests, family fights, divorce, loss of children, loss of job, and adverse health consequences
Opioid withdrawal symptoms	Present when opioids abruptly stopped	Present when opioids abruptly stopped
Opioids often taken to relieve or avoid withdrawal symptoms	Opioid use primarily in response to pain	Opioid withdrawal symptoms precipitate frantic drug seeking behavior
Marked tolerance: need for markedly increased amounts of the opioid to achieve intoxication or desired effect, *or* markedly diminished effect with continued of the same amount	May be present	Usually present

the drug of choice may change. Nevertheless, once it has occurred, addiction may pose a continuing vulnerability. Addicted patients may seek treatment for pain conditions brought about by injury, neglect, or inappropriate drug use and present a great challenge. Alcohol is the most common addiction to a psychoactive substance in our society. Cross-addiction is common and alcoholics are at risk for developing addiction to other substances. Patients addicted to other substances tend to use alcohol and nicotine as substitute drugs at various intervals.

Current research points to various explanations for the causes of addiction. Included among the explanations is that addiction results in part from neurochemical stimulation of reward centers in the limbic system, and different classes of drugs may stimulate different sites. The reward experience may be modified depending on the physicochemical effects of the drugs used, and each reward reinforces further use of the drug.

EXTENT OF THE PROBLEM

General Population

The prevalence of alcoholism in the United States is 3% to 16%. It is highest for men between 18 and 29 and lower (1–6%) among women, although this may not reflect the true prevalence among the latter. The prevalence of other forms of drug addiction is 5% to 6%.

Acute Pain Patients

There is probably a higher incidence of addiction history among hospitalized individuals following trauma, surgery, or medical injury. Alcoholism has been detected in 25% of patients admitted to a medical service, 19% of neurology admissions, and 23% of general surgery patients. Physicians should be aware of the potential for chemical dependency problems among the acute hospital population.

Cancer Patients

The prevalence of addictive disease among cancer patients should not be greater than in the general population, with the possible exception of those with malignancies arising from chronic overuse of alcohol or tobacco.

Chronic Pain Patients

The overall prevalence in this population is unknown, but literature reviews suggest a rate of 3.2% to 18.9%. A higher rate of dependence on opioids would be expected in pain clinics on the basis of greater therapeutic use. Guidelines have been laid down for the use of opioids in nonmalignant pain. As well as complicating treatment, drug addiction can have a direct impact on a patient's pain condition. Addicts experience episodes of increased sympathetic activity during withdrawal from alcohol, opioids, and benzodiazepines and after ingesting cocaine and other stimulants. Increased sympathetic activity aggravates pain states either through neurogenic mechanisms or vascular changes. Alcohol, barbiturate, benzodiazepine, and opioid withdrawal increases skeletal muscle tension, as does cocaine use. Sleep disturbance, a feature of all forms of addiction, also exacerbates many chronic pain conditions.

IDENTIFICATION OF CHEMICAL DEPENDENCY

Addictions tend to be underdiagnosed by physicians because of lack of expertise, uneasiness about discussing such matters with patients, lack of knowledge about treatment resources, belief that the problem is societal rather than medical, or belief that the problem is in itself untreatable. Denial is a cardinal feature of addiction and is difficult to overcome by physicians inexperienced in working with addicted patients. Unless the patient accepts addiction as a problem, withdrawal of medications will not be achieved. When addiction is diagnosed, it is often perceived to be a secondary problem, to be dealt with when the pain condition has been treated. The reality is that pain patients will not improve significantly or overcome their chronic pain behaviors while they continue with addictive behaviors. If one suspects addiction, but the patient will not admit to it, an addiction specialist may help establish the diagnosis by overcoming the patient's denial.

The clinician should identify addiction during the initial visit to avoid therapeutic dilemmas later. Addicts tend to maintain social proprieties and appearances until the later stages; hence, the signs of addiction may be very subtle. The *history* should cover patient and family member use of alcohol, street drugs, and other psychoactive substances. Reports of trauma, hepatitis, HIV infection, and gastrointestinal ulceration, which are often associated with drug and alcohol abuse, and reports of unsatisfactory interactions with multiple physicians or frequent emergency room treatments should alert the clinician. The *physical examination* should focus on psychomotor, neurologic, and cutaneous stigmata of drug and alcohol abuse. *Behaviors* such as missed appointments, reports of multiple drug "allergies," dramatic or histrionic presentation, complaints of conditions such as trigeminal neuralgia for which there are no objective clinical findings, and requests for pain medication in order to tolerate the examination should alert one to the likelihood of addiction. (These are also the behaviors of persons who are not always addicts and who feign similar complaints to obtain drugs for resale. Such individuals generally frequent busy urban emergency rooms and after-hours clinics where they are unlikely to encounter the same physician on repeat visits.) *Laboratory markers* such as raised γGT and increased mean cell volume (MCV) point to alcohol abuse. Some simple screening tests for alcoholism can be incorporated into the physician's history-taking:

1. The two-question screen:
   Has drinking ever been a problem for you?
   When was your last drink?
   ("Yes" and "within 24 hours" = positive screen)
2. The CAGE questions:
   Have you ever felt you ought to **C**ut down on your drinking?
   Have people **A**nnoyed you by criticizing your drinking?
   Have you ever felt bad or **G**uilty about your drinking?
   Have you ever had an **E**ye opener first thing in the morning to steady your nerves?

It is also important to identify patients who are in recovery or abstinent. Most people in recovery will discuss their addictions, but abstinent-only patients may be less open. Both of these groups are at risk of relapse in the course of treatment for pain conditions.

MANAGEMENT OF THE CHEMICALLY DEPENDENT PAIN PATIENT

Assess the Nature of the Dependency

The dependency may be characterized as follows:
- Physical dependence on therapeutic medications without abuse or addictive use, without a history of prior addiction
- Physical dependence on therapeutic medications without abuse or addictive use, with a history of prior addiction
- Addictive use of prescribed drugs
- Addictive use of street drugs or alcohol
- Addictive use of both prescribed and nonprescribed drugs
- Addictive use of prescribed and/or nonprescribed drugs without a history of addiction but with risk factors for addictive disease (so-called "iatrogenic addiction")

The development of tolerance with prolonged use and withdrawal effects on cessation suggest physical dependence, not addiction. Sees and Clark used the DSM-III-R criteria for psychoactive substance dependence to distinguish physical dependence from addiction and to determine whether the individual's use of medication should be seen as either therapeutic physical dependence or an indicator of addiction. Those criteria indicating addiction are as follows:

- Continuing use of a substance despite adverse consequences
- A significant amount of time spent obtaining, using, and thinking about the substance of abuse
- Reduction of social, occupational, or recreational activities due to substance abuse
- Frequent intoxication or recovery from intoxication at times when the individual is expected to fulfill major life roles or when substance abuse is dangerous

Determine the Need for Withdrawal

Patients with disabling nonmalignant pain may benefit from a "drug vacation" or "drug holiday," lasting at least 6 weeks, during which they are free of opioids, benzodiazepines, or other dependency-producing drugs after their initial evaluation. The rationale for the drug vacation is (1) the drugs facilitate or perpetuate pain and (2) chronic use of opioids, cocaine, or alcohol may alter pain modulation by altering epinephrine, GABA, dopamine, and serotonin release. The clinically important effects of chemical dependence in relation to chronic pain tend to be resolved within 6 weeks. Changes in opioid receptors resulting from previous dependency may last indefinitely, and the physical and psychological changes seen with drug dependency may persist for years.

Obtain Agreement for Withdrawal of Medications

The physically dependent patient who does not demonstrate addictive behavior and has no history of addiction will generally agree to a trial period off medication. The individual with a history of addictive disease may resist cessation, and patients recovering from chemical dependence may relapse with a different agent.

Establish a Framework for Change

1. Determine the patient's "Stage of Change":
   Precontemplation: not considering change
   Contemplation: considering change, but ambivalent
   Preparation: wants to change, has made some efforts and had some success
   Action: has had extended periods of abstinence
   Maintenance: stable abstinence
   Relapse: started again after a period of abstinence
2. Acknowledge the patient's thoughts, feelings, fears, and prior efforts.
3. Investigate the patient's reasons for wanting to change.
4. Support the patient's motivation and efforts to change.
5. Explore previous experiences with the drug; what is good and what is bad about using it, and the results of previous attempts to stop.
6. Evaluate the barriers to success and resistance to change.
7. Explore the patient's relationship to the drug.
8. Help identify self-defeating behaviors; clarify what needs to change.
9. Select potentially successful strategies based on the patient's:
   a. Personality
   b. Previous experiences
   c. Willingness
   d. Stage of change

10. Gently move the patient to make a commitment to action: give the patient a clear, consistent, and unequivocal message about stopping drug use.
11. Provide appropriate assistance within your discipline; refer to others for treatment modalities outside your area of expertise.
12. Review progress regularly; continue to assist patients in moving sequentially along the continuum of change, making progressively closer approximations of their goals.

Begin Detoxification

Begin tapering according to the schedules in Detoxification Guidelines by Substance of Abuse, if in accordance with the jurisdiction's legal statutes and practice standards.

STRATEGIES FOR TREATMENT

Patients Who Were Never Addicted

The goal is to minimize the risk of addiction, and the physician must determine whether an opioid is really necessary. A variety of nonopioid approaches can be taken by pain centers. Patients can develop tolerance to opioids after prolonged use, but experience with cancer patients has shown that analgesic requirements tend to remain relatively stable, and increased requirements reflect tumor growth or infection. If opioid therapy is judged to be necessary, an appropriate dose and route of administration must be prescribed. Inadequate dosing by an inappropriate route can increase the patient's risk of developing addiction. Mixed agonist/antagonists, such as pentazocine, or partial agonists, such as buprenorphine, have lower abuse potential with adequate analgesia for some patients. They should not be given to patients receiving pure agonists, as they can precipitate a withdrawal syndrome. As with all patients receiving opioids, the guidelines laid down by Portenoy are a good basis from which to plan opioid prescribing (see Detoxification Guidelines by Substance of Abuse).

Patients Who Are Recovering

Pain or exposure to opioids can trigger craving and relapse to street drug use in this group. The risk is significant, whether it is due to inherent metabolic differences or to a learned response. Addiction specialists consider recovering addicts to be at high risk of relapse, and treatment philosophy for some of them is a "drug-free" one. Strategies for drug-free treatment include either strict avoidance of all psychotropic drugs or controlled access to such agents when they are necessary, in combination with intensive relapse prevention. Patients should increase their recovery activities (e.g., support group or 12-step meetings, frequency of psychotherapy) as soon as possible. The opioid antagonist naltrexone can be taken orally and may offer some protection from relapse.

Patients Who Are Currently Addicted

These individuals may be addicted to prescription drugs, alcohol, street drugs, or to a combination of these. Patients occasionally become addicted because of treatment of acute or chronic pain conditions, but most have a history of alcohol or other drug abuse or have a strong family history of such abuse before their "iatrogenic addiction."

It is important to emphasize again that the treatment of addicted patients requires particular attention to certain matters. Strategies for successful treatment include the following:

1. Work from a written plan, which should be negotiated with the patient. The plan must be specific about medications (amounts and time of day of dosings), replacement of "lost" drugs, and frequency of office visits. The penalty for noncompliance should be stated clearly, and the document should be signed by the physician and the patient. This document becomes part of the patient's chart.

2. One physician should prescribe all psychotropic agents, in cooperation with all other treating physicians, and one pharmacy should be used, if at all possible.
3. Obtain information about drug use from sources other than the patient, including family members, pharmacists, and former physicians.
4. Seek early referral to an addiction specialist if there is a suggestion of addiction.
5. Maintain vigilance with all patients on psychotropic medications.

Detoxification Guidelines by Substance of Abuse

ALCOHOL

1. Up to 200 ml absolute alcohol equivalent daily (one pint spirits or 12 cans of beer):
   Loading dose **chlordiazepoxide** (Librium) 50 mg, *once only*
Day 1:	chlordiazepoxide 25 mg QID
Day 2:	chlordiazepoxide 25 mg TID
Day 3:	chlordiazepoxide 25 mg BID
Day 4:	chlordiazepoxide 25 mg HS
2. 400 ml absolute alcohol or more daily (one quart spirits):
   Loading dose chlordiazepoxide 100 mg, *once only*
Day 1:	chlordiazepoxide 50 mg QID
Day 2:	chlordiazepoxide 50 mg TID
Day 3:	chlordiazepoxide 25 mg QID
Day 4:	chlordiazepoxide 25 mg TID
Day 5:	chlordiazepoxide 25 mg BID
Day 6:	chlordiazepoxide 25 mg HS

One may use chlordiazepoxide, 25 mg every 2 hours, as needed for agitation for the first 24 hours only. Always give oral chlordiazepoxide, as it is erratically and incompletely absorbed by the intramuscular route. **Lorazepam** (Ativan) is well absorbed by both intramuscular and oral routes and does not rely totally on hepatic metabolism. It should be used if the patient's bilirubin is elevated. 25 mg Librium = 1 mg Ativan.

An alternative to the above is **phenobarbital** given orally, substituting 50 mg phenobarbital for each 25 mg of the calculated chlordiazepoxide dose. Other long-acting benzodiazepines, such as **clorazepate** (Tranxene) or **clonazepam** (Klonopin), are also acceptable; **diazepam** (Valium) is more euphorogenic than the others.

OPIOIDS

1. Methadone is a popular detoxifying agent, starting around 30 mg/day and dropping by 2 to 5 mg/day. **Clonidine** (Catapres) can be effective in doses of 0.2-0.3 mg to start, followed with 0.1-0.4 mg TID. **Guanabenz** (Wytensin) has proven more effective with fewer adverse effects than clonidine, with nearly total elimination of the discomfort of opioid withdrawal without using any opioid drugs. Note that Federal law prohibits the use of any scheduled opioid other than methadone for opioid withdrawal.
2. Provide as needed medications that the patient can control to some degree during detoxification:

Loperamide (Imodium), 1 cap after a loose stool, PRN
Dicyclomine (Bentyl), 20 mg, or **propantheline** (Pro-Banthine), 15 mg q 4h PRN for abdominal cramps
Hydroxyzine (Atarax), 25 mg q 4h PRN nausea
Chlordiazepoxide (Librium), 25 mg q 4h PRN for anxiety during the first three to four days
Acetaminophen (Tylenol), 650 mg q 4h PRN for headache
Mylanta, 30 ml q 2h PRN for indigestion
Diphenhydramine (Benadryl), 50 mg QHS PRN for sleep for the first two to three days
Prochlorperazine (Compazine), 25 mg suppository q 6h PRN for *observed* vomiting
Naproxen (Naprosyn), 375 to 500 mg q 8h for back, joint and bone pain (give routinely, *not* PRN)

SEDATIVE-HYPNOTICS (BENZODIAZEPINES, BARBITURATES)

1. **Phenobarbital detoxification**: Start titration with 100 mg every half-hour until patient gets drowsy. The total amount used becomes the total dose for the next 24 hours, in divided doses (usually 400 to 800 mg orally or IM), reducing over 7 to 10 days. This is the agent of choice for patients with a history of seizures.
2. **Chlordiazepoxide** can also be used, as with alcohol detoxification above. Start with a loading dose equivalent to about 25% of the typical 24-hour intake and reduce the daily dose over 10 to 14 days instead of 4 to 6 days with alcohol. Very heavy benzodiazepine users (500 mg/day or greater of diazepam) may require 30 days of gradual detoxification. Detoxification from **alprazolam** (Xanax) is not substantially different from other benzodiazepine detoxification, but the patient may become more confused. If the patient has used alprazolam for panic disorder, clonazepam is probably the safest agent to use. Substitute 1 mg clonazepam for each 1.5 mg alprazolam taken daily, up to a daily dose of 9 mg and give 1 mg clonazepam for each 3 mg alprazolam in excess of 9 mg/day. Start with a loading dose (2–4 mg), divide the rest into TID doses and reduce gradually over 14 days.

Carbamazepine (Tegretol) has also been used successfully. In panic disorder, start an alternative medication (carbamazepine, clonazepam, imipramine, or monoamine oxidase inhibitor) during detoxification, or the patient will not tolerate detoxification. The half-life of alprazolam is 3 to 4 hours, making it a poor agent for detoxification, and seizures are common when it is used.

NICOTINE

1. The nicotine transdermal patch (**Habitrol**, **Nicoderm**, **ProStep**) provides steady- state nicotine levels after 2 to 3 hours. Apply a patch daily to unbroken skin over the arm, back, or chest, making sure to remove the old patch. Base the starting dose on the Fagerström score (Fig. 30-1): a score of 7–10 = 21 mg size; 4–6 = 14 mg size; and < 4 = 7 mg size. Reduce patch size as often as every 3 days, or as seldom as once a month, using the same brand of patch throughout.
2. **Nicotine polacrilex** (Nicorette) contains 2 mg nicotine per piece. The patient identifies physiologic nicotine withdrawal signs and symptoms. When these occur, give 1 piece at a time, to be chewed for 2 to 5 minutes, then discarded. The gum may cause gingivitis if kept in the mouth longer than this. The total number of pieces used is gradually reduced; 25 pieces daily may initially be necessary to match serum nicotine levels. If headaches are a problem, advise patients either to break the gum in half or chew until the nicotine can be tasted and then discard.
3. **Clonidine** (Catapres) may suppress nicotine craving: 0.1 mg TID

1. *How soon after you wake up do you smoke your first cigarette?*

within 5 min	3 points
5–30 min	2 points
31–60 min	1 point
after 60 min	0 points

2. *Do you find it difficult to not smoke in places where it is forbidden, such as in church, in school, in a movie, at the library, on the bus, in court, or in the hospital?*

Yes	1 point
No	0 points

3. *Which cigarette would you hate most to give up?*

The first one in the morning	1 point
Any other one	0 points

4. *How many cigarettes do you smoke each day?*

10 or fewer	0 points
11–20	1 point
21–30	2 points
31 or more	3 points

5. *Do you smoke more frequently during the first hours after waking up than during the rest of the day?*

Yes	1 point
No	0 points

6. *Do you still smoke if you are so sick that you are in bed most of the day?*

Yes	1 point
No	0 points

Fagerström Score   __ points

Fig. 30-1. The Fagerström Questionnaire for nicotine dependence.

Note that medications help the physiologic withdrawal but do nothing for the conditioned responses or the anxiolytic effects of nicotine, and do not substitute for the pleasure of smoking.

PSYCHOSTIMULANTS

Chlordiazepoxide (Librium) is effective for the control of agitation; **haloperidol** (Haldol), **thiothixene** (Navane), or **perphenazine** (Trilafon) for paranoid ideation. Cocaine "craving" is the intense desire to use cocaine and has characteristics of a drive state, *not* clearly a detoxification symptom. If the intensity of the craving interferes with detoxification, it can be alleviated with **bromocriptine** (Parlodel), 2.5 mg, TID or QID, **amantadine** (Symmetrel) 100 mg BID or **carbamazepine** 100–200 mg TID. **Desipramine** (Norpramin) 125–250 mg/day, may help retain patients in treatment. There are no physiologic withdrawal symptoms with abstinence from cocaine or amphetamine; most effects are due to *toxicity*, not withdrawal.

THE PAIN COCKTAIL

A pain cocktail is a drug delivery system that allows medication to be given to the patient on a time-contingent (at a given, fixed time interval, *not* as needed) basis without his or her knowing the exact drug dosages at any given time. The patient is informed of the ingredients. The cocktail consists of up to three major components:

1. A long-acting orally effective opioid (usually methadone).
2. A long-acting orally effective sedative (phenobarbital).
3. A taste- or flavor-masking vehicle (cherry syrup, Maalox, etc.).

These may be enhanced by other ingredients such as acetaminophen (analgesic) or hydroxyzine (sedative and antiemetic).

Pain Cocktail for Tapering Pain Medications

After an evaluation of drug use has been made, equivalent doses of analgesic and/or sedative medications can be calculated using Tables 30-4 and 30-5.

Example: A patient's profile shows that he is taking 12 Percodan (equivalent to 60 mg oxycodone), 30 mg Valium, and 3 oz whiskey per day. His dose of 60 mg of oxycodone is equivalent to 20 mg of methadone (Table 30-5). His dose of 30 mg of Valium is equal to 90 mg of phenobarbital, and 3 oz of whiskey is equal to 30 mg of phenobarbital, making a total of 120 mg of phenobarbital (Table 30-5).

The patient may experience considerable psychological stress when transferred from short-acting, as needed medications to long-acting, time-contingent medications. The long-acting agents in the pain cocktail are slower in onset and longer in duration. Therefore, the patient may miss the "high" feeling associated with the shorter-acting agents. He may feel that he is losing control of his environment and decide that the pain cocktail is of no value. To circumvent this possibility, the initial daily dose of analgesic and/or sedative medications should be **120%** of the patient's calculated daily usage. The pain cocktail for the above example would contain:

Day 1 24 mg methadone   144 mg phenobarbital
Day 2 20 mg methadone   130 mg phenobarbital
Day 3 16 mg methadone   115 mg phenobarbital
etc.

Table 30-4. Opioid Equivalents to Methadone (10 mg PO)

Drug	Oral Dose (mg)	IM Dose (mg)
Alphaprodine		45.0
Anilendine		35.0
Codeine	200.0	130.0
Heroin		3.0
Fentanyl		0.1
Hydromorphone	7.5	1.4
Mependine	400.0	100.0
Methadone		8.0
Morphine	60.0	10.0
Oxycodone	30.0	15.0
Oxymorphone		1.5
Pentazocine	180.0	60.0

Table 30-5. Sedative Equivalents to Phenobarbital (30 mg PO)

Drug	Oral Dose (mg)
Secobarbital	100
Pentobarbital	100
Chlordiazepoxide	25
Diazepam	10
Flurazepam	30
Methaqualone	300
Glutethimide	500
Ethchlorvynol	750
Chloral Hydrate	1000
Hydroxyzine	50–100
Diphenhydramine	50–100
Meprobamate	400
Whiskey (100 proof)	90 ml (3 oz)

The cocktail is ordered as a methadone 6 mg and phenobarbital 36 mg/10 ml vehicle in a syringe and given at 6-hour intervals. The patient must be watched closely for signs of overdosage (e.g., lassitude, drowsiness, decreased respiratory rate) or signs of withdrawal (e.g., increased agitation, seizures). If these occur, the daily dose can be raised and tapering resumed at a slower rate. For detoxification, the methadone dosage can be reduced by 10% to 20% and phenobarbital by 10% of the initial dose every day. Daily phenobarbital reduction should not exceed 10 mg/day.

Opioid withdrawal is usually uncomplicated, but benzodiazepine withdrawal may need to be prolonged because sleep disturbance, anxiety attacks, dizziness, and nausea can continue for several weeks after withdrawal.

GUIDELINES FOR THE MANAGEMENT OF OPIOID MAINTENANCE THERAPY FOR NONMALIGNANT PAIN

1. Opioids should be considered only after all other reasonable attempts at analgesia have failed.
2. A history of substance abuse should be viewed as a relative but not necessarily absolute contraindication.
3. A single practitioner should take primary responsibility for treatment.
4. Patients should give informed consent before the start of therapy; some of the points to be covered include recognition of the low risk of psychological dependence as an outcome, potential for cognitive impairment with the drug alone and in combination with sedative/hypnotics, and understanding by female patients that children born when the mother is on opioid maintenance therapy will likely be physically dependent at birth.
5. After drug selection, doses should be given on a 24-hour basis; several weeks should be agreed on as the period of initial dose titration, and although improvement in function should be continually stressed, all should agree to at least partial analgesia as the appropriate goal of therapy.
6. Failure to achieve at least partial analgesia at relatively low initial doses in the nontolerant patient raises questions about the potential treatability of the pain syndrome with opioids.
7. Emphasis should be given to attempts to capitalize on improved analgesia by gains in physical and social function.

8. In addition to the daily dose determined initially, patients should be permitted to escalate doses transiently on days of increased pain. Two methods are acceptable: (1) prescription of an additional 4–6 "rescue doses" to be taken as needed during the month; or (2) instruction that one or two extra doses may be taken on any day, but must be followed by an equal reduction of dose on subsequent days.

9. Most patients should be seen and drugs prescribed at least monthly. Patients should be assessed for the efficacy of treatment, adverse drug effects, the appearance of either misuse or abuse of the drugs, and psychosocial, including mood and status during each visit. The results of the assessment should be documented clearly in the medical record.

10. Exacerbations of pain not effectively treated by transient, small increases in dose are best managed in the hospital, where dose escalation, if appropriate, can be observed closely, and return to baseline doses can be accomplished in a controlled environment.

11. Evidence of drug hoarding, acquisition of drugs from other physicians, uncontrolled dose escalation, or other aberrant behaviors should be followed by tapering and discontinuation of opioid maintenance therapy.

SUGGESTED READING

American Psychiatric Association: Diagnostic and Statistical Manual of Mental Disorders. 4th Ed. American Psychiatric Association, Washington, DC, 1994

Cyr M, Wartman S: The effectiveness of routine screening questions in the detection of alcoholism. JAMA 259:51–54, 1988

DiClemente CC, Prochaska JO: Processes and stages of change: coping and competence in smoking behavior change. pp. 319–343. In Shiffman S, Wills TA (eds): Coping and Substance Abuse. Academic Press, New York, 1985

Ewing JA: Detecting alcoholism: the CAGE questionnaire. JAMA 252:1905–1907, 1989

Fishbain DA, Rosomoff HL, Rosomoff RS: Drug abuse, dependence and addiction in chronic pain patients. Clin J Pain 8:77–85, 1992

Marlatt GA, Baer JS, Donovan DM, Kivlahan DR: Addictive behaviors: etiology and treatment. Annu Rev Psychol 39:223–252, 1988

Moore RD, Bone LR, Geller G, et al: Prevalence, detection and treatment of alcoholism in hospitalized patients. JAMA 261:403–407, 1989

Portenoy RK: Chronic opioid therapy in non-malignant pain. J Pain Symptom Manage 3:S46–62, 1990

Portenoy RK: Opioid therapy for chronic nonmalignant pain: current status. pp. 247–287. In Fields HL, Liebeskind JC (eds): Progress in Pain Research and Management, Vol. 1. IASP Press, Seattle, 1994

Sees K, Clark HW: Opioid use in the treatment of chronic pain: assessment addiction. J Pain Symptom Manage 8:257–264, 1993

Smith D: Cocaine-alcohol abuse: epidemiology, diagnostic and treatment considerations. J Psychoactive Drugs 18:117–130, 1986

Vailliant GE: The Natural History of Alcoholism. Harvard University Press, Cambridge, 1983

Wesson DR, Ling W, Smith DE: Prescription of opioids for treatment of pain in patients with addictive disease. J Pain Symptom Manage 8:289–296, 1993

Nonpharmacologic pain therapies

Acupuncture/ Dry Needling

The term *acupuncture* is derived from the Latin *acus*, meaning "sharp point" or "needle," and *punctura*, meaning "a pricking." It has been practiced in China for over 5,000 years. Needles of bamboo and bone suggest that it was in use even before the discovery of metal. It was introduced to the United States around 1825. The first and best known form of classical acupuncture is derived from the principles of ancient Chinese medicine. This doctrine taught that human health was created by opposing forces in nature, the yang (light, male) and the yin (dark, female). Vital energy flow was thought to flow through a set of interconnected channels, called meridians, that followed a circadian rhythm. These meridians, which are not defined by physical structures such as nerves, lymphatics, or blood vessels, are named after internal organs. By inserting needles strategically in some of the 365 acupuncture points along individual meridians, the acupuncturists attempted to balance the flow of energy (Qi or chi) throughout the body. There are many variations on classical acupuncture, including ear, scalp, and foot acupuncture. These are based on the belief that the human body can be mapped and treated by points on these peripheral areas.

In chronic pain disorders, trigger points in the muscles appear to correspond closely to classical acupuncture points. Thus, treatment of trigger points may be viewed as treatment of acupuncture points and vice versa.

Acupuncture may work by neuromodulation within the central nervous system. However, the exact mechanism remains to be elucidated. Acupuncture techniques, stripped of their mystique, afford a safe and inexpensive therapeutic alternative to medications. Although the acupuncture research that has been done has its limitations, and it is clear that acupuncture does not offer a miracle cure, acupuncture is reported to be effective in reducing pain in approximately 60% of patients. Following acupuncture with transcutaneous electrical nerve stimulation (TENS) electrode placement over the acupuncture points may increase its efficacy.

The side effects from acupuncture include hyperemia at the site of insertion, vasovagal attacks, hematoma formation, and transmission of infection if disposable or sterile needles are not used. Pneumothoraces and nerve damage have been reported from needles placed without due regard to the underlying anatomy. Most acupuncture needles used in the United States are made of stainless steel, which decreases the incidence of allergic metal reactions. For acupuncture algorithm, see Figure 31-1.

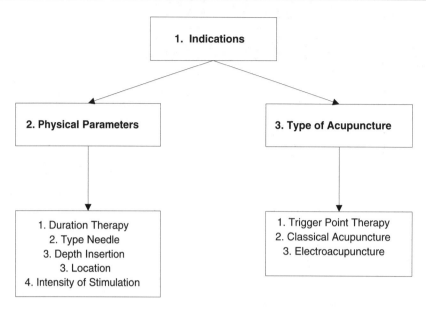

Fig. 31-1. Acupuncture.

INDICATIONS

The World Health Organization has formulated a provisional list of diseases that may be amenable to acupuncture treatment. Unfortunately, this list is based on clinical experience, not controlled clinical trials. However, the indications listed under the neurologic and musculoskeletal disorders include headaches and migraine, trigeminal neuralgia, peripheral neuropathies, intercostal neuralgia, cervicobrachial syndrome, frozen shoulder, tennis elbow, sciatica, low back pain, and osteoarthritis.

PHYSICAL PARAMETERS

Duration of Therapy

The New York Society of Acupuncture for Physicians and Dentists suggest that acupuncture therapy should consist of six treatments, initially twice a week, and later weekly. Of those patients who will respond to acupuncture, 50% will do so within three treatments and 90% within six treatments; 40% of those who subsequently improve with acupuncture may show an initial mild to moderate worsening of their symptoms over the first 48 hours following the first treatment. Patients who respond to acupuncture may require periodic "booster" treatments if flare-ups of pain occurs. Usually the acupuncture on these subsequent visits is as effective as the first time.

Type of Needle

We use size 30- or 32-gauge, disposable, stainless steel needles. These have a beveled point that is less painful for the patient and causes less tissue damage than the cutting edge of a standard injection needle. The needle can be directed through a clear plastic tube or mounted in a guide cylinder equipped with a piston that taps the needle into place at the touch of a finger. These methods help to minimize distress of treatment and to maintain sterility. Needles vary in length from 0.5 inch to 5 inches.

Depth of Insertion

The insertion depth varies considerably with practitioners. Some practitioners will penetrate the skin only over tender points and insert into trigger points at the appropriate depth in the muscle. Others use deep muscle penetration even onto periosteum when a "pecking technique" may be used. If insertion into the muscles is used for trigger point therapy, the underlying muscle should be felt to hold the needle firmly. This is usually associated with the patient complaining of a heaviness or pressure feeling at the needle (te chi). The needle must not be removed until the muscle spasm has relaxed.

Location

The placement of the needle varies, depending on the bias and education of the practitioner. Classical acupuncture includes using points distal from the pain site over so-called "master points." Many Western practitioners use both the tender and trigger points around the painful area.

Intensity of Stimulation

The intensity of stimulation can be effected in the following ways: (1) heating the needle (moxibustion) by lighting a dried herb called mugwort; (2) the needle may be manually lifted, thrust, twisted, or twirled either gently or vigorously, at high or low rates, or (3) the needle may be left in place for 15 to 20 minutes. Electroacupuncture, that is, low-voltage electrodes attached to the needle, can be utilized. The waveform may be square or sinusoidal. The frequency is normally 4–10 Hz, with the intensity, pulse width, and duration varied in a similar fashion to TENS.

TYPE OF ACUPUNCTURE

Trigger Point Therapy

Trigger points and tender points should be carefully palpated with the muscles slightly on stretch. The bandlike trigger point should be fixed with two fingers and the sterile acupuncture needle inserted into the band. A twitch is usually seen, and the patient may complain of a feeling of heaviness, numbness, or pressure. The needle may be left for 15 to 20 minutes, or gently agitated until the muscle is felt to relax. Numerous trigger points and tender points within the painful area can be treated at the same session. After therapy, a full range of stretching exercises and range of movement exercises for the injured area should be practiced by the patient and a home exercise program given. Superficial tender points can be treated by insertion of the needle 1–2 mm under the skin into the subcutaneous tissue. These needles are left for approximately 30 seconds. Many tender points can be treated in one session, which allows a larger painful area to be treated than trigger point treatment alone. Therapy must again be followed by stretching exercises and range of movement exercises.

Classical Acupuncture

Classical acupuncture consists of placing needles in some of the 365 acupuncture points along meridians and attempting to balance the yin and yang. Western practitioners tend to use a cookbook approach, while classical-trained acupuncturists will attempt to individualize treatments for the individual patient independent of their pain syndrome. Gold and silver needles may also be used for stimulating or sedating, although there is little evidence of their efficacy over stainless steel. There are numerous variations of classical acupuncture, but it is not well documented as to the efficacy of one over the other.

Electroacupuncture

Crocodile clips can be attached to the needles, and a low-voltage current run through them. This is similar to TENS except the resistance to the skin is reduced due to the needle penetrating the skin. For chronic pain, low-frequency, sinusoidal current is usually the most effective.

SUGGESTED READINGS

Baldry PE: Acupuncture, trigger points and musculoskeletal pain. Churchill Livingstone, London 1989

Richardson PH, Vincent CA: Acupuncture for the treatment of pain: a review of evaluative research. Pain 24:15–40, 1986

32 | Physical Therapy

Chronic pain usually affects more than one area of the individual's musculoskeletal structure. In the majority of patients seeking treatment for chronic pain, the back or neck is involved. The spine can be likened to a chain where, if one area becomes stiff, the other areas next to it become dysfunctional and painful. For example, when examining and treating pain in the lower back, the neck and thoracic spine must also be examined and, if giving discomfort, must also be treated. Lumbar pain may cause gait abnormalities, which puts abnormal stresses on other areas of the body. If appropriate, there are also many energy-saving devices the physical therapist can recommend that will decrease twisting and bending movements for spinal problems or support a joint during repetitious or painful activities.

Dealing with the patient in chronic pain requires a physical therapist to be "hands on." Ultrasound or other physical modalities should be used before stretching and mobilizing tissues, not as a panacea to make the patient feel "good." While general exercise, such as on a bicycle or treadmill, is to be encouraged, the majority of time in therapy should be spent by the physical therapist working with the chronic pain patient on a one-to-one basis, mobilizing, stretching, retraining, and educating.

The general principles of physical therapy are given in Figure 32-1.

JOINT MOBILIZATION

A joint with a restricted range of movement is passively brought through its full range. Short, sharp thrusts delivered at the end of range are termed a manipulation and are used in an attempt to restore full mobility. A skilled physical therapist can isolate the individual vertebral segments that require mobilization by positioning the patient. Holding the stretch at the point of plastic deformation of connective tissue, or at the point of failure of adhesions or scarring, can produce significant improvements in painful joint range of movements. Oscillation and vibration techniques to stretch connective tissue can cause muscles to further relax. All the above techniques are used to allow normal movement patterns to resume. Mobilization of joints requires expertise and experience on the part of the physical therapist. The effects of any previous surgery must be carefully evaluated before any mobilization techniques. Whenever possible, the patient should be taught self-mobilization techniques.

Contraindication to mobilization includes bone disease such as tuberculosis, malignancy, recent fractures, or acute inflammation.

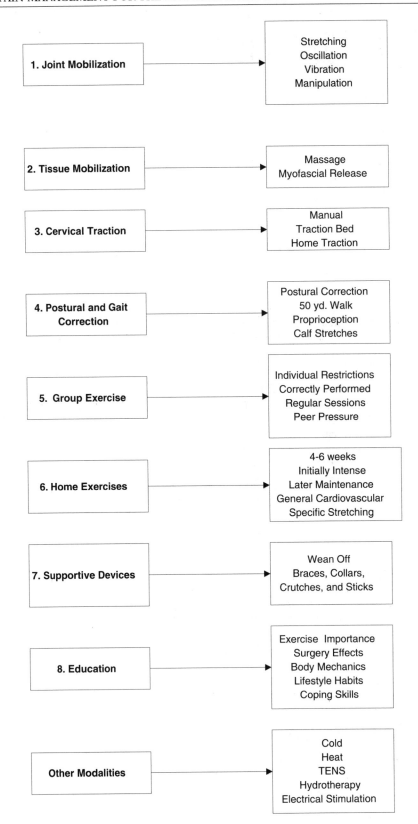

Fig. 32-1. General principles of physical therapy. TENS, transcutaneous electrical nerve stimulation.

TISSUE MOBILIZATION

The most common techniques involve stroking, friction, and kneading. They should be used to break down intramuscular adhesions and decrease edema before stretching and range of movement exercises. Myofascial release is a technique involving stretching along lines of fibers of restricted muscle until the soft tissue is felt to relax or "release." The procedure is repeated several times until the tissues are fully elongated.

TRACTION

Traction is useful for neck pain by distracting the vertebrae with the neck in slight flexion. It is thought to open and mobilize facet joints. This may relieve muscle spasm and improve joint movement. Traction may be done manually by the physical therapist or by a traction adaptation on the bed, using a 10- to 25-lb weight. Lower weights can be used for home traction.

For low back pain "Bat Boots" and other inversion devices have been sold for several years. While they may help milder cases of low back strain, their usefulness in chronic low back pain has not been proved. They can cause acute elevation of intraocular pressure. Glaucoma is a contraindication to their use.

POSTURAL AND GAIT CORRECTION

Abnormal posture and gait may cause problems in other areas not directly affected by the presenting pain syndrome. Poor posture in sitting and standing should be corrected. Gait retraining is extremely important in the rehabilitation of the individual. Timing how long it takes the patient to walk a distance of 50 yards can be used to monitor the progress of the patient. Encouraging the individuals to walk faster as treatment progresses will improve their gait as well as having the secondary benefit of decreasing pain behaviors. Many pain behaviors are related to poor gait and vice versa.

Proprioception or balance should be evaluated by having the patient stand on one leg, initially with eyes opened, subsequently with eyes closed. The therapist should be close by for support. Poor proprioception must be corrected by exercises such as utilizing a wobble board, or having the patient stand on one leg unsupported for increasing periods of time. Once they can "stork stand" with their eyes open for 60 seconds, they may progress to practice it with their eyes closed. Tightness of the calf muscles will also adversely affect gait. Calf-stretching exercises should be part of any gait retraining program. If the patient excessively pronates or has a significant leg length difference, arch supports or heel raises may be necessary.

GROUP EXERCISES

Individuals should be informed of specific restrictions based on the physical therapist's evaluation. Any group fitness program should not be pursued to exhaustion but must be done with the emphasis on doing each exercise correctly. Group exercises can work well because of peer pressure and a sense of friendly competition. The individual's pain problem is deemphasized in a group setting, as there is usually one member of the group who is perceived as being "worse off." This may help put an individual's pain into a more reasonable perspective. Some general rules of exercise are as follows:

1. Initially, an exercise program may worsen the individual's pain as stiffened joints and muscles are used, perhaps for the first time in years. Encouragement is very important in these first days.
2. The reported severity of pain is less important in developing an exercise program than the location, distribution, and characteristics of the pain.
3. The patient must realize that, with chronic pain, hurt does not equal harm. They will be expected to exercise with their pain. This is in contrast to other exercise programs where the sensation of pain may be the limiting factor when prescribing exercise.

HOME EXERCISE PROGRAM

A home exercise program should be developed over the course of treatment. It should include flexibility exercises done daily, strengthening exercises three times a week, and cardiovascular endurance exercise 15 to 20 minutes, 3 to 5 times a week. Initially in a home exercise program, the patient should be encouraged to spend 30 to 60 minutes a day exercising. As the program continues and formal physical therapy sessions decrease, the home exercises should probably not take longer than 5 to 10 minutes twice a day to encourage continued compliance "like brushing one's teeth." Cardiovascular exercise should be incorporated into everyday life such as walking upstairs instead of taking the lift, as well as using it as a stress management technique 3 to 5 times a week.

SUPPORTIVE DEVICES

Supportive devices such as braces, or collars, which restrict joint movement, will, with continued use, lead to muscle weakness, joint capsule contraction, and joint stiffness. This, in turn, causes further pain. Rehabilitation exercises should encourage strengthening of the muscles, stretching, range of movement exercises, and weaning off the supportive device. Braces should only be used where muscle weakness, or joint instability, is permanent or progressive.

Crutches and canes are often used by the chronic pain patient with lower extremity problems. This may consciously, or unconsciously, validate their "sick roles." Gait retraining and speed walking will encourage the abandonment of these devices to which they have become both psychologically and physically dependent.

EDUCATION

The physical therapist often has longer periods of one-on-one contact with the patient than the physician. This enables education to be carried out on an intensive basis. Education should play an important role in any physical therapist's treatment regimen of the chronic pain patient. It should include an explanation of body mechanics, the relevance of prescribed exercises and home exercises, and the effects of any previous surgery. Lifestyle habits should also be emphasized, including a healthy diet and not smoking. The patient must understand the importance of incorporating exercise into his or her daily life. Relaxation techniques, such as imagery, progressive muscle relaxation, and controlled breathing, can be taught or reinforced if the patient has previously been on a stress/pain management program. For education to be effective in the long term, lectures alone are inadequate. Education should be interactive, repetitive, and reinforced.

OTHER MODALITIES

Cold

Cold causes peripheral vasoconstriction, followed by periodic vasodilation (the hunting response), which

1. decreases edema formation due to decreased tissue metabolism, decreased histamine release, and decreased capillary permeability;
2. decreases pain due to slowing of nerve conduction, and possibly by the increased initial peripheral stimulation inhibiting peripheral pain input;
3. decreases spasticity and muscle tone due to decrease in Golgi tendon organ and muscle spindle activity; spasticity may also be decreased by inhibiting the pain–spasm–pain cycle; and
4. attenuates trigger points, allowing less painful stretching and range of movement exercises.

Possibly the most effective way of administering cold therapy is by ice massage. An easy way of doing this is to freeze water in a polystyrene or "Dixie" cup and peel off the upper half inch of the cup. This creates an ice block that can be held relatively comfortably. The ice should be rubbed over the painful area for 5 to 10 minutes until it feels numb. The efficacy of ice in pain management appears to be greater than cold packs. However, cold packs are useful for areas of the body the patient cannot reach. When a cold pack is used, cream should be spread over the skin first and the cold pack not placed directly on the skin but in a paper towel. Both these measures decrease the incidence of ice burns to the unprotected skin. The most effective cold packs are probably those that consist of a polyglycol gel that remains soft even when frozen. This allows the gel to mold to various bony prominences. A vasocoolant spray is another technique of cold therapy.

If cold causes severe pain over the affected area, the possibility of sympathetic maintained pain should be entertained as these syndromes create pain that is exquisitely sensitive to cold.

Contraindications to cold include Raynaud syndrome, certain connective tissue disorders, and cold hypersensitivity syndromes.

Heat

Heat causes

1. an increase in blood flow and nutrition;
2. an increased threshold of the sensory nerve endings, possibly affecting the pain–spasm–pain cycle; and
3. an increase in tissue extensibility, which is useful before massage or stretching exercises (when heat is used, cream should first be placed again on the skin to prevent its drying and damage).

Types of Heat

Conduction. Hot packs and paraffin baths both cause superficial heat penetration. They are useful in joint conditions such as arthritis of the hands or feet.

Convection. Hydrotherapy and whirlpool are useful for their massage effect by agitation. Heat penetration is again superficial.

Conversion. Infrared (superficial), microwave, short-wave diathermy, and ultrasound (deep) are widely used in physical therapy. Ultrasound gives a deep, localized, penetrating heat that may produce more heat at the bone-tissue interface. A close interface between skin and the ultrasound head needs to be made with either gel, water, or oil. Ultrasound cannot be used where there are metal implants, as excessive heat will be produced.

Transcutaneous Electrical Nerve Stimulation

The physical therapist should trial a transcutaneous electrical nerve stimulation (TENS) device if that has not previously been used or it was previously used inappropriately (see Fig. 33-1).

Hydrotherapy

For patients who are extremely deconditioned because of pain, a graded exercise program can be commenced while the patient is immersed in a warm water pool. This unloads the muscles and joints allowing exercise within tissue tolerance levels. Unloading can also be done on the ground with a harness attached to the patient as he or she walks on a treadmill. By a pulley system, the harness takes load off the patient, allowing a normal gait pattern to develop.

Electrical Stimulation

Faradic stimulation is used to stimulate muscle contraction to prevent atrophy. There are home use devices available that may also positively affect the patient's pain. Galvanic stimulation is a direct current that can cause analgesia and vasoconstriction.

Transcutaneous Electrical Nerve Stimulation

There are more than 600 publications supporting the efficacy of transcutaneous electrical nerve stimulation (TENS). It has been used since 1967 with enormous progress being made in both the apparatus and in the understanding of the neurophysiologic mechanisms involved. Yet the Nuprin Pain Report found that fewer than 2% of individuals were offered a TENS for back pain despite a reported efficacy rate of up to 80% in most acute low back pain problems and 50% in most chronic problems. Unfortunately, in chronic pain this efficacy tends to diminish over the course of a year.

Pain relief due to application of TENS may be due to competitive inhibition of small myelinated fibers that block the pain sensation centrally (the gate theory of Melzack and Wall) or due to releasing endorphins and other neuropeptides centrally (neuromodulation). This latter is similar in effect to the postulated mechanism of action of acupuncture. These analgesic effects are reversed by naloxone. There are no side effects to TENS used correctly, with the exception of skin rashes at the site of the electrode pads.

See Figure 33-1 for a TENS algorithm.

EQUIPMENT

The Stimulator

The stimulator is a transistorized, battery-operated pulse generator designed to be worn on a belt or attached to the patient's clothing. It usually has the following features:

1. A control switch for on/off and amplitude (intensity)
2. A frequency control, from a low, 2–5 Hz, to a high, usually 100–250 Hz, frequency.
3. A mode selector, which can be switched between continuous, pulse (burst), modulated, and others specific to the manufacturer.
4. A width or span control (40–400 μs).
5. For dual leads, a second channel can be programmed with the same controls.

Leads

The insulated leads connecting the stimulator to the electrodes should be as supple as possible for patient comfort. Mechanical failure of a TENS usually occurs at the junction of the lead and the jack plug.

Electrodes

Water-impregnated sponge electrodes can be used for trialing a TENS in the clinic. This allows a "search" to be made for the correct electrode placement without the use of more expensive disposable electrodes.

Carbon rubber electrodes make contact with the skin via electrode jelly or, just as effectively (and cheaper), KY jelly. Micropore or hypoallergenic tape can be used to tape the electrodes in place.

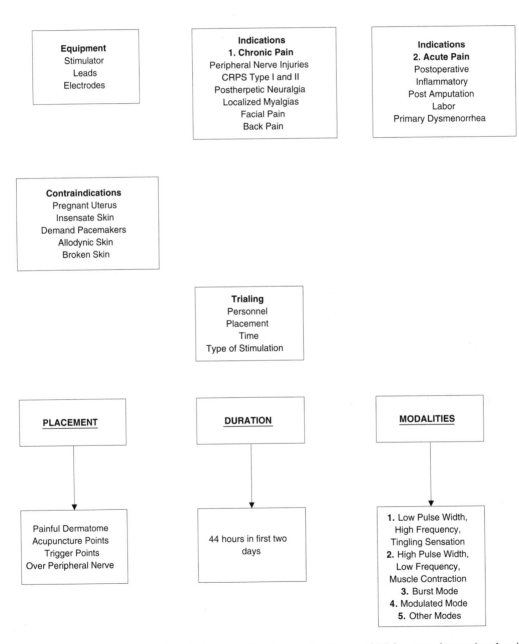

Fig. 33-1. Transcutaneous electrical nerve stimulation algorithm. CRPS, complex regional pain syndrome.

Self-adhesive electrodes are more expensive and often come with their own short lead and socket. When not in use, they should be stored in contact with waxed paper to prevent drying.

Before the application of any electrode, the skin should be clean and dry. The use of an alcohol swab helps to remove excess oil from the skin before the electrode application.

Electrodes should be removed at least once a day to allow the skin to recover.

INDICATIONS

Chronic Pain

It is difficult to predict who will respond to TENS application for chronic pain. Johnson and colleagues in 1991 reported on almost 200 patients who responded to TENS. They reported the following results:

1. No significant relationships were seen between response, diagnosis, or area of body affected.
2. Patients applied the stimulation to create a strong but comfortable paresthesia within the painful area.
3. Almost half the patients had their intensity of pain reduced by more than 50%. The onset of analgesia was within 30 minutes in over 75% and within 60 minutes in over 95% of patients.
4. Pain relief lasted less than 30 minutes in 51% of patients on turning off the TENS. It lasted more than 1 hour in 30% and more than 2 hours in only 20%.
5. About 30% of patients used TENS for more than 7 hours a day; 75% used it on a daily basis.
6. Patients tended to prefer one setting of pulse width, frequency, and amplitude over others; 44% used burst stimulation.
7. Skin reactions to the electrodes, usually due to drying out of the electrode jelly, occurred in 33% of patients.

In general, the chronic pain syndromes that seem to respond best to TENS are peripheral nerve injuries, postherpetic neuralgia, localized myofascial pains, complex regional pain syndromes types I and II, intercostal neuritis, chronic facial pain, and chronic back pain. Chronic pain syndromes that are poorly responsive to TENS include pain mainly of psychogenic origin, headaches, central dysesthetic and central pain syndromes, widespread muscle pains, and pain of visceral origin.

Acute Pain

Postoperative pain often responds well to TENS. Sterile electrodes can be placed on either side of the wound at the end of surgery. It has been used in abdominal surgery, thoracic and spine surgery, for total hip replacements, postcesarean section, and for hand operations.

Acute inflammatory pain due to arthroses, periodontal infections and pulpal inflammation, and muscle injuries responds well to TENS.

After amputation, the incidence of phantom limb pain is decreased over the first few months when TENS is used in the postoperative period. Unfortunately, the studies suggest there is no difference at 12 months in the incidence of phantom limb pain between the patients who received TENS and those who did not.

Labor pain has been successfully reduced with TENS, as has the pain of primary dysmenorrhea.

CONTRAINDICATIONS

Some contraindications to TENS are use over the pregnant uterus, the anterior neck (carotid sinus), and in patients with demand-type pacemakers. Electrodes should not be placed over insensate skin because of the risk of skin damage. Allodynic areas or where the skin is broken should also be avoided for electrode placement.

TRIAL OF TENS

In the Office

Personnel. The individual instructing the patient on the use of TENS should be well trained.

Placement. Adequate time should be spent finding the appropriate placement of the electrodes to give paresthesia over the painful area. The electrodes should be more than 1 cm apart to avoid short circuiting. In general, they are placed in the longitudinal axis of the body, often over the main peripheral nerve going to the painful area. This placement is used for the continuous mode of stimulation.

Time. Initially, the patient should remain in the clinic 30–60 minutes to ensure adequate paresthesia has been obtained over the painful area and that there is no reaction to the electrodes. There is usually a response to the stimulation by this time. This time also allows the patient to familiarize him or herself with the TENS machine.

Type of TENS stimulation. The type of TENS that will be most effective for a particular individual is still a matter of trial and error. Initially, continuous mode is trialed. After setting all controls to zero, the amplitude is slowly increased until a strong but comfortable sensation is felt over the painful area. The frequency and pulse width (when available) is next increased to the maximum comfortable level.

If the continuous stimulation fails to produce any analgesic effects, "acupuncturelike" TENS can be trialed. In this mode the frequency is kept low (5–15 Hz) with the amplitude increased until the muscles underlying the electrode are twitching. The positioning of the electrodes for this mode is best over trigger points or acupuncture points serving the painful area.

One-Week Trial

Having familiarized him- or herself with the TENS, written instructions should be given for a 1-week trial. Many companies will allow up to a 1-week free trial of TENS prior to selling or leasing it.

Day 1: continuous/conventional mode. Use a low-pulse width, 75 µs, high-frequency, 80–110, pps mode. The intensity should be increased until a comfortable tingling is felt, without muscle contraction. Use all day with a 2-hour break.

Day 2. Add burst or modulated modality if present. These are high-frequency pulses at varying pulse widths and rates delivered at intervals that are supposed to decrease the nervous system's accommodation to a fixed pattern of stimulation. Use all day with a 2-hour break.

Day 3. By the third day the patient may experience some hours of carryover relief when the unit is switched off. As pain returns, the patient should turn the unit on and wear for 6 to 8 hours. In the majority of patients relief disappears within 2 hours of switching the unit off.

If minimal or no pain relief is experienced on day 3, the following can be trialed.

Days 4 and 5: acupuncture mode. Use a high-pulse width, 150–200 µs, low-frequency, 2–30 pps. The frequency must be kept low or tetany will occur. Onset of pain relief should be within 20–30 minutes if this mode is going to be effective. Pain reduction may be for several hours. The unit should be turned on again once the pain intensity returns. Different electrode placements can be trialed. A deep aching feeling is often produced if the electrode placement is appropriate.

Other modes on the unit, if present, should be trialed. The electrode placements should be changed with the most effective method of stimulation as found on days 1 to 5.

Noxious-level TENS. If the above trials do not cause significant pain improvement, the electrodes should be placed directly on the painful area. The amplitude intensity is increased to as strong as the patient can tolerate for 20 to 30 minutes. If pain relief occurs, the stimulation should be repeated up to eight times a day for the next 2 weeks. Thereafter, it can be reduced to four times a day or less.

SUGGESTED READINGS

Shealy CN, Mauldin C: Modern medical electricity in the management of pain. Clin Podiatric Med Surg 11:161–175, 1994

Woolf CJ, Thompson JW: Stimulation induced analgesia: transcutaneous electrical nerve stimulation and vibration. In: Wall and Melzack Textbook of Pain. pp. 1191–1208

Future therapies for chronic pain

The Future of Pain Medicine

Through intensive basic science studies, we have gained a better understanding of pain mechanisms and treatment. Basic research continues to be very important in our quest for effective pain management. Unfortunately, pain management has largely been ignored in the clinical arena. This has led to much criticism of medical schools and medical training programs for not instructing medical students and "physicians in training" on proper pain management. Governmental intervention in some states has mandated pain management curricula in medical schools. In the future, we will see more organized courses on pain management given in medical schools. This should lead to a better understanding of pain mechanisms and management and help eliminate the unfounded notion that "pain is all in your head."

PHARMACOLOGIC MANAGEMENT OF PAIN

Because an enormous amount of pain modulation occurs in the dorsal horn of the spinal cord, this area has been the site of intense investigation. It is reasonable, therefore, that drug therapy should be directed at the dorsal horn. This has led to developments in spinal drugs and delivery systems, which continue to play an important role in chronic pain management. A better understanding of dorsal horn pharmacology and physiology has led to the development of new agents for pain management. Most of these agents remain in preclinical studies but have the potential to move into the clinical treatment of pain. Table 34-1 summarizes some of these agents.

MOLECULAR BIOLOGY AND PAIN MANAGEMENT

Magnificent breakthroughs have been made in our understanding of receptors on a molecular level. Pain is a highly complicated phenomenon whereby multiple actions occur at the molecular level. This is true for both acute and chronic pain. Currently, many of the pharmacologic agents used in pain management stimulate multiple receptors, some of which produce pain relief and others that produce unwanted side effects. These side effects prevent optimization of therapy. One aim of molecular biology is to develop drugs that act on specific receptors involved in pain relief. The more specific the agent is for a single receptor, the higher the therapeutic ratio.

Table 34-1. Future Drugs for Spinal Delivery for the Management of Chronic Pain

AGONISTS
  Alpha-2 agonists
  Neuropetide Y agonists
  Adenosine agonists

ANTAGONISTS
  N-Methyl-D-aspartate antagonists
  Neurokinin antagonists

N TYPE CALCIUM CHANNEL BLOCKERS
  Snx-111

ENZYME INHIBITORS
  Acetylcholinase inhibitors
  Nitric oxide synthetase inhibitors
  Cyclo-oxygenase inhibitors

NEUROSTIMULATION

Neurostimulation, both peripheral and central, continues to play a very important role in pain management. Over the years, advances have been made in this area, which have led to more effective techniques. The most common method is spinal column nerve stimulation: an electrode placed in the epidural space stimulates the dorsal column tracts of the spinal cord. This technique has been very effective in managing radicular symptoms in the extremities but ineffective for low back pain. Through modifications of the electrode system, including dual electrodes, it may be possible to provide adequate stimulation for low back pain in the future.

Peripheral nerve stimulation holds much promise in managing peripheral nerve injuries. This technique has the advantage of providing more direct stimulation to painful areas with less chance of electrode migration.

SPINAL ENDOSCOPY

Endoscopy has proved effective for the management of numerous medical conditions. This also seems to hold true for pain management. Spinal endoscopy is a new technique that should be beneficial in the diagnosis and management of spinal abnormalities causing pain. CT scans and MRIs are the gold standard for evaluating spinal contribution to pain. However, these techniques are limited in the information they provide. Many patients have abnormal MRIs with no pain, and many patients have normal MRIs with pain. When a discrepancy is found, spinal endoscopy may provide valuable information. In addition, surgical procedures may be possible with this technique, which would lessen the need for open back procedures. This technique is in the experimental stages but is promising.

NEUROSURGICAL/NEUROABLATION TECHNIQUES

Neurosurgical techniques for the management of pain have largely been eliminated because of poor results. However, with advances and modifications in techniques, this method of pain control may see a resurgence. For example, the use of computers in the performance of dorsal root entry zone lesioning may prove valuable in central dysesthetic pain states. Currently, neurosurgical ablative techniques are largely being reserved for terminally ill patients.

The role of neuroablative procedures in pain management has been met with skepticism because of poor results. Although neuroablative procedures for cancer pain are still commonly performed with good results, the use of this technique for chronic benign pain is controversial. However, the use of radiofrequency techniques has potential for the management of chronic benign pain. Unlike the conventional techniques of neuroablation (i.e., phenol and alcohol injections), radiofrequency ablation techniques allow for a very localized lesion without risk of damaging surrounding structures. This technique has much potential for the management of low back pain.

HOME HEALTH CARE AND HOSPICE LIAISONS

With an increase in managed care comes a push for cost containment. Therefore, fewer patients are being treated in the hospitals and more are being treated in the home and hospice facilities. This also holds true for pain patients—acute, chronic, benign, and cancer. There will be more pain services delivered through nurse practitioners under the direction of physicians. We will also see the development of home postoperative pain services, since many surgeries are performed on an outpatient basis.

SUGGESTED READINGS

Cousins MJ: New horizons. pp. 1139–1147. In Cousins MJ, Bridenbaugh PO (eds): Neural Blockade. Lippincott-Raven, Philadelphia, 1988

Parris WCV: Recent trends and future in pain management. pp. 1005–1018. In Raj PP (ed): Practical Management of Pain. Mosby Year Book, St. Louis, 1992

Index

Note: Page numbers followed by *f* indicate figures; those followed by *t* indicate tables.

FELT ART ACCENTS
for the home

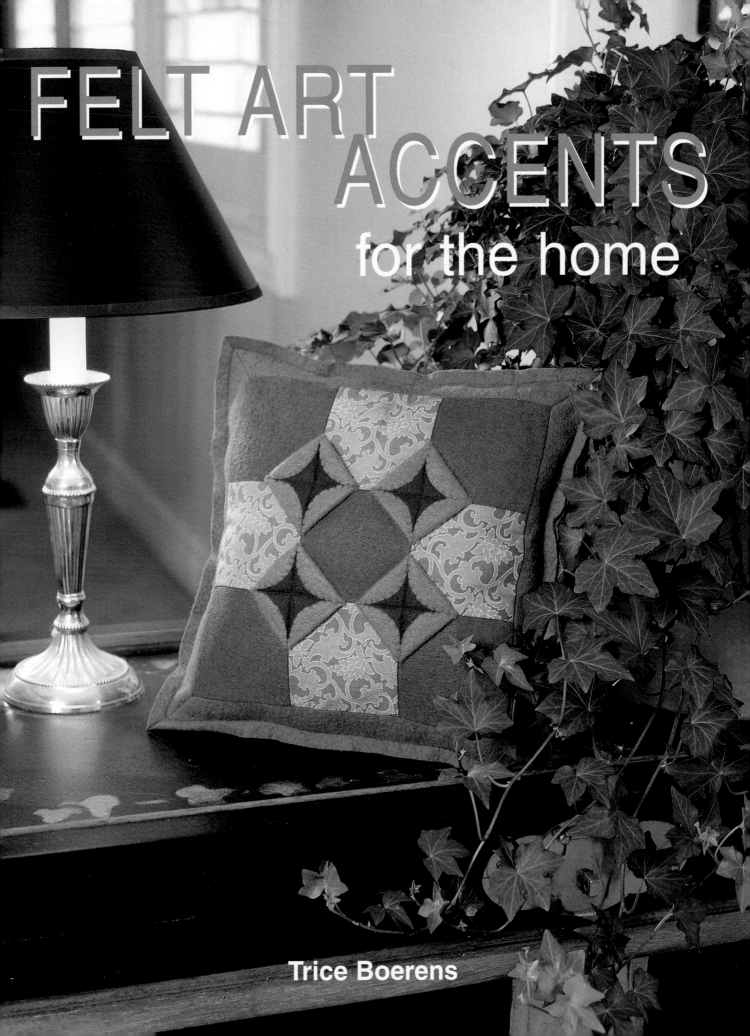

Trice Boerens

Published by

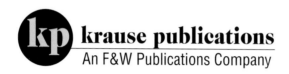

An F&W Publications Company

700 East State Street • Iola, WI 54990-0001
715-445-2214 • 888-457-2873
www.krause.com

Please call or write for our free catalog of publications. Our toll-free number to place an order or obtain a free catalog is (800) 258-0929.

Library of Congress Catalog Number: 2002113122
ISBN: 0-87349-531-4

Photography by Kevin Dilley and illustrations by Cherie Hanson.